# Cardiovascular Risk Factors

# Cardiovascular Risk Factors

Edited by **Janice Hunter**

**FOSTER**
ACADEMICS

New Jersey

Published by Foster Academics,
61 Van Reypen Street,
Jersey City, NJ 07306, USA
www.fosteracademics.com

**Cardiovascular Risk Factors**
Edited by Janice Hunter

International Standard Book Number: 978-1-63242-071-8 (Hardback)

This book contains information obtained from authentic and highly regarded sources. Copyright for all individual chapters remain with the respective authors as indicated. A wide variety of references are listed. Permission and sources are indicated; for detailed attributions, please refer to the permissions page. Reasonable efforts have been made to publish reliable data and information, but the authors, editors and publisher cannot assume any responsibility for the validity of all materials or the consequences of their use.

The publisher's policy is to use permanent paper from mills that operate a sustainable forestry policy. Furthermore, the publisher ensures that the text paper and cover boards used have met acceptable environmental accreditation standards.

**Trademark Notice:** Registered trademark of products or corporate names are used only for explanation and identification without intent to infringe.

Printed in the United States of America.

# Contents

# Preface

It is vital to enforce preventive techniques addressing the burden of cardiovascular disease as early as conceivable. Cardiovascular risk factors lead to the development of cardiovascular disorders from early life. An interdisciplinary approach to the estimation of risk and prevention of vascular events should be adopted at each level of health care. In the past few years, there have been some major advances in this field, with the development of various new markers of heightened cardiovascular risk in particular. With this book, we present some of the emerging concepts and risk elimination factors regarding cardiovascular diseases. It covers some significant issues relating to the impact of stress on specific gender groups, obstructive sleep apnoea syndrome, exposure to lead, and dietary assessment in cardiovascular risks.

The researches compiled throughout the book are authentic and of high quality, combining several disciplines and from very diverse regions from around the world. Drawing on the contributions of many researchers from diverse countries, the book's objective is to provide the readers with the latest achievements in the area of research. This book will surely be a source of knowledge to all interested and researching the field.

In the end, I would like to express my deep sense of gratitude to all the authors for meeting the set deadlines in completing and submitting their research chapters. I would also like to thank the publisher for the support offered to us throughout the course of the book. Finally, I extend my sincere thanks to my family for being a constant source of inspiration and encouragement.

**Editor**

# Nitric Oxide Signalling in Vascular Control and Cardiovascular Risk

Annette Schmidt

*Leibniz-Institute of Arteriosclerosis Research at the University of Muenster,
Germany*

## 1. Introduction

Nitric oxide – a free radical molecule – has been known for many decades, but only since its recognition as endothelium-derived relaxing factor (EDRF) the interest in the molecule has exponentially increased (Moncada, 1991). At the present time NO is an important messenger that regulates numerous functions and also participates in the pathogenesis of various diseases (Lloyd-Jones & Block, 1996). NO is generated from the conversion of arginine to citrulline in a multistep oxidation process by the NO-synthase (NOS), a NADPH-dependent enzyme that requires Calcium-Calmodulin, Flavinadeninedinucleotide, Flavinmononcleotide and Tetrahydro-L-biopterin as cofactors (Förstermann et al., 1994). Three isoforms of NOS have been identified. All isoenzymes, the neuronal NOS (nNOS), the inducible NOS (iNOS) and the endothelial NOS (eNOS) (Liu & Huang, 2008), are homodimers with subunits of 130 – 160 kDa. As major signalling molecule of the vascular system NO is generated by the constitutively expressed eNOS.

## 2. Endothelial nitric oxide synthase (eNOS) and nitric oxide (NO) function

### 2.1 eNOS

The endothelium maintains the balance between vasodilation and vasoconstriction. NO generated by eNOS acts via cGMP-dependent pathway in a paracrine manner on neighbouring smooth muscle cells (SMC) diffusing radially from the production site. NO has a half-life of only a few milliseconds *in vivo* (**Tab. 1**) and rapidly reacts with iron of the heme moiety in the active site of the enzyme guanylate cyclase, stimulating it to produce the intracellular cGMP that in turn enhances the release of neurotransmitters resulting in SMC relaxation and vasodilation (**Fig. 1**). Acting via cGMP-independent pathways it is used in part to S-nitrosylation of intracellular or extracellular proteins (Castel & Vaudry, 2001; Mallis et al., 2001; Sun et al., 2001) or by inhibiting intraendothelial generated superoxide anions (Clancy et al., 1992).

### 2.2 NO functions

Beside its role as vasodilator various other activities of NO have been described: **(I)** NO prevents the expression of cell adhesion molecules thereby preventing leukocytes/monocytes adhering to vascular endothelium and their immigration into the

| Compound | Blood/Plasma Levels, nmol/L | T1/2 |
|---|---|---|
| Nitrate | 20 000 - 50 000 | 5 - 8 hours |
| Nitrite | 100 - 500 | 1 - 5 minutes |
| NO | <1 | 1- 2 milliseconds |
| Hb-NO | <1 - 200 | 15 minutes |
| S-nitroso-Hb | <1 - 200 | -- |
| S-nitroso-albumin | 1 - 200 | -- |

Table 1. Basal blood/plasma levels and half-lifes of some NO-related compounds. Values are approximated from studies in human. For Hb-NO, S-nitroso-Hb and S-nitroso-albumin, no firm agreement about normal values has been reached, and reported values vary greatly. T1/2 for Hb-NO is from pig experiments, values for S-nitroso-Hb and S-nitroso-albumin are unknown (from J.O. Lundberg and E. Weitzberg, Arterioscler Thromb Vasc Biol, 2005;25:915-922).

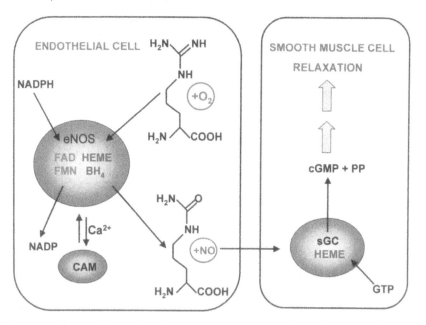

Fig. 1. Nitric oxide signalling axis as therapeutic target in cardiac and vascular disorders. The endothelial eNOS catalyses the formation of NO from L-arginine through two sequential monooxygenation steps. The nitrogen atom of NO is derived from the guanodinogroup of the L-arginine side chain and the oxygen atom of NO derived from molecular oxygen. The cGMP generation in the vascular smooth muscle cell is catalysed by the soluble guanylate cyclase stimulated by the nitric oxide generated by the adjacent endothelial cell.

arterial wall. The monocytes accumulated in the arterial wall can promote local expression or activation of matrixmetalloproteases, which decrease the strength of the cap by degrading collagen and other extracellular matrix components. Furthermore, activated macrophages kill neighbouring SMC by lytic damage leading to necrosis or by inducing apoptosis (Kockx et al., 1996, 1998). **(II)** NO reduces the influx of lipoproteins into the vascular wall and inhibits LDL oxidation. **(III)** NO inhibits DNA synthesis (Förstermann et al., 1994) and proliferation of SMC (Li & Förstermann, 2000; Li et al., 2002a). **(IV)** NO released towards the vascular lumen is a potent inhibitor of platelet aggregation and adhesion (Busse et al., 1987; Radomski et al., 1987). **(V)** NO can react with superoxide anion $O_2^-$ forming the potent peroxynitrite (ONOO-), which causes oxidative damage, nitration and S-nitrosylation of biomolecules. Furthermore, ONOO- oxidizes the NOS cofactor 5,6,7,8-tetrahydrobiopterin with the consequence of uncoupling NOS from NO synthesis thereby leading NOS to a superoxide producing proarteriosclerotic enzyme (Förstermann, 2006). **(VI)** Exogenous NO released from DETA/NONOate causes overexpression of TGF-beta and extracellular matrix in cultured human coronary smooth muscle cells (A. Schmidt et al., 2003).

## 2.3 eNOS-independent sources of NO

The generation of NO is not restricted to NO-synthases. An endothelium-independent source of bioactive NO is the ingestion of dietary (inorganic) nitrate. Naturally occurring dietary nitrate (celery, cress, chervil, beetroot, spinach, rucula contain up to 250 mg NO/100 g fresh weight) elevate the tissue und blood plasma level of nitrite via bioconversion in the entero-salivary circulation. When nitrite is acidified, it yields $HNO_2$, which decomposes to NO and other nitrogen oxides

$$NO_2^- + H^+ \rightleftharpoons HNO_2 \tag{1}$$

$$2\,HNO_2 \rightarrow N_2O_2 + H_2O \tag{2}$$

$$N_2O_2 \rightarrow NO + NO_2 \tag{3}$$

Studies have indicated that acid-catalysed nitrite reduction to NO can also take place in blood vessels and tissues already at a moderately low pH and within nitrite concentrations normally present *in vivo*.

The NO generated by eNOS has a half-life ($T^1/_2$) of 1-2 milliseconds and rapidly oxidizes to nitrate ($NO_2^-$). Nitrate however is not a final end product of NO metabolism but can be a substrate for NOS-independent regeneration to NO (Benjamin et al., 1994; Lundberg et al., 1994). Therefore other sources of nitrate in mammalians can contribute to the formation of NO such as nitrate generated from commensal bacteria in the digestive tract or nitrate present in foodstuff. Thus, in a study of Milkowski (Milkowski et al., 2010) it was shown that the consumption of nitrite- and nitrate-rich food such as fruits, leafy vegetables, and cured meals along with antioxidants can compensate for any disturbance in endogenous NO. Regular intake of nitrate-containing food such as green leafy vegetables may ensure that blood and tissue levels of nitrite and NO pools are maintained at a level sufficient to compensate for any disturbances in endogenous NO synthesis. In several studies (Kapil et al., 2010a, 2010b; Tang et al., 2011) it was shown that nitrate supplementation or vegetable intake (such as beetroot juice) causes dose-dependent elevation in plasma nitrite concentration, elevation of cGMP concentration with a consequent decrease in blood pressure and reduction the risk of ischaemic stroke. The collective body of evidence suggests that food enriched with nitrate and nitrite provide significant health benefits with very little risk. The weak and inconclusive data on the cancer risk of nitrite/nitrate and processed meats are far outweighed by the health benefit of restoring NO homeostasis via dietary nitrite and nitrate (Tang et al., 2011).

## 3. Regulation of eNOS activity

### 3.1 Phosphorylation

eNOS synthesizes NO in a pulsatile $Ca^{2+}$/calmodulin-dependent manner with eNOS activity markedly increasing when intracellular $Ca^{2+}$ increases. $Ca^{2+}$ induces the binding of calmodulin to the enzyme thus increasing the rate of electron transfer from NADPH to heme center (Hemmens & Mayer, 1998). However, eNOS can be activated by other stimuli as increased intracellular $Ca^{2+}$. The best-established stimulus is the shear stress of flowing blood, which can increase enzyme activity. This activation is mediated by phosphorylation of the enzyme (**Fig. 2**). The eNOS protein can be phosphorylated on several Ser, Thr and Tyr residues. Two main changes in enzyme function have been found. Phosphorylation of $Ser^{1177}$ stimulates the flux of electrons within the reductase domain and increases the $Ca^{2+}$ sensitivity of the enzyme (Fleming & Busse, 2003). Several protein kinases participate in phosphorylation of eNOS at $Ser^{1177}$. These kinases include Akt, protein kinase A, 5'-AMP activated protein kinase and calmodulin-dependent kinase II. A negative regulatory site for phosphorylation is $Thr^{495}$ under non-stimulated conditions probably by protein kinase C. $Thr^{495}$ interferes with the binding of calmodulin to the calmodulin-binding domain. Dephosphorylation of $Thr^{495}$ is associated with stimuli such as histamine and bradykinine both elevating intracellular $Ca^{2+}$ concentration. Dephosphorylation of $Thr^{495}$ has also been shown to favour eNOS uncoupling (Lin et al., 2003). Other phosphorylation sites including $Ser^{114}$, $Ser^{633}$ and some Tyr residues are not known to have major consequences for enzyme activity (Fleming & Busse, 2003; Fleming, 2010).

eNOS-associated proteins such as caveolin, heat shock protein 90 or eNOS interacting proteins provide the scaffold for the formation of the eNOS protein complex and its intracellular location (Fleming & Busse, 2003).

eNOS levels in endothelial cells can be regulated by changes in eNOS mRNA stability.

### 3.2 Enhancers of NO availability

**Statins.** Statins are a group of compounds which lower LDL-cholesterol, are inhibiting the enzyme 3-hydroxy-3-methylglutaryl coenzyme A. Beside their lipid lowering property statins improve vascular relaxation, reduce vascular inflammation, reduce oxidative stress, decrease thrombosis and platelet aggregation (E. Schulz et al., 2004; Sowers, 2003). These beneficial effects of statins are in part mediated by an effect on eNOS because they can be blocked by L-NMMA (L-NG-monomethylarginine), an inhibitor of eNOS (John, et al., 1998; Rosenson & Tangney, 1998). Statins increase the expression of eNOS via Rho isoprenylation (Laufs et al., 1998) or posttranslational mechanism (Kureishi et al., 2000).

**Superoxide dismutase (SOD).** Superoxide dismutase has a key antioxidant role by dismutation of $O_2^{-}$ into oxygen and hydrogen peroxide. In humans, three forms of the enzyme are present (SOD1, SOD2 and SOD3). In the cardiovascular system, the action of extracellular SOD3 (Cu–Zn–SOD) lowers $O_2^{-}$ and maintains vascular NO levels (Jung et al., 2007).

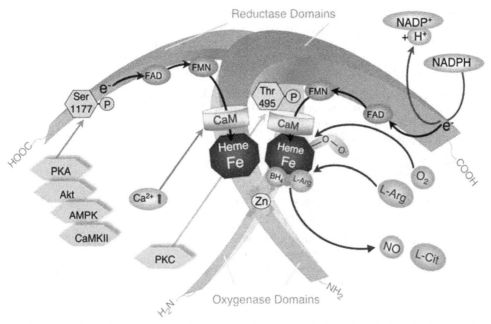

Fig. 2. Regulation of eNOS activity by intracellular $Ca^{2+}$ and phosphorylation. An increase in intracellular $Ca^{2+}$ (as produced by agonists such as histamine or bradykinin) leads to an enhanced binding of CaM (calmodulin) to the enzyme, which in turn displaces an auto-inhibitory loop and facilitates the flow of electrons from NADPH in the reductase domain to the heme in the oxygenase domain. There are several potential phosphorylation sites in eNOS, but most is known about the functional consequences of phosphorylation of Ser[1177] (human eNOS sequence) in the reductase domain and Thr[495] (human eNOS sequence) within the CaM-binding domain. In resting endothelial cells, Ser[1177] is usually not phosphorylated. Phosphorylation is induced when the cells are exposed to fluid shear stress, estrogens, VEGF, insulin, or bradykinin. The kinases responsible for phosphorylation depend on the primary stimulus. Shear stress elicits the phosphorylation of Ser[1177] by activating protein kinase A (PKA), estrogen and VEGF phosphorylate eNOS mainly via Akt, insulin probably activates both Akt and the AMP-activated protein kinase (AMPK), and the bradykinin-induced phosphorylation of Ser[1177] is mediated by CaMKII. Phosphorylation of the Ser[1177] residue increases the flux of electrons through the reductase domain and thus enzyme activity. The Thr[495] residue of human eNOS tends to be constitutively phosphorylated in endothelial cells. Thr[495] is a negative regulatory site, and its phosphorylation is associated with a decrease in enzyme activity. The constitutively active kinase that phosphorylates eNOS Thr[495] is most probably protein kinase C (PKC). The phosphatase that dephosphorylates Thr[495] appears to be protein phosphatase1. (Figure and legend from U. Förstermann, Pflügers Arch - Eur J Physiol, 2010;459:923-933)

**Catalase.** Catalase decomposes hydrogen peroxide to water and oxygen. Overexpression of catalase has protective effects in the cardiovascular system such as delayed development of arteriosclerosis (Yang et al., 2004) and inhibition of angiotensin II-induced aortic wall hypertrophy (Zhang et al., 2005).

**Glutathion peroxidase (GPx).** Several isoenzymes of GPx were found in mammals, the isoenzyme 1 being most abundant. In patients with coronary artery disease the activity of red blood cell GPx1 is inversely associated with the risk of cardiovascular events (Blankenberg et al., 2003). In ApoE-deficient mice, the deficiency of GPx1 leads to arteriosclerotic lesion progression (Torzewski et al., 2007).

**Heme oxygenase (HO).** In break down of heme CO, biliverdin and free ferrous iron are formed. The biliverdin is converted to bilirubin, which has radical-scavenging properties (Jiang et al., 2006). The carbon monoxide has antiproliferative and anti-inflammatory as well as vasodilatory properties (Morita, 2005).

**Thioredoxin (Trx).** Thioredoxin seems to exert most of its ROS-scavenging properties through Trx peroxidase (peroxiredoxin), which uses endogenous SH groups as reducing equivalents. Thioredoxin is present in endothelial- and vascular smooth muscle cells. It exerts its ROS-scavenging properties through Trx peroxidase. Trx scavens ROS and nitric peroxide, ONOO- (Yamawaki et al., 2003).

**Paraoxonase (PON).** The PON family of enzymes acts as vascular antioxidant defense and protects against coronary artery disease (Aviram et al., 1998). The PON1 and PON3 enzymes are synthesized in the liver and circulate in plasma associated with the high-density lipoprotein (HDL) fraction. The capacity of HDL in decreasing HDL and LDL lipid peroxidation largely depends on its PON1 content (Aviram et al., 1998). Deletion of the PON1 gene increases oxidative stress in mouse macrophages and aortae (Rozenberg et al., 2005). The enzyme has been shown to reduce ROS in human endothelial cells, vascular smooth muscle cells, and fibroblasts (Horke et al., 2007).

## 4. eNOS – A multiple cofactors-dependent enzyme

eNOS is a homodimer protein and consists of two subunits: **(I)** the alpha reductase domain which is able to transfer electrons from NADPH to FAD and FMN and can bind calmodulin for stimulation of electron transfer. It has a limited capacity to reduce molecular oxygen to superoxide ($O_2^-$) (Stuehr et al., 2001). **(II)** The oxygenase domain of eNOS is unable to bind the cofactor 5,6,7,8-tetrahydrobiopterin or L-arginine and can not catalyse NO production. The presence of heme allows for NOS dimerization and is the only cofactor that is essential for NOS for the interaction and coupling reductase and oxygenase domains. eNOS monomers are unable to bind the 5,6,7,8-tetrahydrobiopterin or the L-arginine and can not catalyse NO production. Under pathological conditions the molecular oxygen is no longer coupled to L-arginine reduction but results in the production of superoxide. This phenomenon is referred to eNOS uncoupling (Förstermann & Münzel, 2006; Li et al., 2002b).

## 5. eNOS uncoupling

### 5.1 Molecular mechanisms leading to eNOS uncoupling

Various mechanisms can contribute to eNOS uncoupling (**Fig. 3**). Their inbalance causes eNOS dysfunction and cardiovascular risk. This has been shown by numerous clinical studies and for experimental animals. **(I)** Inhibition of eNOS activity. A lack or deficiency of eNOS disrupted at the calmodulin binding site resulted in enhanced arteriosclerosis or peripheral coronary arteriosclerosis and aortic aneurism in ApoE/eNOS double knock out mice (Chen et al., 2001; Hodgin et al., 2002; Knowles et al., 2000; Kuhlencordt et al., 2001).

**(II)** eNOS uncoupling factors such as hypercholesterolemia, diabetes, smoking, hypertension are associated with endothelial dysfunction. Evidence for uncoupling of eNOS has been obtained in endothelial cells treated with LDL (Pritchard et al., 1995) in peroxynitrite-treated rat aorta (Laursen et al., 2001) and in spontaneously hypertensive rats (Li et al., 2006), in human diabetes (Heitzer et al., 2000) and streptozotocin-induced diabetic rats (Hink et al., 2001). **(III)** Arginine deficiency. L-arginine – the physiological substrate of eNOS – is a constituent amino acid and present in human blood plasma in a concentration of $113.6 \pm 14.6$ µM (Psychogios et al., 2011). A decrease of L-arginine induced in hypercholesterolemia below physiological levels favours eNOS uncoupling and formation of ROS. Beside L-arginine the asymmetric dimethylated form of arginine (ADMA) is a major

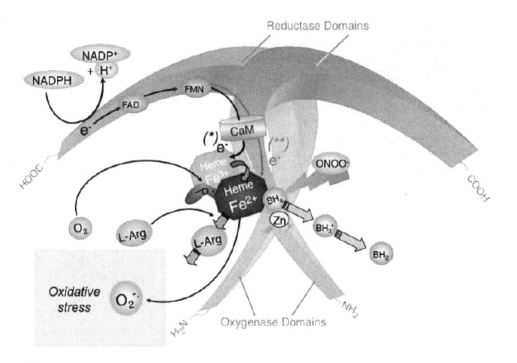

Fig. 3. Scheme of an endothelial NO synthase (eNOS) whose oxygen reduction is uncoupled from NO synthesis. Oxidative stress is associated with endothelial dysfunction. ONOO− can oxidize $BH_4$ to biologically inactive products such as trihydrobiopterin radical ($BH_3 \cdot$) or trihydrobiopterin radical cation protonated at N5 ($BH_3 \cdot H^+$). The $BH_3 \cdot$ radical can be converted to the quinonoid 6,7-[8H]-H2-biopterin ($BH_2$), which also lacks biological activity. When ONOO− overwhelms the cell's capacity to re-reduce these products to $BH_4$, eNOS "uncouples" and reduces oxygen to $O_2$- ; but does not synthesize NO anymore. eNOS then contributes to oxidative stress in the cell. (Figure and legend from U. Förstermann, Pflügers Arch - Eur J Physiol, 2010;459:923-933)

component of blood plasma in a concentration of 0.4-0.8 μM (Billecke et al., 2009) and acts as an endogenous inhibitor of eNOS. ADMA is formed by dimethylation of protein-bound L-arginine and released by proteolysis. ADMA acts as a local competitor of L-arginine (Cooke, 2004; Maas, 2005). Arginase is an ubiquitous enzyme which catalyses the degradation of arginine to ornithine and urea. Two isoenzymes are found in mammals. Arginase I catalyses the final step of the urea cycle in liver. Arginase II is a mitochondrial enzyme that functions in L-arginine homeostasis and can be dysregulated by ox LDL (Ryoo et al., 2006) resulting in eNOS uncoupling. **(IV)** 5,6,7,8-tetrahydrobiopterin deficiency. 5,6,7,8-tetrahydrobiopterin deficiency causes eNOS dysfunction and uncoupling (Moens & Kass, 2006), if the primary function of 5,6,7,8-tetrahydrobiopterin such as both allosteric and redox function, the improvement, the binding affinity of L-arginine for eNOS and providing the second electron to the heme of eNOS are missing. These alterations have the consequence that the reduction of molecular oxygen still occurs at the heme site of eNOS but oxidation of the guanidine nitrogen of L-arginine is prevented so that the reduced oxygen is converted by the uncoupled eNOS to superoxide instead of NO and citrulline (Gao et al., 2007; Xia et al. 1998). Even the partially oxidized 5,6,7,8-tetrahydrobiopterin - the 7,8-tetrahydrobiopterin (BH$_2$) - has no eNOS cofactor activity and is unable to prevent superoxide formation of eNOS (Gao et al., 2007). In addition, BH$_2$ probably competes with BH$_4$ for eNOS binding. Therefore the ratio BH$_4$/BH$_2$ is important for eNOS activity (Shinozaki et al., 1999; Vasquez-Vivar et al., 2002). Apparently a diminished BH$_4$/BH$_2$ level rather than BH$_4$ deficiency is a molecular trigger for eNOS uncoupling (Crabtree et al., 2008). Normally the majority of BH$_4$ is present in vascular endothelial cells (Antoniades et al., 2007; Katusic, 2001) in a concentration of 1.40 pM/10$^6$ cells. Intracellular BH$_4$ concentration has been found under hypercholesterolemic conditions thus aortic BH$_4$ levels are decreased by 50% in hypercholesterolemic ApoE knockout mice compared with wild-type mice (Ozaki et al., 2002), but also discrepant results are described (d'Uscio et al. 2003; d'Uscio & Katusic, 2006) apparently depending on the degree of hypercholesterolemia and differences in the level of oxidative stress. The tissue level of BH$_4$ is determined by the balance of biosynthesis from GTP via de novo synthesis by GTP cyclo hydrolase (GCH-1) or by the salvage pathway from BH$_2$ back to BH$_4$ and degradation by oxidation of BH$_4$ to BH$_2$ (T.S. Schmidt & Alp, 2007) – a process that can be rapidly accelerated by peroxynitrite (Landmesser et al., 2003; Laursen et al., 2001; Zou et al. 2002).

The oxidase-mediated stress of BH$_4$ can be increased by several ROS producing enzyme systems such as NADPH oxidase that plays a major role in vascular cells (Förstermann, 2008; Harrison et al., 2003; Schnabel & Blankenberg, 2007), by xanthine oxidase, cytochrome P450 monooxygenase and enzymes of the respiratory chain. Xanthine oxidase is generated from xanthine dehydrogenase by proteolysis. This enzyme is another potential source of ROS in vascular disease. The enzyme readily donates electrons to molecular oxygen, thereby producing O$_2^{-}$ and hydrogen peroxide. Oxypurinol, an inhibitor of xanthine oxidase decreases O$_2^{-}$ production and improves endothelium-dependent vascular relaxation to acetylcholine in blood vessels from hyperlipidemic animals (Ohara et al., 1993). This suggests a contribution of xanthine oxidase to endothelial dysfunction in early hypercholesterolemia. Experimental evidence suggests that endothelial cells themselves can express xanthine dehydrogenase (xanthine oxidase) and that this expression is regulated in a redox sensitive way depending on endothelial NADPH oxidase (McNally et al., 2003).

All these cited cofactors required for regulation eNOS activity depend on the physiological transcription and translation of the corresponding genes. These processes, however, are regulated by epigenetics. Epigentics refer to chromatin-based pathways including three distinct but highly interrelated mechanisms: DNA methylation, Histone density and posttranslational modifications. These factors together offer new perspectives on transcriptional control paradigm in vascular endothelial cells and provide a molecular basis for understanding how the environment impacts the genome to modified function and disease susceptibility (Yan et al., 2010).

## 5.2 Mechanisms leading to a loss of function of eNOS

Oxidative stress is associated with endothelial dysfunction. Mechanistically, superoxide derived from NADPH oxidases and/or xanthine oxidase may combine with NO formed by a still functional eNOS. This would lead to increased formation of peroxinitrite (Laursen et al., 2001). Peroxynitrite has been shown to oxidize $BH_4$ to biological inactive products. Significant $O_2^-$ production also occurs when concentrations of L-arginine fall below the levels required to saturate the enzyme. In these circumstances eNOS catalysis the uncoupled reduction to $O_2$ leading to the production of $O_2^-$ and/or $H_2O_2$. Whether L-arginine concentration ever becomes critical as a substrate *in vivo* appears questionable since the $K_m$ of eNOS for L-arginine is ~3 µM while the L-arginine plasma concentration is ~100 µM and a ~10-fold accumulation of L-arginine within cells (Closs et al., 2000).

## 5.3 eNOS uncoupling in arteriosclerosis

Under cardiovascular risk factors such as diabetes, hypertension, smoking, the enzymatic reduction of molecular oxygen by eNOS is no longer used for L-arginine conversion to citrulline and NO, but the uncoupling of oxidase and reductase chain of eNOS produced ROS via the NADPH domains. The cardiovascular risk factors initiate the eNOS uncoupling and this can occur before arteriosclerotic lesions can be detected. The eNOS uncoupling can be triggered by various mechanisms which include $BH_4$ deficiency, shortage of L-arginine or HSP 90, inhibitory phosphorylation of eNOS on $Thr^{495}$ (see above) eNOS redistribution to the cytosolic fraction of the cell, oxidation of the zinc-thiolate cluster in eNOS or elevated ADMA levels (Sud et al. 2008). Among all of these mechanisms the reaction $BH_4$ to $BH_2$ is probably a dominant factor, and $BH_4$ deficiency seems to be the primary cause for eNOS uncoupling in pathophysiology. Some researchers have postulated that eNOS may exist in two separate pools: a coupled form and an uncoupled form. The coupled enzyme is associated with the membrane and is readily accessible to the "signalome" for activation and NO production, whereas the uncoupled enzyme may reside in the cytosol and produces superoxide (Gharavi et al., 2006; Sullivan et al., 2006). In eNOS overexpressing mice for example, there is clear evidence for eNOS uncoupling (i.e. eNOS-mediated ROS production). In the same mice, however, NO-generating activity is elevated 2-fold when compared with wild-type mice (the total eNOS protein levels are elevated 8-fold) (Bendall et al., 2005). Thus, it is possible that coupled eNOS and uncoupled eNOS may exist in the same tissue at the same time.

The principle mechanisms of vascular protection by eNOS-derived NO and the consequences of endothelial dysfunction and the concomitant eNOS uncoupling are listed in **Tab. 2.**

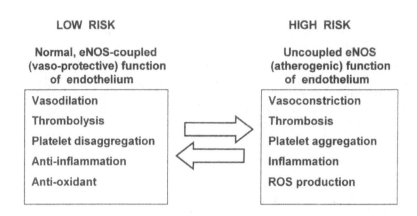

Table 2. The vaso-protective effect of eNOS is not restricted to the control of arterial dilation and constriction. The NO released towards the vascular lumen is a potent inhibitor of platelet aggregation and adhesion. The expression and formation of the alpha and beta component of various integrins including the cell adhesion molecules ICAM and VCAM can also be inhibited and reduce the transendothelial migration of macrophages and T-lymphocytes known to be an early event in the development of arteriosclerosis and characteristic for its inflammatory phases. The uncoupled eNOS leads to an excessive production of superoxide ($O_2^-$) and in turn to the formation of highly toxic peroxynitrite (Förstermann & Münzel, 2006).

## 6. eNOS-independent production of reactive oxygen species in vascular disease

Beside the eNOS there are several enzymes that can produce ROS in the endothelial cells: NADPH oxidase, xanthine oxidase, and enzymes of the mitochondrial respiratory chain are of major importance.

**NADPH oxidases.** Several isoforms of ROS producing NADPH oxidase are present and active in the vascular wall. In arteriosclerotic arteries the NADPH oxidase subunits NOX 2 and NOX 4 (Sorescu et al., 2002) have been identified.

**Xanthine oxidase (XO).** Increased cholesterol levels have been shown to stimulate the release of xanthine oxidase from the liver into the circulation. The circulating xanthine oxidase than can associate with endothelial glycosaminoglycans (White et al., 1996) however endothelial cells themselves can express xanthine oxidase and the expression is regulated in a redox sensitive pathway depending on endothelial NADPH oxidase (McNally et al., 2003) (**Fig. 4**).

**Respiratory chain of the mitochondria.** The molecular oxygen is consumed by mitochondria thereby forming $O_2^-$. Evidence has been provided that some cardiovascular diseases are associated with mitochondrial dysfunction (Ramachandran et al., 2002) and the mitochondrial production of ROS may be linked to the development of early arteriosclerotic lesions.

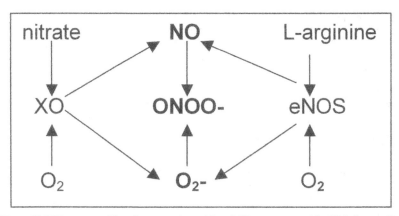

Fig. 4. XO and NOS are capable of generating either NO or superoxide ($O_2$) depending on the conditions. When the supply of L-arginine and oxygen is good, NOS makes NO, whereas the same enzyme may generate considerable amounts of superoxide when L-arginine or cofactors are limited. XO generates superoxide, for example, during reperfusion after ischemia, whereas nitrite reduction to NO occurs preferentially during hypoxia. NO generation from XO can be beneficial and works as a backup system to supply NO during hypoxia when NO synthesis from NOS is compromised. Detrimental effects of these 2 enzyme systems can also be foreseen, for example, in a situation in which NO and superoxide are generated simultaneously and react to form potentially harmful peroxynitrite. (Figure and legend from J.O. Lundberg and E. Weitzberg, Arterioscler Thromb Vasc Biol, 2005;25:915 – 922)

## 7. Factors protecting against eNOS uncoupling and oxidative stress

### 7.1 Nitric oxide donors

NO-delivering drugs (NO donors) are used for their potential therapeutic benefit in coronary heart disease risk patients (D.J. Lefer & A.M. Lefer, 1988) by increasing coronary blood flow and dilating coronary arteries. Several studies have described the action of NO donors on vascular smooth muscle cells (Sarkar et al., 1997; A. Schmidt et al. 2003; Young et al., 2000). The pathway leading to NO formation differs among individual NO donor classes: indirect NO donors such as organic nitrates (nitroglycerol, isosorbide mononitrate, isosorbide dinitrate) require enzymatic catalysis, other NO donors require interaction with thiols to release NO, some have to undergo oxidation or reduction. In contrast, direct NO donors generate NO non-enzymatically. Examples are nicorandil, SIN-1 (the active metabolite of molsidomine) and the group of 1-substituted diazen-1-ium-1,2-diolates that releases NO spontaneously with a half-life from minutes to hours (Mooradian et al., 1995).

### 7.2 The NO donor DETA/NONOate

The compound (Z)-1-[2-Aminoethyl]-N-(2-ammonioethyl) amino] diazen-1-ium-1,2-diolate (in the following detNO) belongs to the class of direct NO donors. Under cell culture conditions detNO releases spontaneously NO with a half-life of about 20 h at 37° C in a strictly first order reaction (Hrabie et al., 1993; Keefer et al., 1996; Mooradian et al., 1995), thereby disintegrating to two NO and diethylentriamine. Diethylentriamine, the byproduct of detNO disintegration, is known to be effectiveless (Mooradian et al., 1995; Sarkar et al., 1997). detNO has been successful used (Boyle et al., 2002; Ishimaru et al., 2001; A. Schmidt et al., 2003). In experimental studies (A. Schmidt et al., 2008) on cultured endothelial cells exogenously applied NO released from the NO donor detNO has a dual function in the regulation of eNOS expression. During short–term exposure of endothelial cells, exogenous detNO enhances the phosphorylation of the protein kinase Akt that in turn activates eNOS of endothelial cells by increasing its phosphorylation leading to a higher release of endogenous NO.

Phosphorylation can be achieved by exposure of human vascular endothelial cells to 150 μmol/L detNO. In short-term experiments in Western blot analysis detNO shows a clear increase of eNOS phosphorylation at $Ser^{1177}$ after a short lag phase, detectable 20 min after detNO addition. The phosphorylation is mediated by the protein kinase Akt that is converted into p-Akt within 10 min after addition of detNO in a concentration-dependent manner. The phosphorylated Akt increases in turn $Ser^{1177}$ phosphorylation of eNOS. This phosphorylation cascade could be reverted by preincubation of the cells with the PI-3 kinase inhibitor LY294002 that prevents phosphorylation of both Akt and eNOS. $Thr^{495}$ is constitutively phosphorylated in all endothelial cells (Fleming & Busse, 2003) and is a negative regulatory site, i.e. phosphorylation leads to a decrease of eNOS activity. The release of endogenous NO in response to exogenous detNO was confirmed by L-[2,3,4,5-$^3$H]arginine as indicator. The eNOS-mediated conversion of [$^3$H]arginine to NO and [$^3$H]citrulline was measured and the results are given in [$^3$H]citrulline equivalents. A statistically significant increase of endogenous NO production after 20 and 30 min exposure to detNO is shown. N-nitro-L-arginine methyl ester HCl (NAME), a competitive NOS inhibitor, verifies the reaction conditions of the assay. Taking this reaction sequence into account, the effect of the NO donor could be considered partially a trigger for the acceleration of endogenous NO production that finally effects vasodilation via the physiologic pathway. This leads to the hypothesis of a potential switch from an exogenously applied to an endogenously generated NO stimulation (**Fig. 5**).

### 7.3 Long-term application of detNO and other NO donors

In contrast an exposure of endothelial cells to detNO for 24 and 48 h reduces the eNOS protein content as compared with controls. Densitometry revealed a reduced eNOS protein content after 24 h and 48 h. Real-time RT-PCR confirmed the reduced transcription of eNOS-specific mRNA. For direct determination of the reduced eNOS enzyme activity after long-term exposure to detNO, [2,3,4,5-$^3$H]arginine was added to the culture medium. The radioactivity of [$^3$H]citrulline formed by the NADPH-dependent NOS oxidoreductase is direct proportional to the NO produced and released by the endothelial cells. Under these conditions the results show a significant reduction of NO production expressed as [$^3$H]citrulline equivalents in accordance to the reduced $Ser^{1177}$ phosphorylation of eNOS. Taken together, these results emphasize a limitation of NO donors as long-term therapeutics owing to the inhibition of eNOS synthesis. However, whether exogenous NO donors are operative and effective in a similar way also in humans is still uncertain. In numerous clinical studies the outcome of repeated administration of indirect or direct NO donors to patients with coronary artery disease were ambiguous and the potential benefit of long-acting nitrates has remained controversial. Pathways leading to NO formation differ significantly among individual NO donor classes. In the Fourth International Study of

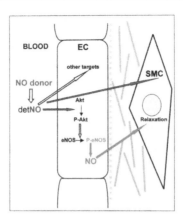

Fig. 5. Scheme of the new mechanism of action of the NO-donor DETA/NONOate in cultured human vascular endothelial cells. During short-term exposure the exogenous NO donor enhances the phosphorylation of the protein kinase Akt (PKB) that in turn activates eNOS of the endothelial cells by increasing its phosphorylation of Ser[1177] leading to a higher release of the physiological endogenous NO as judged by the conversion of [3H]arginine to [3H]citrulline. The NOS-released NO reaches the smooth muscle cell and effects vasodilation.

Infarct Survival (ISIS-4), there was no significant reduction in five-week mortality and no survival advantage (ISIS-4 (Fourth International Study of Infarct Survival) Collaborative Group, 1995). Chronic administration of long acting nitrates in patients with healed myocardial infarction resulted in an increased number of patients with cardiac events (Ishikawa et al., 1996) and an increased risk of cardiac deaths occurred in CAD patients with long acting nitrates (Nakamura et al., 1999). Furthermore, a study on 19 healthy volunteers documented that isosorbide mononitrate given over 7 days impaired endothelial function due to formation of free radicals (Thomas et al., 2007). In total, epidemiological evidence indicates that chronic administration of long acting nitrates increase rather than decreases fatal and non-fatal events (Ishikawa et al., 1996; Nakamura et al., 1999). This view is confirmed by experiments on human vascular endothelial cells, which show detNO-induced cell cycle arrest and hypertrophy. Cultured quiescent EC released from the $G_0$-phase by seeding at a low density re-enter the cell cycle and proliferate up to confluence. In this phase detNO causes a dose-dependent suppression of proliferation of EC indicated by a decreased incorporation of [3H]thymidine and a cell cycle arrest. The antiproliferative effect of detNO was associated with a remarkable increase of cell protein content that continued up to a 2-3-fold amount of control cells within 3 days while the cell number indicates an inhibition of cell proliferation and shows neither increase nor decrease. The elevated total cell protein was the result of *de novo* synthesis indicated by measurements of [3H]leucine incorporation into total cellular protein. After 48 h incubation of subconfluent cultures in the presence of [4,5-3H]leucine the incorporated radioactivity was 24.8 x $10^3$ dpm/$10^5$ control cells and 34.6 x $10^3$ dpm/$10^5$ cells exposed to detNO. The concomitant upregulation of p21 refers to a block at the $G_1$-phase of the cell cycle. The detNO-induced metabolic alterations convert the cells into a hypertrophic phenotype. Measurements of cell volume show an increase from $2.49 \pm 0.18$ up to $3.38 \pm 0.36$ (200 µmol/L detNO) fL /cell.

The inhibition of proliferation is cytostatic but not cytotoxic as evaluated by cell death determination and is reversible. A quantitative determination of mono- and oligonucleosomes revealed no significant apoptotic cell death in detNO-pretreated cells. When the medium of detNO-induced growth-arrested cells is replaced by a standard medium, cell proliferation recovers within the following 48 h with continuous increase of cell number.

### 7.4 Antioxidant compounds potentially protecting against vascular oxidative stress

Important antioxidant enzymes include superoxide dismutase (SOD), glutathione peroxidase (GPx), catalase, heme oxygenase (HO), and the thioredoxin (Trx) peroxidase and perhaps also paraoxonases (PON) (see Chapter 3.2).

**Pentaerythritol tetranitrate (PETN)** is a NO donor that does not induce significant nitrate tolerance and reduces oxidative stress (probably by inducing heme oxygenase). **Sepiapterin** can be reduced in cells by sepiapterin reductase (SR) to 7,8-BH$_2$, sepiapterin reductase catalyses the following reaction

$$7,8\text{-dihydrobiopterin} + NADP^+ \rightleftharpoons \text{tetrahydrobiopterin} + NADPH + H^+$$

**Midostaurin, betulinic acid and ursolic acid** upregulate eNOS and concomitantly decrease NADPH oxidase expression (Li & Förstermann, 2009).

**AVE9488 and AVE3085**, a new class of eNOS enhancers, upregulated the promotor activity of eNOS *in vitro* and *in vivo*. Application to wild type and ApoE-knockout mice over 12 weeks enhanced vascular eNOS expression at mRNA and protein level (Xue et al., 2010). The hybrid NO-releasing prodrug PABA/NO can be stabilized as nanoparticle with significant stability in mice circulation over 24h (Kumar et al., 2010).

**Nebivolol** - a NO-releasing beta-blocker induced a consistent increase of aortic eNOS expression rabbits receiving high-cholesterol diet (de Nigris et al., 2008). NO-releasing S-nitrosothiol-modified xerogels are capable of generating NO for up to 2 weeks (Riccio et al., 2009). These new generation of NO donors might be a rational approach to develop a new generation of antiatherogenic and anti-inflammatory NO donors. AVE9488 and AVE3085 are eNOS transcription enhancers that reverse eNOS uncoupling and preserve eNOS functionality.

**Angiotensin II type 1-receptor blockers (ARBs),** estrogens and erythropoietin (EPO) enhance (6R)-5,6,7,8-BH$_4$ synthesis by stimulating GCH1 expression or activity (Li & Förstermann, 2009.)

Angiotensin-converting enzyme (ACE) inhibitors, the aldosterone antagonist eplerenone and the renin inhibitor aliskiren prevent (6R)-5,6,7,8-BH$_4$ oxidation by decreasing the expression and/or activity of NADPH oxidase.

### 8. Clinical implications

Cardiovascular risk factors cause oxidative stress that alters the endothelial cells capacity and leads to endothelial dysfunction. The term „endothelial dysfunction" is used to refer to an incompetence of endothelial cell-dependent vasorelaxation resulting from eNOS uncoupling but a molecular or biochemical basis for biomarkers indicating uncoupled eNOS has not been established. A biomarker is a characteristic that is objectively measured and evaluated as an indicator for normal or pathogenic processes or pharmacological response to a therapeutic intervention. As biomarkers for cardiovascular diseases oxLDL, CRP, IL-6, fibrinogen, TNF-alpha, MMP-9, MPO and cell adhesion molecules have been proposed (Vasan, 2006). Indirect biomarkers for eNOS uncoupling are a number of pharmaceuticals that have been shown to act as vaso-protective agents. Such agents listed by Förstermann (Förstermann, 2010) are: pentaerythritol tetranitrate, a NO donor that does not induce significant nitrate tolerance and reduces oxidative stress probably by inducing heme oxygenase 1, L-arginine stimulates NO release from eNOS, folic acid may improve eNOS functionality by stabilising $BH_4$ and stimulating the endogenous regeneration of $BH_2$ back to $BH_4$, sepiapterin can be reduced in cells by sepiapterin reductase to $BH_2$ and further dihydrofolate reductase to form $BH_4$, midostaurin, betulinic acid and ursolic acid upregulate eNOS and concomitantly decrease NADPH oxidase expression, AVE9488 and AVE3085 are eNOS transcription enhancers that reverse eNOS uncoupling and preserve eNOS functionality, statins, angiotensin II type 1-receptor blockers, estrogens and erythropoietin enhance $BH_4$ synthesis by stimulating GTP cyclohydrolase1 expression or activities. Statins, angiotensin converting enzyme inhibitors, the aldosterone antagonist eplerenone and the renin inhibitor prevent $BH_4$ oxidation by decreasing the expression and/or activity of NADPH oxidase. All these compounds are secondary biomarkers indicating a pharmacological response to a therapeutic intervention.

Clinically, endothelial function can be assessed by invasive or non-invasive techniques (for review see Esper et al., 2006). These techniques evaluate the endothelial functional capacity depending on the amount of NO produced and the resulting vasodilation effect. The percentage of vasodilation with respect to the basal value represents the endothelial functional capacity. A non-invasive technique most often used is the transient flow-modulate endothelium-dependent post-ischemic vasodilation performed on conductance arteries such as the brachial, radial or femoral arteries. This vasodilation is compared with the vasodilation produced by NO donors. The vasodilation is quantified by measuring the arterial diameter with high-resolution ultrasonography. Laser-Doppler techniques are used to consider tissue perfusion. There is no doubt that endothelial dysfunction contributes to the initiation and progression of arteriosclerosis and could be considered an independent vascular risk factor.

## 9. Conclusion

Nitric oxide produced in vascular endothelial cells by the nitric oxide synthase is a major signalling molecule for maintaining vascular homeostasis. The nitric oxide synthase - constitutionally expressed by endothelial cells – is a dimeric enzyme molecule depending on multiple cofactors for its physiological activity and optimal endothelial function. Any imbalance of reductase and NADPH oxygenase or deficient supply of the enzyme substrate L-arginine or of cofactors leads to an upregulation of endothelial nitric oxide synthase and oxygenase activity with the consequence of an uncoupling of the nitric oxide synthase and production of detrimental reactive oxygen species and/or highly toxic peroxinitrate instead of nitric oxide. The resulting endothelial dysfunction implies a high cardiovascular risk. Several drugs reverting endothelial nitric oxide synthase uncoupling and/or improving endothelial dysfunction are in clinical use. Nitric oxide delivering drugs (NO donors) show potential therapeutical benefit and are used to relief or prevent acute episodes of angina pectoris by activating the endothelial nitric oxide synthase – a new mechanism found for the NO donor DETA/NONOate. However, a long-term administration of NO donors has been found to reduce endothelial nitric oxide synthase of endothelial cells drastically (in cell culture experiments). This could be the basis for development of a new generation of NO donors that mimics the low continuous pulsatile stress-induced release of endogenous nitric oxide.

## 10. Acknowledgment

The author wishes to thank Prof. Dr. E. Buddecke, Muenster, for critical discussion and revising the manuscript.

## 11. References

Antoniades, C., Shirodaria, C., Crabtree, M., Rinze, R., Alp, N., Cunnington, C., Diesch, J., Tousoulis, D., Stefanadis, C., Leeson, P., Ratnatunga, C., Pillai, R., & Channon, K.M. (2007). Altered plasma versus vascular biopterins in human atherosclerosis reveal relationships between endothelial nitric oxide synthase coupling, endothelial function, and inflammation. *Circulation*, 116(24):2851-2859

Aviram, M., Rosenblat, M., Bisgaier, C.L., Newton, R.S., Primo-Parmo, S.L., & La Du, B.N. (1998). Paraoxonase inhibits high-density lipoprotein oxidation and preserves its functions. A possible peroxidative role for paraoxonase. *J Clin Invest*, 101:1581–1590

Bendall, J.K., Alp, N.J., Warrick, N., Cai, S., Adlam, D., Rockett, K., Yokoyama, M., Kawashima, S., & Channon, K.M. (2005). Stoichiometric relationships between endothelial tetrahydrobiopterin, endothelial NO synthase (eNOS) activity, and eNOS coupling in vivo: insights from transgenic mice with endothelialtargeted GTP cyclohydrolase 1 and eNOS overexpression. *Circ Res*, 97(9):864-871

Benjamin, N., O'Driscoll, F., Dougall, H., Duncan, C., Smith, L., Golden, M., & McKenzie, H. (1994). Stomach NO synthesis. *Nature*, 368:502

Billecke, S.S., D'Alecy, L.G., Platel, R., Whitesall, S.E., Jamerson, K.A., Perlman, .L., & Gadegbeku, C.A. (2009). Blood content of asymmetric dimethylarginine: new insights into its dysregulation in renal disease. *Nephrol Dial Transplant*, 24(2):489-496

Blankenberg, S., Rupprecht, H.J., Bickel, C., Torzewski, M., Hafner, G., Tiret, L., Smieja, M., Cambien, F., Meyer, J., Lackner, K.J., & AtheroGene Investigators. (2003). Glutathione peroxidase 1 activity and cardiovascular events in patients with coronary artery disease. *N Engl J Med*, 349(17):1605–1613

Boyle, J.J., Weissberg, P.L., & Bennett, M.R. (2002). Human macrophage- induced vascular smooth muscle cell apoptosis requires NO enhancement of Fas/Fas–L interactions. *Arterioscler Thromb Vasc Biol*, 22:1624–1630

Busse, R., Luckhoff, A., & Bassenge, E. (1987). Endotheliumderived relaxant factor inhibits platelet activation. *Naunyn-Schmiedeberg's Arch Pharmacol*, 336:566–571

Castel, H., & Vaudry, H. (2001). Nitric oxide directly activates GABA (A) receptor function through a cGMP/protein kinase-independent pathway in frog pituitary melanotrophs. *J Neuroendocrinol*, 13:695–705

Chen, J., Kuhlencordt, P.J., Astern, J., Gyurko, R., & Huang, P.L. (2001). Hypertension does not account for the accelerated atherosclerosis and development of aneurysms in male apolipoprotein e/endothelial nitric oxide synthase double knockout mice. *Circulation,* 04(20):2391-2394

Clancy, R.M., Leszczynska, P., Piziak, J., & Abramson, S.B. (1992). Nitric oxide, an endothelial cell relaxation factor, inhibits neutrophil superoxide anion production via a direct action on NADPH oxidase. *J Clin Invest,* 90:1116–1121

Closs, EI., Scheld, J.S., Sharafi, M., & Förstermann, U. (2000). Substrate supply for nitric-oxide synthase in macrophages and endothelial ells: role of cationic amino acid transporters. *Mol Pharmacol,* 57:68–74

Cooke, J.P. (2004). Asymmetrical dimethylarginine: the Uber marker? *Circulation,* 109(15): 1813-1818

Crabtree, M.J., Smith, C..L, Lam, G., Goligorsky, M.S., & Gross, S.S. (2008). Ratio of 5,6,7,8-tetrahydrobiopterin to 7,8-dihydrobiopterin in endothelial cells determines glucose-elicited changes in NO vs. superoxide production by eNOS. *Am J Physiol Heart Circ Physiol,* 294:H1530-1540

de Nigris, F., Mancini, F.P., Balestrieri, M.L., Byrns, R., Fiorito, C., Wiiliams- Ignarro, S., Palagiano, A., Crimi, E., Ignarro, L.J., & Napoli, C. (2008). Therapeutic dose of nebivolol, a nitric oxide-releasing beta-blocker, reduces atherosclerosis in cholesterol-fed rabbits. *Nitric Oxide,* 19(1):57–63

d'Uscio, L.V., Milstien, S., Richardson, D., Smith, L., & Katusic, Z.S. (2003). Longterm vitamin C treatment increases vascular tetrahydrobiopterin levels and nitric oxide synthase activity. *Circ Res,* 92:88-95

d'Uscio, L.V., & Katusic, Z.S. (2006). Increased vascular biosynthesis of tetrahydrobiopterin in apolipoprotein E-deficient mice. *Am J Physiol Heart Circ Physiol,* 290:H2466-2471

Esper, R.J., Nordaby, R.A., Vilarino, J.O., Paragano, A., Cacharrón, J.L. & Machado, R.A. (2006). Endothelial dysfunction: a comprehensive appraisal. *Cardiovasc Diabetol,* 5:4 doi:10.1186/1475-2840-5-4

Fleming, I. & Busse, R. (2003). Molecular mechanisms involved in the regulation of the endothelial nitric oxide synthase. *Am J Physiol Regul Integr Comp Physiol,* 284:R1–12

Fleming, I. (2010). Molecular mechanisms underlying the activation of eNOS. *Pflügers Arch - Eur J Physiol,* 459:793-806

Förstermann, U., Closs, EI., Pollock, JS., Nakane, M., Schwarz, P., Gath, I., & Kleinert, H. (1994). Nitric oxide synthase isozymes. Characterization, purification, molecular cloning, and functions. *Hypertension,.*23(6, Part 2):1121-1131

Förstermann, U., & Münzel, T. (2006). Endothelial nitric oxide synthase in vascular disease: from marvel to menace. *Circulation,* 113:1708-1714

Förstermann, U. (2006). Janus-faced role of endothelial NO synthase in vascular disease: uncoupling of oxygen reduction from NO synthesis and its pharmacological reversal. *Biol Chem,* 387:1521–1533

Förstermann, U. (2008). Oxidative stress in vascular disease: causes, defense mechanisms and potential therapies. *Nat Clin Pract Cardiovasc Med,* 5:338-349

Förstermann, U. (2010). Nitric oxide and oxidative stress in vascular disease *Pflügers Arch - Eur J Physiol,* 459:923–939

Gao, Y.T., Roman, L.J., Martasek, P., Panda, S.P., Ishimura, Y., & Masters, B.S. (2007).Oxygen metabolism by endothelial nitric-oxide synthase. *J Biol Chem,* 282:28557- 28565

Gharavi, N.M., Baker, N.A., Mouillesseaux, K.P., Yeung, W., Honda, H.M., Hsieh, X., Yeh, M., Smart, E.J., & Berliner, J.A. (2006). Role of endothelial nitric oxide synthase in the regulation of SREBP activation by oxidized phospholipids. *Circ Res,* 98(6):768-776

Harrison, D., Griendling, K.K., Landmesser, U., Hornig, B., & Drexler, H. (2003). Role of oxidative stress in atherosclerosis. *Am J Cardiol,* 91:7A-11A

Heitzer, T., Krohn, K., Albers, S., & Meinertz, T. (2000). Tetrahydrobiopterin improves endothelium-dependent vasodilation by increasing nitric oxide activity in patients with Type II diabetes mellitus. *Diabetologia*, 43:1435-1438

Hemmens, B. & Mayer, B. (1998). Enzymology of nitric oxide synthases. *Methods Mol Biol*, 100:1–32

Herman, A. G., & Moncada, S. (2005). Therapeutic potential of nitric oxide donors in the prevention and treatment of atherosclerosis. *Eur Heart J*, 26(19):1945–1955

Hink, U., Li, H., Mollnau, H., Oelze, M., Matheis, E., Hartmann, M., Skatchkov, M., Thaiss, F., Stahl, R.A.K., Warnholtz, A., Meinertz, T., Griendling, K., Harrison, D.G., Förstermann, U., & Münzel, T. (2001). Mechanisms underlying endothelial dysfunction in diabetes mellitus. *Circ Res*, 88(2):E14-E22

Hodgin, J.B., Knowles, J.W., Kim, H.S., Smithies, O., & Maeda, N. (2002). Interactions between endothelial nitric oxide synthase and sex hormones in vascular protection in mice. *J Clin Invest*, 109:541-548

Horke, S., Witte, I., Wilgenbus, P., Kruger, M., Strand, D., & Förstermann, U. (2007). Paraoxonase-2 reduces oxidative stress in vascular cells and decreases endoplasmic reticulum stress-induced caspase activation. *Circulation*, 115:2055–2064

Hrabie, J.A., Klose, J.R., Wink, D.A., & Keefer, L.K. (1993). New nitric oxide- releasing zwitterions derived from polyamines. *J Org Chem*, 58:1472–1476

Ishikawa, K., Kanamasa, K., Ogawa, I., Takenaka, T., Naito, T., Kamata, N., Yamamoto, T., Nakai, S., Hama, J., Oyaizu, M., Kimura, A., Yamamoto, K., Aso, N., Arai, M., Yabushita, & H., Katori, Y. (1996). Long-term nitrate treatment increases cardiac events in patients with healed myocardial infarction. Secondary Prevention Group. *Jpn Circ J*, 60(10):779-788

Ishimaru, R.S., Leung, K., Hong, L., & LaPolt, P.S. (2001). Inhibitory effects of nitric oxide on estrogen production and cAMP levels in rat granulose cell cultures. *J Endocrinol*, 168:249–255 ISIS-4 (Fourth International Study of Infarct Survival) Collaborative Group. (1995). ISIS-4: arandomised factorial trial assessing early oral captopril, oral mononitrate, and intravenous magnesium sulphate in 58,050 patients with suspected acute myocardial infarction. *Lancet*, 345:669–685

Jiang, F., Roberts, S.J., Datla, S., & Dusting, G.J. (2006). NO modulates NADPH oxidasefunction via heme oxygenase-1 in human endothelial cells. *Hypertension* 48:950–957

John, S., Schlaich, M., Langenfeld, M., Weihprecht, H., Schmitz, G., Weidinger, G., &Schmieder, R.E.(1998). Increased bioavailability of nitric oxide after lipidlowering therapy in hypercholesterolemic patients: a randomized, placebo-controlled, double-blind study. *Circulation*,211–216

Jung, O., Marklund, S.L., Xia, N., Busse, R., & Brandes, R.P. (2007). Inactivation of extracellular superoxide dismutase contributes to the development of high-volume hypertension. *Arterioscler Thromb Vasc Biol*, 27:470–477

Kapil, V., Milsom, A.B., Okorie, M., Maleki-Toyserkani, S., Akram, F., Rehman, F.,Arghandawi, S., Pearl, V., Benjamin, N., Loukogeorgakis, S., Macallister, R., Hobbs, A.J., Webb, A.J., & Ahluwalia, A. (2010a). Inorganic nitrate supplementation lowers blood pressure in humans: role for nitrite-derived NO. *Hypertension*, 56(2):274-281

Kapil,V., Webb, A.J., & Ahluwalia, A. (2010b). Inorganic nitrate and the cardiovascularsystem. *Heart*, 96(21):1703-1709

Katusic, Z.S. (2001). Vascular endothelial dysfunction: does tetrahydrobiopterin play a role?*Am J Physiol Heart Circ Physiol*, 281: H981-986

Keefer, L.K., Nims, R.W., Davies, K.M., & Wink, D.A. (1996). 'NONOates' (1-substituteddiazen-1-ium-1,2-diolates) as nitric oxide donors: convenient nitric oxide dosage forms. *Meth Enzymol*, 268:281–293

Knowles, J.W., Reddick, R.L., Jennette, J.C., Shesely, E.G., Smithies, O., & Maeda N. (2000).Enhanced atherosclerosis and kidney dysfunction in eNOS(-/-)Apoe(-/-) mice are ameliorated by enalapril treatment. *J Clin Invest*, 105:451-845

Kockx, M.M., de Meyer, G.R., Muhring, J., Bult, H., Bultinck, J., & Herman, A.G. (1996).Distribution of cell replication and apoptosis in atherosclerotic plaques of cholesterol-fed rabbits. *Atherosclerosis*, 120:115–124

Kockx M.M. (1998). Apoptosis in the atherosclerotic plaque: quantitative and qualitativeaspects. *Arterioscler Thromb Vasc Biol*, 18:1519–1522

Kuhlencordt, P.J., Gyurko, R., Han, F., Scherrer-Crosbie, M., Aretz, T.H., Hajjar, R., Picard,M.H., & Huang, P.L. (2001). Accelerated atherosclerosis, aortic aneurysm formation, and ischemic heart disease in apolipoprotein E/endothelial nitric oxide synthase double-knockout mice. *Circulation*, 104(4):448-454

Kumar, V., Hong, S.Y., Maciag, A.E., Saavedra, J.E., Adamson, D.H., Prud' homme, R.K., Keefer, L.K., & Chakrapani, H. (2010). Stabilization of the nitric oxide (NO) prodrugs and anticancer leads, PABA/NO and double JS-K, through incorporation into PEG-protected nanoparticles. *Mol Pharm*, 7(1):291–298

Kureishi, Y., Luo, Z., Shiojima, I., Bialik, A., Fulton, D., Lefer, D.J., Sessa, W. C., & Walsh, K. (2000). The HMG-CoA reductase inhibitor simvastatin activates the protein kinase Akt and promotes angiogenesis in normocholesterolemic animals. *Nat Med*, 6:1004–1010

Landmesser, U., Dikalov, S., Price, S.R., McCann, L., Fukai, T., Holland, S.M., Mitch, W.E., &Harrison, D.G. (2003). Oxidation of tetrahydrobiopterin leads to uncoupling of endothelial cell nitric oxide synthase in hypertension. *J Clin Invest*, 111(8):1201-1209

Laufs, U., La Fata, V., Plutzky, J., & Liao, J.K. (1998). Upregulation of endothelial nitric oxidesynthase by HMG CoA reductase inhibitors. *Circulation*, 97:1129–1135

Laursen, J.B., Somers, M., Kurz, S., McCann, L., Warnholtz, A., Freeman, B.A., Tarpey, M., Fukai, T., & Harrison D.G. (2001). Endothelial regulation of vasomotion in apoE-deficient mice: implications for interactions between peroxynitrite and tetrahydrobiopterin. *Circulation*, 103(9):1282-1288

Lefer, D.J., & Lefer, A.M. (1988). Studies on the mechanism of the vasodilator action ofnicorandil. *Life Sci*, 42:1907–1914

Li, H., & Förstermann, U. (2000). Nitric oxide in the pathogenesis of vascular disease. *JPathol*, 190:244-254

Li, H., Wallerath, T., & Förstermann, U. (2002a). Physiological mechanisms regulating theexpression of endothelial-type NO synthase. *Nitric Oxide*, 7:132-147

Li, H., Wallerath, T., Münzel, T., & Förstermann, U. (2002b). Regulation of endothelial-typeNO synthase expression in pathophysiology and in response to drugs. *Nitric Oxide*, 7:149-164

Li, H., Witte, K., August, M., Brausch, I., Godtel-Armbrust, U., Habermeier, A., Closs, El.,Oelze, M., Münzel, T., & Förstermann, U. (2006). Reversal of endothelial nitric oxide synthase uncoupling and up-regulation of endothelial nitric oxide synthase expression lowers blood pressure in hypertensive rats. *J Am Coll Cardiol*, 47(12):2536-2544

Li, H., & Förstermann, U. (2009). Prevention of Atherosclerosis by Interference with theVascular Nitric Oxide System. *Curr Pharm Des*, 15(27):3133-3145

Lin, M.I., Fulton, D., Babbitt, R., Fleming, I., Busse, R., Pritchard, K.A. Jr., & Sessa, W.C. (2003). Phosphorylation of threonine 497 in endothelial nitric-oxide synthase coordinates the coupling of L-arginine metabolism to efficient nitric oxide production. *J Biol Chem*, 278: 44719–44726

Lloyd-Jones, IM., & Block, KD. (1996). The vascular biology of nitric oxide and its role inatherogenesis. *Annu Rev Med,*.47:365–375

Liu, VW., & Huang, PL. (2008). Cardiovascular roles of nitric oxide: a review of insightsfrom nitric oxide synthase gene disrupted mice. *Cardiovasc Res,*.77(1):19-29

Lundberg, J.O, Weitzberg, E., Lundberg, J.M., & Alving, K. (1994). Intragastric nitric oxideproduction in humans: measurements in expelled air. *Gut*. 35:1543–1546

Lundberg, J.O., & Weitzberg, E. (2005). NO Generation From Nitrite and Its Role in VascularControl. *Arterioscler Thromb Vasc Biol*, 25(5):915-922

Maas, R. (2005). Pharmacotherapies and their influence on asymmetric dimethylargine(ADMA). *Vasc Med*, 10(Suppl 1): S49-57

Mallis, R.J., Buss, J.E., & Thomas J.A. (2001). Oxidative modification of H-ras: S-thiolationand S-nitrosylation of reactive cysteines. *Biochem J*, 355:145–153

McNally, J.S., Davis, M.E., Giddens, D.P., Saha, A., Hwang, J., Dikalov, S., Jo, H., Harrison,D.G. (2003). Role of xanthine oxidoreductase and NAD(P)H oxidase in endothelial superoxide production in response to oscillatory shear stress. *Am J Physiol Heart Circ Physiol*, 285:H2290–H2297

Milkowski, A., Garg, H.K., Coughlin, J.R. & Bryan, N.S. (2010). Nutritional epidemiology inthe context of nitric oxide biology: A risk–benefit evaluation for dietary nitrite and nitrate. *Nitric Oxide*, 22(2):110-119

Moens, A.L., & Kass, D.A. (2006). Tetrahydrobiopterin and cardiovascular disease.*Arterioscler Thromb Vasc Biol*, 26:2439-2444

Moncada, S., Palmer, RM., & Higgs EA. (1991). Nitric oxide: physiology, pathophysiology,and pharmacology. *Pharmacol Rev*, 43(2):109–142

Mooradian, D.L., Hutsell, T.C., & Keefer, L.K. (1995). Nitric oxide (NO) donor molecules:effect of NO release rate on vascular smooth muscle cell proliferation in vitro. *J Cardiovasc Pharmacol*, 25:674–678

Morita, T. (2005). Heme oxygenase and atherosclerosis. *Arterioscler Thromb Vasc Biol*, 25: 1786–1795

Nakamura, Y., Moss, A.J., Brown, M.W., Kinoshita, M., & Kawai, C. (1999). Longterm nitrateuse may be deleterious in ischemic heart disease: A study using the databases from two large-scale postinfarction studies. Multicenter Myocardial Ischemia Research Group. *Am Heart J*, 138:577-585

Ohara, Y., Peterson, T.E., & Harrison, D.G. (1993). Hypercholesterolemia increasesendothelial superoxide anion production. *J Clin Invest*, 91:2546–2551

Ozaki, M., Kawashima, S., Yamashita, T., Hirase, T., Namiki, M., Inoue, N., Hirata, K., Yasui,H., Sakurai, H., Yoshida,Y., Masada, M., & Yokoyama, M. (2002). Overexpression of endothelial nitric oxide synthase accelerates atherosclerotic lesion formation in apoE-deficient mice. *J Clin Invest*, 110(3):331-340

Pritchard, K.A., Jr., Groszek, L., Smalley, D.M., Sessa, W.C., Wu, M., Villalon, P., Wolin,M.S., & Stemerman, M.B. (1995). Native low-density lipoprotein increases endothelial cell nitric oxide synthase generation of superoxide anion. *Circ Res*, 77(3):510-518

Psychogios, N., Hau, D.D., Peng, J., Guo, A.C., Mandal, R., Bouatra, S., Sinelnikov, I.,Krishnamurthy, R., Eisner, R., Gautam, B., Young, N., Xia, J., Knox, C., Dong, E., Huang, P., Hollander, Z., Pedersen, T.L., Smith, S.R., Bamforth, F., Greiner, R., McManus, B., Newman, J.W., Goodfriend, T., & Wishart, D.S. (2011). The human serum metabolome. *PLoS One*,16;6(2):e16957

Radomski, M.W., Palmer, R.M., & Moncada, S. (1987). The anti- aggregating properties ofvascular endothelium: interactions between prostacyclin and nitric oxide. *Br J Pharmacol*, 92:639–646

Ramachandran, A., Levonen, A.L., Brookes, P.S., Ceaser, E., Shiva, S., Barone, M.C., &Darley-Usmar, V. (2002). Mitochondria, nitric oxide, and cardiovascular dysfunction. *Free Radic Biol Med*, 33:1465–1474

Riccio, D.A., Dobmeier, K.P., Hetrick, E.M., Privett, B.J., Paul, H.S., & Schoenfisch, M.H. (2009). Nitric oxide-releasing S-nitrosothiol-modified xerogels. *Biomaterials*, 30:4494–502

Rosenson, R.S., & Tangney, C.C. (1998). Antiatherothrombotic properties of statins:implications for cardiovascular event reduction. *JAMA*, 279:1643–1650

Rozenberg, O., Shih, D.M., & Aviram, M. (2005). Paraoxonase 1 (PON1) attenuatesmacrophage oxidative status: studies in PON1 transfected cells and in PON1 transgenic mice. *Atherosclerosis*, 181:9–18

Ryoo, S., Lemmon, C.A., Soucy, K.G., Gupta, G., White, A.R., Nyhan, D., Shoukas, A.,Romer, L.H., & Berkowitz, D.E. (2006). Oxidized low-density lipoprotein-dependent endothelial arginase II activation contributes to impaired nitric oxide signaling. *Circ Res*, 99(9):951-960

Sarkar, R., Gordon, D., Stanley, J.C., & Webb, R.C. (1997). Cell cycle effects of nitric oxide onvascular smooth muscle cells. *Am J Physiol*, 272:H1810–1818

Schmidt, A., Geigenmüller, S., Völker, W., Seiler, P., & Buddecke, E. (2003). Exogenousnitric oxide causes overexpression of TGF-beta1 and overproduction of extracellular matrix in human coronary smooth muscle cells. *Cardiovasc Res*, 58: 671–678

Schmidt, A., Bilgasem, S., Lorkowski, S., Vischer, P., Völker, W., Breithardt, G., Siegel, G., &Buddecke, E. (2008). Exogenous nitric oxide regulates activity and synthesis of vascular endothelial nitric oxide synthase. *Eur J Clin Invest*, 38(7):476–485

Schmidt, T.S., & Alp, N.J. (2007). Mechanisms for the role of tetrahydrobiopterin inendothelial function and vascular disease. *Clin Sci (Lond)*, 113:47-63

Schnabel, R., & Blankenberg, S. (2007). Oxidative stress in cardiovascular disease: successfultranslation from bench to bedside? *Circulation*, 116:1338-1340

Schulz, E., Anter, E., & Keaney, J.F. Jr. (2004).Oxidative stress, antioxidants, and endothelialfunction. *Curr Med Chem*, 11:1093–1104

Schulz, R., Kelm, M., & Heusch, G. (2004). Nitric oxide in myocardial ischemia/reperfusioninjury. *Cardiovasc Res*, 61(3):402– 413

Shinozaki, K., Kashiwagi, A., Nishio, Y., Okamura, T., Yoshida, Y., Masada, M., Toda, N., & Kikkawa, R. (1999). Abnormal biopterin metabolism is a major cause of impaired endothelium-dependent relaxation through nitric oxide/O2- imbalance in insulin-resistant rat aorta. *Diabetes*, 48(12):2437-2445

Sorescu, D., Weiss, D., Lassegue, B., Clempus, R.E., Szocs, K., Sorescu, G.P., Valppu, L.,Quinn, M.T., Lambeth, J.D., Vega, J.D., Taylor, W.R., & Griendling, K.K. (2002). Superoxide production and expression of nox family proteins in human atherosclerosis. *Circulation*, 105:1429–1435

Sowers, J.R. (2003). Effects of statins on the vasculature: implications for aggressive lipidmanagement in the cardiovascular metabolic syndrome. *Am J Cardiol*, 91:14B–22B

Stuehr, D., Pou, S., & Rosen, G.M. (2001). Oxygen reduction by nitric- oxide synthases. *J BiolChem*, 276:14533–14536

Sud, N., Wells, S.M., Sharma, S., Wiseman, D.A., Wilham, J., & Black, S.M. (2008).Asymmetric dimethylarginine inhibits HSP90 activity in pulmonary arterial endothelial cells: role of mitochondrial dysfunction. *Am J Physiol Cell Physiol*, 294:C1407-1418

Sullivan, J.C., Pollock, J.S. (2006). Coupled and uncoupled NOS: separate but equal?Uncoupled NOS in endothelial cells is a critical pathway for intracellular signaling. *Circ Res*, 98:717-719

Sun, J., Xin, C., Eu, J.P., Stamler, J.S., & Meissner, G. (2001). Cysteine-3635 is responsible forskeletal muscle ryanodine receptor modulation by NO. *Proc Natl Acad Sci USA*, 98:1158-1162

Tang, Y., Jiang, H., & Bryan, N.S. (2011). Nitrite and nitrate: cardiovascular risk-benefit andmetabolic effect. *Curr Opin Lipidol*, 22(1):11-15

Thomas, G.R., DiFabio, J.M., Gori, T., & Parker, J.D. (2007). Once daily Therapy WithIsosorbide-5-Mononitrate Causes Endothelial Dysfunction in Humans. *J Am Coll Cardiol*, 49:1289-1295

Torzewski, M., Ochsenhirt, V., Kleschyov, A.L., Oelze, M., Daiber, A., Li, H., Rossmann, H., Tsimikas, S., Reifenberg, K., Cheng, F., Lehr, H.A., Blankenberg, S., Förstermann, U., Münzel, T., & Lackner, K.J. (2007). Deficiency of glutathione peroxidase-1 accelerates the progression of atherosclerosis in apolipoprotein E-deficient mice. *Arterioscler Thromb Vasc Biol*, 27:850-857

Vasan, R.S. (2006). Biomarkers of Cardiovascular Disease: Molecular Basis and PracticalConsiderations. *Circulation*, 113:2335-23362

Vasquez-Vivar, J., Duquaine, D., Whitsett, J., Kalyanaraman, B. & Rajagopalan, S. (2002).Altered tetrahydrobiopterin metabolism in atherosclerosis: implications for use of oxidized tetrahydrobiopterin analogues and thiol antioxidants. *Arterioscler Thromb Vasc Biol*, 22:1655-1661

White, C.R., Darley-Usmar, V., Berrington, W.R., McAdams, M., Gore, J.Z., Thompson, J.A.,Parks, D.A., Tarpey, M.M., & Freeman, B.A. (1996). Circulating plasma xanthine oxidase contributes to vascular dysfunction in hypercholesterolemic rabbits. *Proc Natl Acad Sci USA*, 93:8745-8749

Xia, Y., Tsai, A.L., Berka, V., & Zweier, J.L. (1998). Superoxide Generation from endothelialnitric-oxide synthase. A a2+/calmodulin-dependent and tetrahydrobiopterin regulatory process. *J Biol Chem*, 273:25804-25808

Xue, H.M., He, G.W., Huang, J.H., & Yang, Q. (2010). New strategy of endothelial protectionin cardiac surgery: use of enhancer of endothelial nitric oxide synthase. *World J Surg*, 34:1461-1469

Yamawaki, H., Haendeler, J., & Berk, B.C. (2003). Thioredoxin: a key regulator ofcardiovascular homeostasis. *Circ Res*, 93:1029-1033

Yan, M.S., Matouk, C.C., & Marsden, P.A. (2010). Epigenetics of the vascular endothelium. *JAppl Physiol*, 109(3):916-926

Yang, H., Roberts, L.J., Shi, M.J., Zhou, L.C., Ballard, B.R., Richardson, A., & Guo, Z.M.(2004). Retardation of atherosclerosis by overexpression of catalase or both Cu/Zn-superoxide dismutase and catalase in mice lacking apolipoprotein E. *Circ Res*, 95:1075-1081

Young, D.V., Serebryanik, D., Janero, D.R., & Tam, S.W. (2000). Suppression of proliferationof human coronary artery smooth muscle cells by the nitric oxide donor, S-nitrosoglutathione, is cGMP-independent. *Mol Cell Biol Res Commun*, 4:32-36

Zhang, Y., Griendling, K.K., Dikalova, A., Owens, G.K., & Taylor, W.R. (2005). Vascularhypertrophy in angiotensin II-induced hypertension is mediated by vascular smooth muscle cell-derived H2O2. *Hypertension*. 46:732-737

Zou, M.H., Shi, C.,& Cohen, R.A. (2002). Oxidation of the zinc- thiolate complex anduncoupling of endothelial nitric oxide synthase by peroxynitrite. *J Clin Invest*, 109:817-826

# 2

# The Role of Stress in a Pathogenesis of CHD

Taina Hintsa[1], Mirka Hintsanen[1,2],
Tom Rosenström[1] and Liisa Keltikangas-Järvinen[1]
*[1]IBS, Unit of Personality Work and Health Psychology, University of Helsinki*
*[2]Helsinki Collegium for Advanced Studies, University of Helsinki*
*Finland*

## 1. Introduction

Stress has been commonly seen as a risk factor of diseases of major public health relevance including Type 2 diabetes and coronary heart disease (CHD). An influence of stress in their development has been considered a "well-known fact" even to the extent that a pathogenesis of those diseases has been widely attributed to stress. Empirical evidence is, however, somewhat conflicting. Even though studies showing an association between work stress and CHD are great in number, negative findings also exist. Thus, there is no consensus on the clinical importance of work stress in a development of CHD. Consequently, work stress is currently not included in the list of established risk factors of CHD (www.americanheart.org).

There are, however, several reasons explaining the conflicting findings, and several aspects have been omitted in stress research. Even an assessment of stress is far from unambiquity. The present paper was taken with a purpose to highlight complicated associations between different kind of stress reactions and risk factors of CHD.

This review will capitalize on the longitudinal population based birth cohort study of the *Young Finns Study*. Here, the representative, population based sample of 3596 healthy subjects from six age cohorts have been followed for 30 years and monitored in 9 study phases in order to discover the lifelong development of risk factors of coronary heart disease. From the great multidisciplinary reservoir of risk factors available in the Young Finns settings, stress is the focus of the current paper.

In this chapter we focus on different types of stress, e.g. psychological, psychosocial, physiological stress and work stress. Special issues to be highlighted here are as follows: Do the origins of stress proneness lie in childhood? Is stress vulnerability inherited?, Which is worse in regard to health: chronic or acute stress?, Does stress really have health consequences? Do genetic predispositions explain an association between stress and its health outcomes? What are the problems with statistical analyses in epidemiological studies?

## 2. Coronary heart disease

Coronary artery disease (CAD) which gradually progresses to coronary heart disease (CHD) is still the leading cause of death in industrialized countries. According to World Health

Organization cardiovascular diseases are the number one cause of death globally. In 2004, cardiovascular diseases were globally the cause of death of 29% of all deaths. Of those deaths, approximately 7.2 million were due to CHD (www.who.int/mediacentre/factsheets/fs317/en/index.html). In Finland, among the working aged population, in men there were 1218 and in women 231 deaths due to CHD in 2008 (http://www3.ktl.fi/stat/).

Atherosclerosis is the pathogenic process that underlies most cardiovascular diseases including CHD. Recently, a non-invasive technique such as an ultrasound measure of intima-media thickness has been developed to assess early stages of atherosclerosis. Carotid artery intima-media thickness (IMT) is a marker of subclinical atherosclerosis and increased IMT has been shown to predict CHD (O'Leary & Polak 2002).

Although the inherited, even a genetic disposition to CHD has been documented, CHD is seen as a lifestyle disease. Certain lifestyle factors may contribute to the manifestation of genetic disposition, and eventually have an effect on the onset of CHD. American Heart Association lists traditional risk factors for CHD: increasing age, male sex and heredity; smoking, high blood cholesterol, high blood pressure, physical inactivity and obesity (modifiable risk factors), and stress, alcohol and diet/nutrition as other risk factors of CHD.The traditional behavioural risk factors of CHD include smoking, alcohol consumption and physical inactivity. Behavioural and personality characteristics may be seen as lifestyle factors too, because they contribute to significant choices and decisions that individuals make during their lives. A systematic review of the epidemiological literature of prospective cohort studies, that is articles between 1966-1997 identify four psychosocial or behavioural risk factors of CHD: Type A behaviour,/hostility, depression, psychosocial work characteristics, and social support (Hemingway & Marmot 1999). According to a prognosis of World Health Organization stressful life events and psychosocial stress will the most detrimental risk factors for the development of cardiovascular diseases in the near future (http://www.who.int/en/).

In this chapter we introduce some recent findings about childhood and adolescent origins of stress, stress-health associations, e.g. temperament and early atherosclerosis (Hintsanen et. al., 2009a), the association between chronic stress and preclinical atherosclerosis (Chumaeva et. al., 2009a), and long-lasting chronic stress strengthening the physiological stress reactions in acute stress (Chumaeva et. al., 2010a). Furthermore, the topic whether stress has implications for CHD risk and what are the potential mechanisms are discussed.

## 3. The Young Finns study

In the literature, The Bogalusa Heart Study and the Young Finns Study are the only population-based prospective follow-up studies that have examined cardiovascular disease and CHD risks since childhood that have collected psychological information. The collection of psychological information in the Bogalusa Heart Study continued until the end of 1980s, and since then the Young Finns Study has been collecting psychological data. Thus, the Young Finns data is worldwide quite unique and it makes possible to study psychological risk factors of CHD from childhood on.

The Young Finns Study is a multi-centre study which was carried out in five university cities in Finland which have medical schools (Helsinki, Kuopio, Oulu, Tampere and Turku), and in rural municipalities nearby (Fig. 1). The areas of Helsinki, Tampere and Turku represented the west of the country, and the Kuopio and Oulu areas represented eastern Finland. The rural municipalities were chosen using the criteria of correspondence of industrial structure with average municipalities in the province, the age cohort being sufficiently large. The sample included an equal number of urban and rural populations in the area (Åkerblom et. al., 1991).To ensure equal and sufficiently large samples from east and west, and to include some communities in the extreme east, the sample size in Kuopio was twice that in other cities, with four instead of two rural municipalities included in the study (Åkerblom et al 1991). Two of the easternmost rural municipalities studied in the Kuopio area belonged to the province of North Karelia, where CHD morbidity and mortality among adults have been especially high (Menotti et. al., 1989). In 1980 the baseline study sample consisted of 4326 invited participants of which over 3500 children and adolescents aged from 3 to 18 participated (83.1%). The study included medical examinations and questionnaires (both self- and parent reports). These participants have had medical examinations and have filled questionnaires including demographic, socioeconomic/social and psychological information in the follow-up studies conducted in 1983, 1986, 1989, 1992, 1997, 2001, 2007 and 2011. The study design and the number of participants and the response rates at each data collection phases are outlined in Figure 2.

The participants have reported several aspects of their lives during 31 years, at several time points. These aspects include a wide range of CHD risk factors such as socioeconomic conditions, social life, health behaviour, dietary habits, environmental factors and personality.

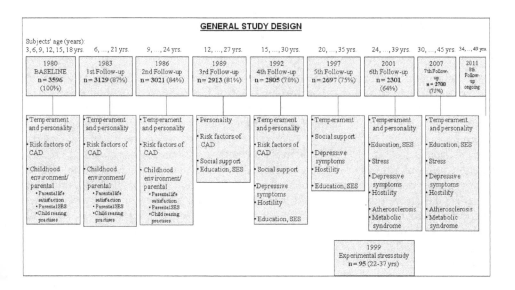

Fig. 1. The general study desing of the Young Finns Study.

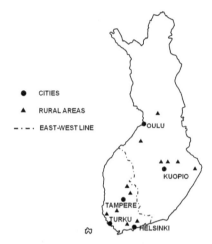

Fig. 2. The Young Finns Study: participating universities in Finland.

## 4. Stress

The purpose of this chapter is to highlight complicated associations between different kind of stress reactions and risk factors of CHD. Generally the term stress refers to experiences of endangering one's physical or psychological wellbeing. Physiological stress refers to bodily adaptation processes and the maintenance of body's balance (McEwen 1998; Selye 1973). Selye (1973) defined stress as a function of elevated corticosteroid levels and used the term stress to refer to the effects of any agent that threatens the homeostasis of the organism. McEwen and Stellar introduced (1993) the term allostasis which refers to the body's ability to achieve stability. The allostatic load is assumed to be caused by frequent stress, lack of adaptation to repeated stress, and inability to shut down the allostatic response when the stress is over and inadequate response or dysfunction of the stress systems (McEwen 1998).

In the behavioural sciences, stress refers to a mental experience of distress caused by the evaluation of the imbalance between available personal resources (individual appraisals of stressful encounters) and environmental demands (e.g. stressful life events). Thus, psychological stress can be defined as a discrepancy between personal capacities and environmental demands (Lazarus & Folkman 1984). Somatic stress symptoms are related to both physiological and psychological stress (Lazarus & Folkman 1984; Lovallo 1997). The different types of stressors are likely to elicit divergent stress reactions. The multifaceted nature of stress and various sources of stress must also be taken into account. It is important to define the stress precisely in epidemiological studies. Consequently, stress has been determined here in terms of stressful life events, experience of chronic stress, experimentally induced mental and physiological stress reactions and work stress.

### 4.1 Work stress

European Foundation for the improvement of living and working conditions (2007) reports that work stress is affecting more than 40 million individuals across the European Union, and is among the most often reported cause of illness by employees. Work stress has been suggested to increase the CHD risk via several different pathways and mechanisms. Therefore it is important to focus also on psychosocial characteristics at work in regard to cardiovascular health. The work stress models that are presented here have been used extensively in studies of occupational and cardiovascular health (Belkic et. al., 2004; van Vegchel et. al., 2005).

Theories of work stress focus on various aspects in the work environment. Contemporary models on work stress include factors that are long-term harmful stressors at work. There are several work stress models, but the scientifically most tested concepts include The Job Demands-Job control Model (Karasek & Theorell 1990) and the Effort-Reward Imbalance (ERI) model (Siegrist et. al., 2004). More recently organisational justice has been hypothesized to form an important source of stress at work (Elovainio et. al., 2010; Kivimäki et. al., 2005).

The two-dimensional Job Demands-Job Control model involves work-related aspects of job demands and job control. Job demands refer to time pressures and an excessive work load, and job control involves employees' decision latitude and opportunities to use social, organisational and personal resources in their work. The model proposes that employees who have high job demands together with low job control are suffering from job strain, and if prolonged, have increased risk of stress-related diseases. The ERI model of work stress is based on social exchange theory and it has broadened the view from proximal work aspects into descriptive and evaluative information on job demands, i.e. efforts, and more distant aspects of work, i.e. rewards. Efforts denote quantative and qualitative load, and increase in total load at work. Rewards refer to financial reward, esteem reward, reward related to promotion aspects and job security (Siegrist et al 2004).

Research on the psychosocial health determinants has recently extended the focus also to organizational justice, that is, social relations, decision making and managerial procedures at work (Colquitt 2001; Kivimäkii et. al., 2005). Organizational justice can be defined as "the extent to which employees are treated with justice at their workplace" (Colquitt 2001; Moorman 1991). Organisational justice includes four components: 1) procedural justice, 2) interpersonal justice, 3) informational justice and (4) distributive justice. Procedural justice refers to being able to express your views and feelings during organisational procedures, perceiving that they have been consistently applied. Interpersonal justice denotes aspects of supervisors' behaviour, i.e. have they treated the person with respect and dignity. Informational justice consists of communicating and giving details about the decisions. Distributive justice refers to the perception of whether outcomes at work reflect the effort one has put into work and whether the outcome is appropriate.

## 5. Do the origins of stress-proneness lie in childhood?

It may be suggested that origins of one's stress proneness lie in childhood. This has not been studied a lot in humans, but rationale for this suggestion has been derived from animal studies. Several studies conducted on rats and nonhuman primates have shown that lack of nurturing behavior does affect the stress systems of the pups so that pups that have received less nurturing develop altered physiological stress responsiveness and show increased behavioral stress reactivity in adulthood (Caldji et. al., 1998; Coplan et. al., 1996; Ladd et. al., 1996; Liu et. al., 1997).

The effect of maternal care to the development of offspring stress responsiveness has been examined with various research designs. For example, by handling the pups it is possible to increase the nurturing behaviors performed by the mother such as licking and grooming, and this makes it possible to compare pups that have received high nurturing by the mother and pups who have received normal care (Liu et al 1997). Studies have also used maternal separation for instant by comparing the physiological stress responsiveness of pups that have not been separated and pups that have been separated from their mother for varying periods of time (Stanton et. al., 1988). However, this kind of design might be suspected to reflect effects of food deprivation rather than deprivation of maternal nurturing. To examine whether this is the case, a study by Stanton, Gutierrez and Levine (1988) specifically examined whether increased stress responsiveness is related to lack of maternal nurturing or to lack of nutrition offered by the lactating mother. Their results showed that the association was partly dependent on the age of the examined rat pups so that in younger ages (12 and 16 days of age), lack of maternal nurturing increased stress reactivity, whereas when the pups grew somewhat older (20 days of age), the lack of maternal nurturing as well as the lack of nutrition increased stress reactivity assessed as elevated corticoid levels in response to novelty situation (Stanton et al 1988). Based on these results, it seems that maternal nurturing has an independent effect that cannot be explained by food deprivation.

Still other design was used by Coplan and colleagues (1996) who compared offspring of mother monkeys (bonnet macaques) who had differing conditions in which they foraged for food. One group of mothers foraged in uncertain conditions (the amount of needed foraging varied) whereas the other group foraged in predictable conditions (the amount of needed foraging was either constantly low or constantly high) (Coplan et al 1996). As it has been shown that unpredictable need for foraging lowers the amount of grooming the mother directs towards the monkey infants (Rosenblum & Paully 1984), comparing different foraging groups allows to compare the effects of higher and lower maternal nurturing behaviors.

In general, the studies conducted on animals that have examined effects of maternal nurturing to the stress responsiveness of the infants in their adulthood, have shown that those infants who have received less nurturing from their mothers show various alterations in their hypothalamic-pituitary-adrenal (HPA) -axis functioning later in life (Caldji et al 1998; Coplan et al 1996; Liu et al 1997). For instance, in response to acute stressors, offspring have shown changed physiological stress reactivity measured with plasma levels of adrenocorticotrophin hormone (ACTH), levels of corticosterone, glucocorticoid feedback sensitivity, and levels of hypothalamic corticotrophin-releasing hormone messenger RNA (Liu et al 1997). Furthermore, stable increases in corticotrophin releasing factor (CRF) in the cerebrospinal fluid have been found in grown up offspring of less nurturing mothers (Coplan et al 1996). Also changes in behaviour are observable, and offspring of less nurturing mothers show higher rates of behaviours reflecting stress (e.g. fearfulness) (Caldji et al 1998).

There are also several other findings that show that changes in stress reactivity in response to lower maternal nurturing can be found also in humans. For instance, Repetti, Taylor and Seeman (2002) have reviewed the literature and concluded that childhood unsupportive family relations (e.g. high rate of conflicts in the family and low nurturing) affect physiological stress responsiveness of HPA-axis functioning and sympathetic-adrenomedullary (SAM) functioning as well as emotion regulation and coping with stress. However, long-term prospective studies are rare.

## 6. Is stress vulnerability inherited?

Temperament refers to biologically rooted, partly inherited, relatively stable individual differences in reactivity to stimuli (Cloninger et. al., 1993; Gray 1991; Lewis & Haviland 1993; Strelau 1998). The inheritance of stress refers here to an innate temperament. Rationale is as follows: temperament a) has a biological basis, b) is highly inherited, and c) explains what one experiences as a stress and partly determines what the health consequences are. The common assumption in several temperament theories is that temperament plays important role in moderating stress (Strelau 1998). Temperament traits are closely related to emotions that have been suggested to be a possible source of stress-related individual differences (Lovallo 1997). Temperament is considered to be an important determinant in what one indentifies as a stressor, a state of stress, in how one copes with stress and therefore also the physiological consequences of stress (Strelau 1998). Temperament may explain a perception of stress and may predispose to negative emotional stress reactions.

## 7. Acute stress vs. chronic stress

Acute stress refers to a very short-time stress that can both be positive (eustress) and more distressing experience such as daily hassles or stressful encounters in day-to-day life. Chronic stress is the type of stress that is ongoing for a longer period of time and often feels unmanageable. Both acute and chronic stress may be detrimental to health (Lovallo 1997). It is not clear which is more detrimental to health, acute or chronic stress. What is likely that they may have different effects on health.

Acute stress is a normal adaptive reaction to threat of the sympathetic-adrenal-medullary axis (SAM) releasing catecholamines and the hypothalamic-pituitary-adrenal (HPA) axis secretion of glucocorticoids (Sapolsky et. al., 2000). Even though acute stress reaction is adaptive and necessary, it may have detrimental influences on cardiac health. Acute stress may trigger cardiac events or lead to sudden death (Culic 2007; Hemingway et. al., 2001).

Chronic stress is likely to influence the autonomic nervous system function, and may alter the endocrine system and the immune system function. If a person is exposed to chronic stress, the SAM and HPA axis are continuously over-activated or in imbalance, and overcompensation or collapse of these systems may leave the individual susceptible to stress-related diseases (Korte et. al., 2005). Prolonged secretion of epinephrine, norepinephrine and cortisol, i.e. primary stress mediators, may affect the stress system so that their ability to protect the organism is compromised and instead starting to damage the brain and the body (McEwen 2008). The secondary outcomes of the wear and tear condition processes are the metabolic parameters such as insulin, cholesterol, triglycerides which may reach sub-clinical level at this stage of stress. The final stage of stress may include the wear and tear of the body, i.e. allostatic exhaustion (McEwen 1998; 2008).

## 8. Work stress

Several epidemiological studies have shown the association between work stress and CHD risk (Belkic et al 2004; Kivimäki et. al., 2006; van Vegchel et al 2005). Job strain has been suggested to be a risk factor for CHD and cardiac events (Belkic et al 2004; Kivimäki et. al., 2002; Kivimäkii et. al., 2006). A review of 45 empirical studies on effort-reward imbalance between 1986-2003 reports that the extrinsic effort-reward hypothesis (high effort combined with low rewards increase disease risk) has shown a good explanatory power for the incidence of CHD (van Vegchel et al 2005).

Previous studies report lower levels of organisational justice to be associated with lower wellbeing, higher self reported morbidity, higher medically certified absence from work, and increased mental health problems (Elovainio et. al., 2000; Elovainio et. al., 2001; Kivimäki et. al., 2003; Kivimäki et. al., 2005). Injustice at work has been related to impaired cardiovascular regulation among women (Elovainio et. al., 2006b), and cardiovascular mortality (Elovainio et al 2006b). Low organizational justice has been reported to be a risk to the health of employees (Elovainio et. al., 2006a). Furthermore, it has been reported that employees who experience high organisational justice at work had lower risk of incident CHD than those with low or an intermediate level of justice (Kivimäki et. al., 2005).

When studying work stress-CHD risk associations, it is important to examine the role of third variables such as pre-employment origins of work stress. We have examined the childhood origins of work stress which is a novel perspective in work stress research. Furthermore, it is also important to extend work stress research towards taking individual differences and genetic influences into account.

## 9. Does stress have implications for CHD risk and what are the potential mechanisms?

Showing the causal link between stress and the outcome requires evidence and knowledge about the potential mechanisms. The research of the Young Finns Study provides epidemiological and experimental evidence on the importance of stress in early atherosclerosis and in the pathogenesis of CHD, and also shows that the associations between stress and cardiovascular risk are complicated.

Stress may influence health via several different pathways, i.e. alterations in autonomic nervous system, neuroendocrine activity, immune system functions, behavioral and cognitive functions (Lovallo 1997). Prolonged stress may alter the function of autonomic nervous system, neuroendocrine functions and inflammation systems (McEwen 1998; Sapolsky 1996; Sapolsky et al 2000), and it may affect individuals' health-behaviour in terms of increased smoking and alcohol consumption, and decreased physical activity, and may increase anxiety, depression and psychological distress and include alterations in memory functions and attention (Hemingway & Marmot 1999; Lovallo 1997). Being exposed to chronic stress may lead to different types of health problems such as mental disorders, vital exhaustion, burnout and increase of CHD disease risk via several different pathways (Lovallo 1997).

### 9.1 Epidemiological evidence

The findings presented in this chapter are mainly from the Young Finns study (YFS) and they focus on early atherosclerosis. The results of a smaller sample of men describe the associations between psychological factors and hormonal variables and Insulin resistance syndrome risk factors.

In the YFS, an association between job strain and IMT has been documented among men aged 32.3 years on average (Hintsanen et. al., 2005). This implies that among men job strain may be linked to atherosclerosis in its early non-symptomatic stages. A recent longitudinal study on the association between job strain and IMT reports that large decreases in job strain from 2001 to 2007 in men was associated with slower progression of IMT and decreases in both job control and demands (a change towards passive jobs) were associated with greater IMT progression (Rosenström et. al., 2011). These results imply that temporal changes in job demands and control are linked with IMT.

Our research has focused in three temperament theories: Gray's neurobiological model of temperament, Cloninger's psychobiological theory of temperament, and the EAS theory of temperament by Buss and Plomin. Gray's temperamental model assumes three fundamental systems with independent neurobiological mechanisms in the mammalian central nervous system (CNS): the behavioral inhibition system (BIS), the behavioral approach system (BAS) and the fight/flight system (FFS). The BIS is activated by aversive stimuli and is assumed to cause behavioral inhibition, and increase in attention levels and negative affects. The BAS is primarily activated by appetitive stimuli causing approach behavior and positive affects. There are individual differences in the sensitivity or functioning strength of these systems. Thus, some individuals are more prone to react to incentives and to experience positive affects, that is BAS sensitive, while some are fixed to threats in the environment and more likely to experience negative affects than others (Corr 2008; Gray 1991).

Cloninger's psychobiological theory of temperament, measured by temperament and character inventory (TCI) includes three genetically independent dimensions of temperament: novelty seeking (NS), harm avoidance (HA) and reward dependence (RD) (Cloninger et al 1993). Persistence (P) was added to the model a little bit later (Cloninger et al 1993). Novelty seeking, linked with dopaminergic activity, refers to tendency to respond strongly to novelty. High novelty seeking is characterized by exploratory behaviors, impulsivity, excitability and disorderliness. Harm avoidance, related to serotonergic activity, denotes that high harm avoidant persons are cautious, fearful, inhibited and prone to anxiety and fatigue. Reward dependence, associated with noradrenalin activity, refers to sensitivity to social cues, empathy and sentimentality. Persistence is a tendency to act persistently regardless of weariness and frustration, and high persistence is characterized by perseverance.

The emotionality-activity-sociability (EAS) theory of temperament focuses on broad temperament traits that are likely to be present in majority of situations (Buss & Plomin 1984). The temperament traits are negative emotionality, sociability and activity. Negative emotionality is characterized by tendency to get upset easily and equals to stress sensitivity. Sociability is a preference to be in a company of other people. Activity refers to the tempo of physical actions and vigor referring to the strength with which these actions are performed.

*Temperament and early atherosclerosis.* Temperament traits in terms of Cloninger's temperament theory explain between-individual variation in atherosclerosis (Hintsanen et al 2009a). Higher NS and RD, and lower HA were associated with preclinical atherosclerosis. The effect sizes of the associations found were comparable to those of traditional risk factors of CHD, which is an important finding. Novelty seekers are likely to seek for novel situations and environments, and via that encounter stressful situations continuously, i.e. be exposed to stress frequently. High RD persons seek for approval and have desire to please others, potentially even at the expense of their own wellbeing. Harm avoidant persons are characterised by stress-proneness and therefore a positive relation between high HA and higher IMT would have been expected. Stress reactions of highly harm avoidant persons increase in experimental settings, but in real life, however, they may have successfully learned to avoid stressful situations and thus be less exposed to stress.

In women, childhood hyperactivity has been shown to predict IMT in adulthood (Keltikangas-Järvinen et. al., 2006). It was concluded that childhood temperament may directly contribute to the development on IMT in women. This association might partly be explained by different environmental expectations for boys and girls. The same temperament plays a different roles in boys and girls (Kerr et. al., 1997). The association between childhood hyperactivity and adulthood IMT among women might be due to that high hyperactivity in girls may enhance the misfit with the environment which, in turn, may be related to chronic stress (Keltikangas-Järvinen et. al., 2006).

We have found an association between active temperament and early atherosclerosis among men. The results of a study on emotionality-activity-sociability temperament and preclinical atherosclerosis showed that a highly active temperament may contribute to early atherosclerosis in men, and that body mass may mediate this association (Pulkki-Råback et. al., 2011).

*Chronic stress and cardiac responsiveness.* Endothelial dysfunction is a marker of atherosclerotic risk (Bonetti et. al., 2003), and arterial elasticity indicated by carotid arterial compliance (CAC) may be an additional indicator of early atherosclerosis (Anderson 2006). We studied the role of chronic stress, endothelial dysfunction and arterial elasticity in regard to IMT. Chronic stress was indexed by vital exhaustion which is a state of unusual fatigue, a loss of mental and physical energy and increased irritability (Appels et. al., 1987), and has been referred as an indicator of long-term mental stress (Ingles et. al., 1999). Endothelial dysfunction was indexed by brachial flow-mediated dilation (FMD), and carotid elasticity by CAC. A significant VE and FMD, and VE and CAC interactions on IMT were found in participants with the very lowest FMD and CAC. It was concluded that chronic stress may especially harmful if the endothelium is not working properly (Chumaeva et al 2009a). Chronic stress was negatively related to FMD, which may imply that chronic stress may contribute to endothelial dysfunction. A study on the possible sex differences in the combined effect of chronic stress with impaired vascular endothelium functioning and the development of early atherosclerosis showed a significant VE x CAC interaction on IMT among men. High VE level was related to higher IMT among those men with low CAC (Chumaeva et. al., 2010b). These results imply that vital exhaustion is a risk only if it has resulted in ineffective cardiac stress reactivity. Chronic stress may induce imbalance of the autonomic function which may be the mechanism linking vital exhaustion and cardiac responsiveness to an increased risk of atherosclerosis.

Chronic stress in terms of major stressful life events and vital exhaustion has been related to arrhythmic events (Hintsa et. al., 2010c). A history of stressful life events and prolonged mental stress have been associated with arrhythmic events among subjects who are genetically predisposed to cardiac vulnerability (a sample of molecularly defined patients with long QT syndrome). In this group of patients the interaction of a gene defect and the environmental loading may contribute to the manifestation of arrhythmic events.

*Psychological factors and IRS.* Stress may be a trigger for the neuroendocrine and metabolic abnormalities characteristic to the metabolic syndrome. It has been shown that chronic stress may exert effects on waist-hip –ratio (WHR) and on subsequent metabolic alterations.

Chronic stress is suggested to exert a pathophysiological effect on WHR, on alterations in insulin and lipid metabolism, in fibrinolysis and in blood pressure. Perceived stress modifies an association between neuroendocrine mechanisms and metabolic syndrome. The associations may be explained by HPA-axis dysfunction, that is, a failure to adrenal hypoactivity to prevent overshooting of reactions to stress (Räikkönen et. al., 1997). Psychological factors may explain a proportion of HPA-axis responses that are related to Insulin resistance syndrome (IRS). Type A behavior was related to a high level of mean basal ACTH and a low level of cortisol response to ACTH stimulation after dexamethasone suppression. Hostility was linked to a high level of mean basal cortisol and a high cortisol in cortisol/ACTH –ratio. Vital exhaustion that indexes chronic stress was related to a low level of mean basal ACTH and a decreased ACTH in relation to cortisol (Keltikangas-Järvinen et. al., 1997; Keltikangas-Järvinen et. al., 1996b). Stress modulated adrenal responsiveness may partly explain the IRS risk, and the risk of atherosclerosis, too. Chronic stress and stressful life-style have been related to the IRS (Räikkönen et. al., 1996b). Chronic stress in terms of vital exhaustion, and a stressful life-style (Type A behavior, hostility and anger) were associated with hyperinsulinemia, hyperglycemia, dyslipidemia, hypertension, and increased abdominal obesity. The secondary outcomes of allostatic load include metabolic, cardiovascular and immune parameters' alterations and potential to reach sub-clinical levels of these (McEwen 1998; 2008; McEwen & Stellar 1993). Therefore it is important to further investigate the role of stress-related personality and behavioral factors in regard to metabolic alterations.

*Psychological factors and HPA-axis responses.* The studies presented in this paragraph have been conducted among middle-aged male managers who responded questionnaires, participated in laboratory analyses, and were clinically examined in Helsinki University Central hospital (n=64-90). Results of a study on the relationships between the pituitary adrenal hormones, insulin and glucose in regard to chronic stress showed that basal ACTH level during oral glucose tolerance test was positively related to the cortisol response to ACTH at 60 minutes, the fasting insulin level, and the insulin to glucose ratio among chronically stressed men (Keltikangas-Järvinen et. al., 1998).

A neuroendocrine pattern characterized by an elevation in cortisol response to ACTH stimulation and dominance of cortisol in the ratio of mean basal cortisol level to mean basal ACTH level denoting a defeat type of reaction to stress differentiated borderline hypertensive men from normotensive men (Räikkönen et. al., 1996a). The results may imply that the variance shared by chronic stress, emotional distress and pituitary-adrenocortical hormones could be the mechanism by which stress influences and increased risk for hypertension.

| Author, year | Study focus | Main findings |
|---|---|---|
| Hintsanen et. al., 2005 | IMT: job strain and social support | In men, job strain was related to higher IMT. |
| Rosenström et al., 2010 | IMT and job strain (2001 and 2007) | An association between job strain and IMT in 2001 among men. In men with large decreases in job strain-slower progression of IMT. |
| Hintsanen et. al., 2009a | IMT and Cloninger temperament | Higher NS and RD, and lower HA was associated with IMT. |
| Keltikangas-Jarvinen et. al., 2006 | IMT and childhood temperament | In women, childhood hyperactivity predicted adulthood IMT. |

| Author, year | Study focus | Main findings |
|---|---|---|
| Pulkki-Råback et. al., 2011 | IMT and EAS temperament | A highly active temperament may contribute to early atherosclerosis in men, and that body mass may mediated this association. |
| Chumaeva et. al., 2009a | IMT and chronic stress (VE) and endothelial dysfunction (FMD) | Significant VE and FMD, and VE and CAC interactions on IMT were found in participants with the very lowest FMD and CAC. |
| Chumaeva et. al., 2010b | IMT and chronic stress (VE), flow-mediated dilation (FMD), Carotid elasticity (CAC) | In men, a significant VE x CAC interaction on IMT. High VE level was related to higher IMT among those men with low CAC. |
| Hintsa et. al., 2010c | Arrhythmic events and chronic stress | A history of stressful life events and prolonged mental stress are associated with arrhythmic events in LQTS patients. The association between stressful life events and arrhythmic events was independent of age, sex, specifically focused drugs and LQTS subtype. |
| Räikkönen et. al., 1997 | IRS and chronic stress (VE) | Chronic stress excerted effects on WHR and on subsequent metabolic alterations which denote a chance of adrenal steroid biosynthesis. |
| Keltikangas-Järvinen et. al., 1996b | IRS and psychological factors | A link between VE-anger out and net-increment of cortisol and the IRS. |
| Räikkönen et. al., 1996b | IRS and stress inducing life style (Type A behaviour, hostility and anger) | Chronic stress in terms of vital exhaustion, and a stressful life-style (Type A behavior, hostility and anger) were associated with hyperinsulinemia, hyperglycemia, dyslipidemia, hypertension, and increased abdominal obesity. |
| Keltikangas-Järvinen et. al., 1998 | HPA-axis and chronic stress | Basal ACTH level during OGTT was positively related to the cortisol response to ACTH at 60 minutes, the fasting insulin level, and the insulin to glucose ratio among exhausted men. |
| Keltikangas-Järvinen et. al., 1997 | HPA-axis responses and Type A behaviour (TABP), hostility, chronic stress (VE) | TABP was related to a high level of mean basal ACTH and a low level of cortisol response to ACTH stimulation after dexamethasone suppression; Hostility was related to a high level of mean basal cortisol and a high cortisol in cortisol/ACTH ratio, and VE was related to a low level of mean basal ACTH and a decreased ACTH in relation to cortisol. |
| *Räikkönen et.al., 1996a | HPA-axis and Chronic stress (VE), anger | A neuroendocrine pattern characterized by an elevation in cortisol response to ACTH stimulation and dominance of cortisol in the ratio of mean basal cortisol level to mean basal ACTH level denoting a defeat type of reaction to stress differentiated borderline hypertensive men from normotensive men. |

Table 1. Summary of results of the epidemiological studies.

## 9.2 Experimental studies

In the series of our studies on experimental stress we have found that psychological factors are related to experimentally induced stress. The typical psychological stressors in the laboratory are an acoustic startle probe, a mental arithmetic task, and a public speaking task. The experimental stressors in the laboratory in our studies were a mental arithmetic (the three best participants would be awarded a prize of $40, appetitive task), and a startle and a reaction time tasks (aversive tasks). Exaggerated heart rate reactivity to stress may imply disease proneness. It has been suggested that heightened heart rate responses to stress may be a risk for development of atherosclerosis and coronary heart disease (Matthews, 1986, Krantz & Manuck, 1984). Temperament may also be important in regard to stress-related cardiac reactivity and may even predispose the individual to elevated risk profile of the metabolic parameters. Temperament refers to individual differences in arousability of behavioural and physiological systems. There are prominent individual differences in the mode of autonomic response to stress (Cacioppo 1994).

The self-reported emotions have been measured according to the Larsen and Diener (1992) circumplex model of affects (Larsen & Diener 1992). Emotions can be defined as action tendencies or action dispositions (Lewis & Haviland 1993). Two general dimensions of affects are valence (pleasant/unpleasant) and activation or arousal (Larsen & Diener 1992). The two-dimensional circumplex model of affect consists of eight sections which are: high/low activation, unpleasant/pleasant, activated/ unactivated unpleasant, and activated/unactivated pleasant. We have also used the Watson's and Tellegen's model of positive affectivity (PA) and negative affectivity (NA) to measure the general affective orientation during laboratory tasks (Watson et. al., 1988) in our studies.

Temperament may predispose the person to stress and negatively biased environmental and personal interpretations. In an experimental study it has been reported that temperament in terms of Gray's concept explains emotional reactions during laboratory stress (Heponiemi et. al., 2003). This model was used to structure the self-reported affects in our study. The experimental stressors in the laboratory were a mental arithmetic, a startle and a reaction time tasks. The main finding was that BIS sensitivity was related to activated unpleasant affects (e.g. anxious, fearful, tense) during reaction time and startle tasks whereas BAS sensitivity was associated with activated pleasant affects (e.g. vigorous, lively) during mental arithmetic task. BIS sensitivity is, thus, likely to predispose a person to emotional distress in stressful situation regardless of the nature of the stressor, and also probably to a higher stress proneness. Thus, BIS sensitivity may increase one's stress vulnerability by predisposing the person to poor and inactive coping. BIS has been previously related to negative affectivity (Heponiemi et al 2003). BIS sensitivity may also influence person's focus of attention and predispose to bias towards negative cues of the environment because it has been suggested that high BIS-persons would be negatively biased in environmental interpretations.

We have found that temperament trait persistency (in terms of Cloninger's concept) interacted with chronic stress predisposing to a high physiological stress reactivity (Keltikangas-Järvinen & Heponiemi 2004). Chronic stress was indexed by vital exhaustion. Vital exhaustion was associated with parasympathetic withdrawal, i.e. low RSA magnitude, during stressful tasks in laboratory. Temperament trait persistence was likely to strengthen cardiac stress reactivity of exhausted women. Findings suggest that background stress may decrease one's capacity to cope with acute stress and be related to continuous physiological stress.

According to Gray's theory, BAS sensitivity refers to strong reaction to incentives and thus BAS is assumed to primarily be activated by appetitive stimuli such as reward and termination of punishment (Gray 1991). We found that BAS sensitivity was related to heart rate reactivity and parasympathetic withdrawal during the tasks (Heponiemi et. al., 2004). The relationship between BAS temperament and cardiac reactivity might be mediated by the parasympathetic nervous system. HR expresses the balance between the parasympathetic and sympathetic nervous system. Normal parasympathetic control of heart is suggested to promote good health, may protect the heart and dampen the sympathetic reactions to stress (Porges 1992) whereas low parasympathetic control of HR has been associated with cardiovascular diseases (Tsuji et. al., 1996).

Temperament in terms of Cloninger's concept, that is HA, has been related to chronic stress, and when associated with vital exhaustion, likely to predispose negative affects when accompanied by exhaustion (Heponiemi et. al., 2005). The level of vital exhaustion among healthy persons was related to unpleasant affects such as sadness, fear, anxiety and anger. In other words, the participants with high level of vital exhaustion felt more tense, fearful, anxious, sad, depressed, angry and irritated during stress, and less lively than participants with low levels of vital exhaustion. Furthermore, inherited temperament may increase proneness to exhaustion and predispose to negative affects when feeling exhausted. The results imply that temperamental tendency to perseverance combined with stressful environmental loading may predispose to exhaustion. Temperament may predispose an exhausted person to negative affects and lead to individual differences in stress vulnerability.

Cloninger's psychobiological model of temperament and character postulates that each of the temperament dimensions is associated with a specific emotional experience. We tested this assumption and found that NS was associated with dullness during monotonous and aversive situations and with a higher level of pleasantness during the initial baseline period and the appetitive situation. HA was associated with higher levels of fear and unpleasant emotions and lower levels of positive emotions, depending on the situational cues. The study provides support for the validity of Cloninger's temperament dimensions as predictors of emotional responses during different challenges. Especially, novelty seeking and harm avoidance appear to have a significant influence on emotional experience (Puttonen et. al., 2005).

Temperament in terms of Cloninger's concept is related to a perception of stress during experimentally induced stress (Ravaja et. al., 2006). HA was consistently associated with high anticipated threat prior to stressors and high perceived stress after the stressors. In addition, the interaction of HA and NS predicted threat appraisals prior the task. Low HA and high NS was associated with higher threat before the social task (public speech). Individual differences in perceived threat may be important because it is assumed that the primary appraisal of threat affects psychological and physiological responses to stressors (Lazarus & Folkman 1984).

Novelty seeking temperament has been associated with higher IMT (Hintsanen et. al., 2009b). Cardiac stress reactivity and recovery was studied among extremely high and extremely low scorers of novelty seeking. We examined whether novelty seeking is associated with cardiac reactions to a laboratory challenge. The results suggest that, that high novelty seekers may be more stress resilient because they might have faster cardiac recovery after stress (Hintsanen et. al., 2009b).

A study of hemodynamic and other autonomically mediated responses to mental stress in laboratory and the parameters of IRS among adolescent boys showed that a high level and an increasing trend of heart rate (HR) and finger blood volume (FBV)were related during challenging tasks (Keltikangas-Järvinen et. al., 1996a). Automatically mediated physiological responses (HR, HRV, FBV and skin conductance level, SCL) to experimentally induced stress are related to serum insulin level and other parameters of IRS in adolescent boys. The finding suggests that trends of psychophysiological responses to task-induced stress implicate important individual differences in stress modulation. In addition, results imply a relationship between stress-induced sympathetically mediated physiological responses and the metabolic and anthropometric parameters constituting IRS in healthy adolescent boys.

Individuals differ widely in the extent to which they are prone to experience normal daily challenges as positive or negative. Watson's and Tellegen's model of positive affectivity (PA) and negative affectivity (NA) was used to measure the general affective orientation during laboratory tasks (Watson et al 1988). PA included emotions such as active, enthusiastic and energetic, and NA refers to being distressed, fearful and nervous. A study examining the relationship between PA and NA to autonomic cardiac reactivity during laboratory tasks reports that participants with high levels of PA during varying laboratory tasks exhibited high parasympathetic reactivity and heart rate reactivity (Heponiemi et. al., 2006). However, against expectations, high levels of NA were not related to sympathetic arousal. It was concluded that cardiac reactivity may be associated with positive involvement and enthusiasm, and thus, should not be automatically considered as pathological.

Acute mental stress may contribute to the cardiovascular disease progression via autonomic nervous system controlled negative effects on the endothelium. We examined the interactive effect of acute mental stress-induced cardiac reactivity/recovery and endothelial function on the prevalence of carotid atherosclerosis. The results showed a significant interaction of FMD and cardiac RSA recovery for IMT, and a significant interaction of FMD and pre-ejection period (PEP). P recovery for IMT. Among participants with low FMD, slower PEP recovery was related to higher IMT. Among individuals with high FMD, slow RSA recovery predicted higher IMT. It seems that the development of endothelial dysfunction may be one possible mechanism linking slow cardiac recovery and atherosclerosis via autonomic nervous system mediated effect. Cardiac recovery plays a role in progression of atherosclerosis in persons with high and low FMD. The role of sympathetically mediated cardiac activity seems to be more important in those with impaired FMD, and parasympathetically mediated in those with relatively high FMD (Chumaeva et al 2010a; Chumaeva et. al., 2009b).

High parasympathetic reactivity during stress is considered as appropriate stress response whereas an inability to suppress parasympathetic tone is related to experienced stress and stress vulnerability (Porges 1992). When considering the potential mechanisms (summary over all our findings including the temperament-related experiments) between stress and CHD risk slow cardiac recovery is of high importance. It seems that the important role of stress in CHD risk is played rather by parasympathetic underactivity than sympathetic overactivity.

| Author, year | Study focus | Main findings |
|---|---|---|
| Heponiemi et. al., 2003 | Self-rated affects and BIS-BAS temperament (n= 95) | BAS was related to pleasant affects with an especially great increase of activated pleasant affect (vigorous, peppy, lively) during an appetitive task. BIS was related to unpleasant affects with a great increase of activated unpleasant affects (anxious, fearful, tense) during an aversive task. |
| Keltikangas-Järvinen et. al., 1996 | Cardiac reactivity, chronic stress (VE) and temperament (n=76) | Chronic stress was related to parasympathetic withdrawal. Chronically stressed women expressed the highest level of physiological reactivity. Among the chronically stressed the initial parasympathetic tone had no effect whereas in the non-chronically stressed parasympathetic reactivity was greatest when initial parasympathetic tone was high. |
| Heponiemi et. al., 2004 | Cardiac autonomic stress profiles and BIS-BAS temperament (n=65) | BAS was related to HR reactivity and parasympathetic withdrawal during the tasks. |
| Heponiemi et. al., 2005 | Affects, chronic stress and temperament (n=76) | Chronic stress was related to unpleasant state affects other than state fatigue. Temperament modified the relationship between chronic stress and affects. Chronic stress was related to harm avoidance. |
| Puttonen et. el., 2005 | Affective responses during challenge and temperament | NS was associated with dullness during monotonous and aversive situations and with a higher level of pleasantness during the initial baseline period and the appetitive situation. HA was associated with higher levels of fear and unpleasant emotions and lower levels of positive emotions. |
| Ravaja et. al., 2006 | Threat, stress and performance appraisalsand temperament (n= 97) | Temperament traits are related to threat, stress and performance appraisals. HA was related to high anticipated threat prior to the stressors. |
| Hintsanen et. al., 2009b | Cardiac stress reactivity and recovery and temperament (n= 29) | High novelty seekers may be more stress resilient because they had faster cardiac recovery than others. |
| Keltikangas-Järvinen et. al., 1996a | IRS parameters (insulin, HDL, TG, SBP, SSF, STR) and mental stress (n=48) | Automatically mediated physiological responses (HR, HRV, FBV and SCL) to experimentally induced stress are related to serum insulin level and other parameters of IRS in adolescent boys. |
| Heponiemi et. al., 2006 | Cardiac reactivity, facial muscle movements and positive and negative affects (n=77) | Experiencing positive affects was related to more pronounced parasympathetic, heart rate, and orbicularis oculi reactivity. |
| Chumaeva et. al., 2009b | IMT and chronic stress (VE), cardiac stress reactivity and recovery (n=69) | Among the highly exhausted men aged 28-37, lower HR reactivity was related to greater IMT. |
| Chumaeva et. al., 2010a | IMT and chronic stress (VE), cardiac stress reactivity and recovery, flow-mediated dilation (FMD) (n= 81) | A FMD and cardiac RSA interaction, and FMD and PEP recovery for IMT. Among participants with low FMD, slower PEP recovery was related to higher IMT. Among individuals with high FMD, slow RSA recovery predicted thicker IMT. |

Table 2. Summary of the results of experimental studies.

## 9.3 Work stress

Several epidemiological studies have shown the association between work stress and CHD risk but there are also non-significant findings (Belkic et al 2004; Lange et al 2003; van Vegchel et al 2005). To explain conflicting findings, it is important to study whether the excess CHD risk among employees with high job strain is confounded by the pre-employment, personality and genetic effects. Therefore, we have focused on a novel perspective of examining effects of biological, psychological and socioeconomic factors in early life and adolescence, i.e. the period before entering work life, on perceptions of work stress and early atherosclerosis.

*Pre-employment factors and work stress.* We have examined whether pre-employment factors influence perceptions of work stress in adulthood. The socioeconomic conditions in childhood and adolescence may also contribute to perceptions of work stress in adulthood. Lower parental socioeconomic position (SEP), that is low paternal and maternal education and low family income, has been shown to predict increased job strain of the offspring in adulthood (Hintsa et. al., 2006). Part of the effect of low parental SEP on job strain and job control was mediated by participants' education. In addition, high parental SEP in the childhood family predicted higher rewards at work in adulthood among women (Hintsa et. al., 2007). We also found a strong positive relationship between parental SEP and the participants' educational attainment. A potential explanation for the predictive relationship between parental SEP and participants' education is that highly educated parents may offer good educational resources and through that enhance the educational attainment of their offspring. These findings indicate that pre-employment factors should be taken into account as potential confounders in future research on job strain-CHD risk associations.

Stressful childhood environments are suggested to contribute to later stress vulnerability. It has been shown that deficient nurturing attitudes in childhood predict offspring's work stress and low job control in adulthood (Hintsanen et. al., 2010). Deficient nurturing attitudes were indicated by intolerance of the mother towards the normal activity of the child, and low emotional warmth by the mother towards to the child. Deficient nurturance may also have indirect stress-inducing effects: the development of social skills has previously been related to child-rearing styles (Steelman et. al., 2002). Social skills are very important in the contemporary work as team work and personal networks have become increasingly important. Furthermore, inadequate social skills are likely to be sources of stress.

*Temperament and personality in perceptions of work stress.* Temperament traits may predispose the individual to experience work stress. Temperament in terms of Cloninger's concept is related to work stress, also to the components that are expected to reflect environmental loading by characteristics at work (Hintsa et. al., 2010a). Low NS and high HA predicted higher job strain. High NS, low HA and high P predicted higher long-term job control. Partly inherited, quite stable temperamental tendencies seem to contribute to job strain and its components. High NS seems to protect from job strain whereas high HA may predispose the individual to long-term work stress. HA may increase the number of stressful encounters at work because the individual predisposition to experience stress more easily. HA has previously been related to inefficient coping strategies such as rumination, resignation and escaping from stressful situations. Therefore, HA may lead to the selection of less efficient coping strategies and subsequently influence the time it takes to recover from stress.

Furthermore, it has been documented that temperament traits negative emotionality and sociability predict work stress. Negative emotionality refers to tendency to easily react with anger or fear and sociability a tendency to enjoy being in the company of others and to search for others company (Buss & Plomin 1984). The results have shown that higher negative emotionality and lower sociability systematically predict higher perceived job strain and effort-reward imbalance (ERI) (Hintsanen et. al., 2011).

*Type A behaviour – work stress.* Personality may also predispose a person to experience work stress. Type A behaviour is a stress—related personality type originally found by Friedman and Rosenman, and it has been related to risk of CHD. Type behaviour is characterized by aggressiveness, feelings of time urgency, competitiveness, easily aroused anger/hostility, and hard-driving elements. Ambition and competitiveness are very relevant traits in regard to work context. Type A persons have high need for control, and demanding and challenging situations are likely to elicit Type A behaviour. Of the components of Type A behaviour, high leadership was found to predict low long-term work stress while high hard-driving (taking things seriously, high responsibility and competitiveness,) predicted higher long-term work stress (Hintsa et. al., 2010b). Furthermore, high aggression and eagerness-energy may predispose the employee to unfavourable effort-reward condition. Thus, it seems that different Type A behaviour components may have divergent influence on long-term work stress. These results suggest that more attention should be paid to individual factors and stress vulnerability in work stress research. Our findings strongly suggest that stress sensitivity may have childhood roots.

*Do pre-employment factors explain work stress-CHD risk association?* We have also aimed at examining the possible explanation for conflicting findings in work stress – CHD risk research. Therefore a series of studies examining the role of confounding factors in the work stress – CHD risk associations have been conducted. A prospective study on the contribution of biological, familial and socioeconomic risk factors in adolescence to the association between adulthood job strain and IMT reported that these pre-employment factors did not confound the relationship between job strain and early atherosclerosis in men (Kivimäki et. al., 2007). The findings of this study support the role of job strain as a risk factor for increased CHD risk.

In a study among Finnish men, it was found that personality trait leadership (willingness to always win, being selected as a leader in group activities, being socially active and having many hobbies), which is a component of Type A behaviour, attenuated the association between job strain and IMT (Hintsa et. al., 2008). Low leadership in adolescence predicted higher job strain 15 years later, and this personality characteristic attenuated the association between job strain and IMT by 17% to nonsignificant. It was concluded that leadership component of Type A behaviour may represent a non-risk component of Type A behaviour, and that personality characteristics might also be important to include in work stress-CHD risk studies.

A study among British male civil servants showed that selected pre-employment factors such as family history of CHD, height, paternal education and social class, and number of siblings were related to increased risk for CHD. The significant hazard ratios (HR) for CHD found were 1.33 for family history of CHD, 1.18 for each quartile decrease in height, and 1.16 for each category increase in number of siblings. Psychosocial factors at work also predicted CHD: the significant HR was 1.72 both for low job control and low organisational justice (Hintsa et. al., 2010d). However, the association between psychosocial factors at work and CHD incidence was largely independent of selected pre-employment factors.

| Author, year | Study focus | Main findings |
|---|---|---|
| Hintsa et. al., 2006 | Job strain and pre-employment factors | Lower parental SEP and higher parental life dissatisfaction independently of the number of siblings and educational level predicted job strain in adulthood 18 years later. The effects were partly mediated by participants' education. |
| Hintsa et. al., 2007 | ERI and pre-employment factors | High rewards were predicted by high parental life satisfaction in men and by high parental SEP in women. |
| Hintsanen et. al., 2010 | Job strain, ERI and maternal nurturing attitudes | Deficient emotional warmth in childhood predicted lower adulthood job control and higher job strain. |
| Kivimäki et. al., 2007 | Job strain-IMT association and early risk factors | Pre-employment influences did not confound the association between job strain and IMT. |
| Hintsa et. al., 2008 | Job strain-IMT association and pre-employment factors | Type A personality leadership component attenuated the association between job strain and IMT by 17% to non-significant. Pre-employment family factors had only modest effect on this association. |
| Hintsanen et. al., 2007 | Job strain-IMT association and NRG-1 | Job strain was associated with increased IMT among men with T/T genotype of NRG-1. A direct association between NRG-1 and IMT was found in women. |
| Hintsanen et. al., 2008 | Job strain-IMT association and COMT | In men, job strain was associated with increased IMT in Val/Val carriers. |
| Hintsa et. al., 2010d | Psychosocial factors at work and CHD, and pre-employment factors | The association between psychosocial factors at work (low job control and organisational justice) and CHD was largely independent of the selected pre-employment factors. Increase in number of siblings, quartile decrease in height and family history of CHD predicted development of CHD. |
| Hintsanen et. al., 2010 | Job strain, ERI and maternal nurturing attitudes | Deficient emotional warmth in childhood predicted lower job control and higher job strain in adulthood independently of age, sex, SES in childhood, maternal mental problems, and participants' hostility and depressive symptoms. |
| Hintsa et. al., 2010a | Long-term job strain, job control and job demands (6 years) and temperament | Low NS and high HA predicted higher long-term job strain. Higher NS, lower HA and higher P predicted higher long-term job control. Higher HA and higher P predicted higher long-term job demands. |
| Hintsanen et. al., 2011 | Job strain, ERI and temperament | Higher negative emotionality and lower sociability systematically predicted higher perceived job strain and ERI. Activity predicted higher perceived ERI. |
| Hintsa et. al., 2010b | Job strain, ERI and personality (Type A behaviour) | High leadership (Type A dimension) predicted lower long-term job strain and higher long-term job control. High hard-driving predicted higher long-term job strain. High aggression, hard-driving and eagerness-energy predicted ERI. |

Table 3. Summary of results of the work stress studies.

*Do genetic factors contribute to the association between work stress and IMT?* We have extended our research to clarify whether genetic predispositions explain an association between stress and its health outcomes. When trying to indentify groups at risk, examining whether an interaction between genotype and job strain may predispose to increased atherosclerotic processes is important. Another study reports that the association between job strain and greater IMT was found only among men with the T/T genotype of NRG-1 gene (Hintsanen et. al., 2007). Thus, the T/T genotype may be a marker of genetic susceptibility to the negative health effects of job strain on early atherosclerosis in men. Job strain has been related to higher IMT among men with Val/Val genotype of the catechol-O-methyltranferase (COMT) gene (Hintsanen et. al., 2008). This implies that Val/Val carriers may be at higher risk for negative health effects of job strain. It seems that the new study strategy of taking the genetic influences into account in identifying groups at risk for negative effects of work stress on cardiovascular risk may be worthwhile.

In sum, all the findings described here imply that although work stress seems to increase the CHD risk, there are some pre-employment factors that should be taken into account in work stress-CHD risk studies. In addition, this evidence should motivate the development of systematic intervention strategies for large-scale studies testing whether reducing work stress, giving employees a stronger say in decisions about their work and enhancing a righteous manner of treating employees at work would reduce CHD.

### 9.4 Statistical problems

In this section we discuss shortly three general problems in statistical modelling of population data that we think are particularly central for behavioural epidemiology. If objective of science is to go beyond what can be seen with naked eyes, implication is that our observations depend on the instruments we use. One such instrument is the statistical model. Careful scrutiny of instrument limitations is every bit as important as the results they provide.

Linear models between behavioural variables are most frequently used in epidemiological studies, while psychological theories rarely assume independency or linearity, and also many of the above cited studies demonstrated some interaction effects. Questionnaire-based measures are typically thought to contain measurement error. Measurement error makes the estimation of nonlinear and interactive effects between variables notoriously hard (Carroll et. al., 2006; Griliches & Ringstad 1970). A lot of methodological development is warranted regarding modelling of general nonlinearities in this context, and either more precise measurements or more precise models of measurement error may be the prerequisite. Also, exponentially increasing amounts of data are required for the data-driven exploration of increasingly high dimensional interactions (Wasserman 2006). In below, we turn to problems that are present even when linear approximation is reasonable.

Often questionnaire-based measurement instruments entertain floor/ceiling-effect (inadequate sampling of true variation) and/or measurement error. Using a variable suffering from either one as a covariate in ordinary (and generalized) linear regression model can results in bias and false findings if the covariate is correlated with another 'independent' (predictor) variable (Austin & Brunner 2003; Brunner & Austin 2009; Carroll et al 2006). These problems could be addressed, along with those arising from more familiar overfitting problem (Babyak 2004), from the point of view of combined cross-validation and partial least squares regression (Abdi 2010; Rosipal & Kramer 2006).

In this young field of science, often little is known about precise type of measurement error, and model assumptions rarely are firmly established. Partial least squares regression handles well a range of error types (Reis & Saraiva 2004) and cross-validation is able to control for errors in assumptions (Arlot & Celisse 2010). For these (and other) reasons this combination holds promise beyond many more commonly encountered choices of explorative data analysis.

Finally, both linear and nonlinear models typically assume that model holds over entire study population, whereas often only a part of the study population displays an effect. Genetic vulnerability and gene-environment interactions are clear examples of interacting variables that may not always be available in the data (Caspi et. al., 2010; Keltikangas-Järvinen & Jokela 2010). A statistical null finding can thus result from an inappropriate combination of heterogeneous groups instead of the lack of association. Such grouping of data according to latent (unobserved) variable can be modelled with mixture (weighted sum) of statistical models (McLahlan & Peel 2000).

Although mixture models are frequently referred as readily available and their utility is apparent, they are not a similarly well-researched topic as many other familiar statistical models. Their estimation actually involves technical difficulties known as singularities of parameter space (Watanabe 2009). This is a way of saying that more than one set of model parameters can result in the exact same model and that miniscule chances in parameters may cause drastic changes in the resulting model. This is undesirable phenomenon because one often interprets the data in terms of model parameters (e.g. regression slope). Mathematical theories that are most frequently used to analyze statistical models cannot cope with these difficulties, and new developments seem important (Watanabe 2009).

Above we discussed of some pertinent difficulties that still hinder most statistical modelling attempts in the field, from linear to nonlinear and mixture models. We feel that scientists applying these methods are not always sufficiently informed about involved difficulties. Current section attempted to fill this gap to a small degree and point some important methodological research topics, not to discourage researchers from doing their best possible work.

## 10. Conclusions

The findings of the Young Finns Study imply that stress is related to an increase of CHD risk through several pathways. The results also imply that more attention should be paid to pre-employment factors and individual differences in work stress research.

Stress affects people differently, that is, there are differences in individuals in stress proneness and what is considered as a stressor. These individual differences in stress experience stem from inherited characteristics and life experiences from childhood on. The influence of stress on cardiovascular health may be mediated through several different mechanisms. Based on our research it seems that the important role of stress in CHD risk is played rather by parasympathetic underactivity than sympathetic overactivity. Stress has to be measured appropriately and accurately keeping several different aspects of stress in mind: source of stress, the duration of stress, and individual vulnerability to stress have to be kept in mind when studying the role of stress in pathogenesis of CHD.

However, the research also shows that studying stress-health associations and the etiological role of stress in CHD is complicated and needs accurate measuring, appropriate statistical methods and population-based longitudinal study designs.

## 11. References

Abdi H. 2010. Partial least squares regression and projection on latent structure regression (PLS-regression) *Wiley Interdisciplinary Reviews: Computational Statistics* 2:97-106.

Anderson TJ. 2006. Arterial stiffness or endothelial dysfunction as a surrogate marker of vascular risk. *Canadian Journal of Cardiology* 22 Suppl B:72B-80B.

Appels A, Hoppener P & Mulder P. 1987. A questionnaire to assess premonitory symptoms of myocardial infarction. *International Journal of Cardiology* 17:15-24.

Arlot S & Celisse A. 2010. A survey of cross-validation procedures for model selection. *Statistics Surveys* 4 40-79.

Austin PC & Brunner LJ. 2003. Type I error inflation in the presence of a ceiling effect *The American Statistician* 57:97-104.

Babyak MA. 2004. What you see may not be what you get: a brief, nontechnical introduction to overfitting in regression-type models. *Psychosomatic Medicine* 66:411-21.

Belkic KL, Landsbergis PA, Schnall PL & Baker D. 2004. Is job strain a major source of cardiovascular disease risk? *Scandinavian Journal of Work, Environment & Health* 30:85-128.

Bonetti PO, Lerman LO & Lerman A. 2003. Endothelial dysfunction: a marker of atherosclerotic risk. *Arteriosclerosis, Thrombosis and Vascular Biology* 23:168-75.

Brunner J & Austin PC. 2009. Inflation of type I error rate in multiple regression when independent variables are measured with error. *Canadian Journal of Statistics* 37:33-46.

Buss AH & Plomin R. 1984. *Temperament: Early developing personality traits.* Hillsdale, NJ: Lawrence Erlbaum Associates Inc.

Cacioppo JT. 1994. Social neuroscience: autonomic, neuroendocrine, and immune responses to stress. *Psychophysiology* 31:113-28.

Caldji C, Tannenbaum B, Sharma S, Francis D, Plotsky PM & Meaney MJ. 1998. Maternal care during infancy regulates the development of neural systems mediating the expression of fearfulness in the rat. *Proceedings of the National Academy of Sciences of the United States of America* 95:5335-40.

Carroll RJ, Ruppert D, Stefanski LA & Crainiceanu CM. 2006. *Measurement error in nonlinear models: A modern perspective* Boca Raton, USA: Chapman & Hall/CRC.

Caspi A, Hariri AR, Holmes A, Uher R & Moffitt TE. 2010. Genetic sensitivity to the environment: the case of the serotonin transporter gene and its implications for studying complex diseases and traits. *American Journal of Psychiatry* 167:509-27.

Chumaeva N, Hintsanen M, Hintsa T, Ravaja N, Juonala M, Raitakari OT & Keltikangas-JärvinenL. 2010a. Early atherosclerosis and cardiac autonomic responses to mental stress: a population-based study of the moderating influence of impaired endothelial function. *BMC Cardiovascular Disorders* 10:16.

Chumaeva N, Hintsanen M, Juonala M, Raitakari OT & Keltikangas-Järvinen L. 2010b. Sex differences in the combined effect of chronic stress with impaired vascular endothelium functioning and the development of early atherosclerosis: the Cardiovascular Risk in Young Finns study. *BMC Cardiovascular Disorders* 10:34.

Chumaeva N, Hintsanen M, Ravaja N, Juonala M, Raitakari OT & Keltikangas-Järvinen L. 2009a. Chronic stress and the development of early atherosclerosis: moderating effect of endothelial dysfunction and impaired arterial elasticity. *International Journal of Environmental Research and Public Health* 6:2934-49.

Chumaeva N, Hintsanen M, Ravaja N, Puttonen S, Heponiemi T, Pulkki-Råback L, Juonala M, Raitakari OT, Viikari JS & Keltikangas-Järvinen L. 2009b. Interactive effect of long-term mental stress and cardiac stress reactivity on carotid intima-media thickness: The Cardiovascular Risk in Young Finns study. *Stress* 12:1.

Cloninger CR, Svrakic DM & Przybeck TR. 1993. A psychobiological model of temperament and character. *Archives of General Psychiatry* 50:975-90.

Colquitt JA. 2001. On the dimensionality of organizational justice: a construct validation of a measure. *Journal of Applied Psychology* 86:386-400.

Coplan JD, Andrews MW, Rosenblum LA, Owens MJ, Friedman S, Gorman JM & Nemeroff CB. 1996. Persistent elevations of cerebrospinal fluid concentrations of corticotrophin-releasing factor in adult nonhuman primates exposed to early-life stressors: Implications for the pathophysiology of mood and anxiety disorders. *Proceedings of the National Academy of Sciences of the United States of America* 93:1619-23.

Corr PJ. 2008. Reinforcement sensitivity theory: introduction. In *The reinforcement sensitivity theory of personality*, ed. PJ Corr. Cambridge: Cambridge University Press.

Culic V. 2007. Acute risk factors for myocardial infarction. *International Journal of Cardiol* 117:260-9.

Elovainio M, Heponiemi T, Kuusio H, Sinervo T, Hintsa T & Aalto AM. 2010. Developing a short measure of organizational justice: a multisample health professionals study. *J Occupational and Environmental Medicine* 52:1068-74.

Elovainio M, Kivimäki M, Puttonen S, Lindholm H, Pohjonen T & Sinervo T. 2006a. Organisational injustice and impaired cardiovascular regulation among female employees. *Occupational and Environmental Medicine* 63:141-4.

Elovainio M, Kivimäki M, Steen N & Kalliomaki-Levanto T. 2000. Organizational and individual factors affecting mental health and job satisfaction: a multilevel analysis of job control and personality. *Journal of Occupational Health Psychology* 5:269-77.

Elovainio M, Kivimäki M & Helkama K. 2001. Organizational justice evaluations, job control and occupational strain. *Journal of Applied Psychology* 86:418-24.

Elovainio M, Leino-Arjas P, Vahtera J & Kivimäki M. 2006b. Justice at work and cardiovascular mortality: a prospective cohort study. *Journal of Psychosomatic Research* 61:271-4.

Gray JA. 1991. The neuropsychology of temperament. In *Explorations in temperament: International perspectives on theory and measurement. Perspectives on individual differences.*, ed. J Strelau, A Angleitner, pp. 105-28.

Griliches Z & Ringstad V. 1970. Error-in-the-variables bias in nonlinear contexts. . *Econometrica: Journal of the Econometric Society*, 38:368-70.

Hemingway H, Malik M & Marmot M. 2001. Social and psychosocial influences on sudden cardiac death, ventricular arrhythmia and cardiac autonomic function. *European Heart Journal* 22:1082-101.

Hemingway H & Marmot MG. 1999. Psychosocial factors in the aetiology and prognosis of coronary heart disease: systematic review of prospective cohort studies. *British Medical Journal* 318:1460-7.

Heponiemi T, Keltikangas-Järvinen L, Kettunen J, Puttonen S & Ravaja N. 2004. BIS-BAS sensitivity and cardiac autonomic stress profiles. *Psychophysiology* 41:37-45.

Heponiemi T, Keltikangas-Järvinen L, Puttonen S & Ravaja N. 2003. BIS/BAS sensitivity and self-rated affects during experimentally induced stress. *Personality and Individual Differences* 34:943-57.

Heponiemi T, Keltikangas-Järvinen L, Puttonen S & Ravaja N. 2005. Vital exhaustion, temperament, and the circumplex model of affect during laboratory-induced stress. *Cognition & Emotion* 19:879-97.

Heponiemi T, Ravaja N, Elovainio M, Näätänen P & Keltikangas-Järvinen L. 2006. Experiencing positive affect and negative affect during stress: relationships to cardiac reactivity and to facial expressions. *Scandinavian Journal of Psychology* 47:327-37.

Hintsa T, Hintsanen M, Jokela M, Elovainio M, Raitakari OT & Keltikangas-Järvinen L. 2010a. The influence of temperament on long-term job strain and its components: The Cardiovascular Risk in Young Finns Study. *Personality and Individual Differences* 49:700-5.

Hintsa T, Hintsanen M, Jokela M, Pulkki-Råback L & Keltikangas-Järvinen L. 2010b. Divergent influence of different type a dimensions on job strain and effort-reward imbalance. *Journal of Occupational and Environmental Medicine* 52:1-7.

Hintsa T, Kivimäki M, Elovainio M, Hintsanen M, Pulkki-Råback L & Keltikangas-JärvinenL. 2007. Pre-employment family factors as predictors of effort/reward imbalance in adulthood: a prospective 18-year follow-up in the Cardiovascular Risk in Young Finns study. *Journal of Occupational and Environmental Medicine* 49:659-66.

Hintsa T, Kivimäki M, Elovainio M, Keskivaara P, Hintsanen M, Pulkki-Råback L & Keltikangas-Järvinen L. 2006. Parental socioeconomic position and parental life satisfaction as predictors of job strain in adulthood: 18-year follow-up of the Cardiovascular Risk in Young Finns Study. *Journal of Psychosomatic Research* 61:243-9.

Hintsa T, Kivimäki M, Elovainio M, Vahtera J, Hintsanen M, Viikari JS, Raitakari OT & Keltikangas-Järvinen L. 2008. Is the association between job strain and carotid intima-media thickness attributable to pre-employment environmental and dispositional factors? The Cardiovascular Risk in Young Finns Study. *Occupational and Environmental Medicine* 65:676-82.

Hintsa T, Puttonen S, Toivonen L, Kontula K, Swan H & Keltikangas-Järvinen L. 2010c. A history of stressful life events, prolonged mental stress and arrhythmic events in inherited long QT syndrome. *Heart* 96:1281-6.

Hintsa T, Shipley M, Gimeno D, Elovainio M, Chandola T, Jokela M, Keltikangas-Järvinen L, Vahtera J, Marmot MG & Kivimäki M. 2010d. Do pre-employment influences explain the association between psychosocial factors at work and coronary heart disease? The Whitehall II study. *Occupational and Environmental Medicine* 67:330-4.

Hintsanen M, Elovainio M, Puttonen S, Kivimäki M, Lehtimaki T, Kahonen M, Juonala M, Rontu R, Viikari JS, Raitakari OT & Keltikangas-Järvinen L. 2008. Val/Met polymorphism of the COMT gene moderates the association between job strain and early atherosclerosis in young men. *Journal of Occupational and Environmental Medicine* 50:649-57.

Hintsanen M, Elovainio M, Puttonen S, Kivimäki M, Raitakari OT, Lehtimäki T , Rontu R, Juonala M, Kahonen M, Viikari J & Keltikangas-Järvinen L. 2007. Neuregulin-1 genotype moderates the association between job strain and early atherosclerosis in young men. *Annals of Behavioral Medicine* 33:148-55.

Hintsanen M, Hintsa T, Widell A, Kivimäki M, Raitakari OT & Keltikangas-Järvinen L. 2011. Negative emotionality, activity, and sociability temperaments predicting long-term job strain and effort-reward imbalance: A 15-year prospective follow-up study. *Journal of Psychosomatic Research* 71:90-6.

Hintsanen M, Kivimäki M, Elovainio M, Pulkki-Råback L, Keskivaara P, Juonala M, Raitakari OT & Keltikangas-Järvinenn L. 2005. Job strain and early atherosclerosis: the Cardiovascular Risk in Young Finns study. *Psychosomatic Medicine* 67:740-7.

Hintsanen M, Kivimäki M, Hintsa T, Theorell T, Elovainio M, Raitakari OT, Viikari JSA & Keltikangas-Järvinen L. 2010. A prospective cohort study of deficient maternal nurturing attitudes predicting adulthood work stress independent of adulthood hostility and depressive symptoms. *Stress*:1-10.

Hintsanen M, Pulkki-Råback L, Juonala M, Viikari JS, Raitakari OT & Keltikangas-Järvinen L. 2009a. Cloninger's temperament traits and preclinical atherosclerosis: the Cardiovascular Risk in Young Finns Study. *Journal of Psychosomatic Research* 67:77-84.

Hintsanen M, Puttonen S, Järvinen P, Pulkki-Råback L, Elovainio M, Merjonen P & Keltikangas-Järvinen L. 2009b. Cardiac Stress Reactivity and Recovery of Novelty Seekers. *International Journal of Behavioral Medicine*:16:236-40.

Ingles JL, Eskes GA & Phillips SJ. 1999. Fatigue after stroke. *Archives of Physical Medical Rehabilitation* 80:173-8.

Karasek RA & Theorell T. 1990. *Healthy work: Stress, productivity and the reconstruction of working life.* New York: Basic Books.

Keltikangas-Järvinen L & Jokela M. 2010. Nature and nurture in personality *Focus* 8:180-6.

Keltikangas-Järvinen L & Heponiemi T. 2004. Vital exhaustion, temperament, and cardiac reactivity in task-induced stress. *Biological Psychology* 65:121-35.

Keltikangas-Järvinen L, Pulkki-Råback L, Puttonen S, Viikari J & Raitakari OT. 2006. Childhood hyperactivity as a predictor of carotid artery intima media thickness over a period of 21 years: the cardiovascular risk in young Finns study. *Psychosomatic Medicine* 68:509-16.

Keltikangas-Järvinen L, Ravaja N, Räikkönen K, Hautanen A & Adlercreutz H. 1998. Relationships between the pituitary-adrenal hormones, insulin, and glucose in middle-aged men: moderating influence of psychosocial stress. *Metabolism* 47:1440-9.

Keltikangas-Järvinen L, Ravaja N, Räikkönen K & Lyytinen H. 1996a. Insulin resistance syndrome and autonomically mediated physiological responses to experimentally induced mental stress in adolescent boys. *Metabolism* 45:614-21.

Keltikangas-Järvinen L, Räikkönen K & Adlerkreutz H. 1997. Response of the pituitary-adrenal axis in terms of Type A behavior, hostility and vital exhaustion in healthy middle aged men. *Psychology and Health* 12:533-42.

Keltikangas-Järvinen L, Räikkönen K, Hautanen A & Adlercreutz H. 1996b. Vital exhaustion, anger expression, and pituitary and adrenocortical hormones. Implications for the insulin resistance syndrome. *Arteriosclerosis, Thrombosis and Vascular Biology* 16:275-80.

Kerr M, Tremblay RE, Pagani L & Vitaro F. 1997. Boys' behavioral inhibition and the risk of later delinquency. *Archives of General Psychiatry* 54:809-16.

Kivimäki M, Elovainio M, Vahtera J & Ferrie JE. 2003. Organisational justice and health of employees: prospective cohort study. *Occupational & Environmental Medicine* 60:27-34.

Kivimäki M, Ferrie JE, Brunner E, Head J, Shipley MJ, Vahtera J & Marmot MG. 2005. Justice at work and reduced risk of coronary heart disease among employees: the Whitehall II Study. *Archives of Internal Medicine* 165:2245-51.

Kivimäki M, Hintsanen M, Keltikangas-Järvinen L, Elovainio M, Pulkki-Råback L, Vahtera J, Viikari JSA & Raitakari OT. 2007. Early risk factors, job strain, and atherosclerosis among men in their 30s: the Cardiovascular Risk in Young Finns Study. *American Journal of Public Health* 97:450-2.

Kivimäki M, Leino-Arjas P, Luukkonen R, Riihimäki H, Vahtera J & Kirjonen J. 2002. Work stress and risk of cardiovascular mortality: prospective cohort study of industrial employees. *British Medical Journal* 325:857-61.

Kivimäki M, Virtanen M, Elovainio M, Kouvonen A, Väänänen A & Vahtera J. 2006. Work stress in the etiology of coronary heart disease--a meta-analysis. *Scandinavian Journal of Work, Environment and Health* 32:431-42.

Korte SM, Koolhaas JM, Wingfield JC & McEwen BS. 2005. The Darwinian concept of stress: benefits of allostasis and costs of allostatic load and the trade-offs in health and disease. *Neuroscience and Biobehavioral Reviews* 29:3-38.

Ladd CO, Owens MJ & Nemeroff CB. 1996. Persistent changes in corticotrophin-releasing factor neuronal systems induced by maternal deprivation. *Endocrinology* 137:1212-8.

Larsen RJ & Diener E. 1992. Promises and problems with the circumplex model of emotion. In *Review of personality and social psychology: Emotion*, ed. MS Clark. Newbury Park, CA: Sage.

Lazarus RS & Folkman S. 1984. *Stress, appraisal and coping.* New York: Springer Publishing Company

Lewis M & Haviland JM. 1993. *Handbook of emotions.* New York, NY: Guilford Press

Liu D, Diorio J, Tannenbaum B, Caldji C, Francis D, Freedman A, Sharma S, Pearson D, Plotsky PM & Meaney MJ. 1997. Maternal care, hippocampal glucocorticoid receptors, and hypothalamic-pituitary-adrenal responses to stress. *Science* 277:1659-62.

Lovallo WR. 1997. *Stress & Health. Biological and Psychological interactions.* Thousand Oaks: SAGE publications, Inc.

McEwen BS. 1998. Protective and damaging effects of stress mediators. *New England Journal of Medicine* 338:171-9.

McEwen BS. 2008. Central effects of stress hormones in health and disease: Understanding the protective and damaging effects of stress and stress mediators. *European Journal of Pharmacology* 583:174-85.

McEwen BS & Stellar E. 1993. Stress and the individual. Mechanisms leading to disease. *Arch Intern Med* 153:2093-101.

McLahlan G & Peel D. 2000. *Finite mixture models.* . New York, USA John Wiley & Sons, Inc.

Menotti A, Keys A, Aravanis C, Blackburn H, Dontas A, Fidanza F, Karvonen MJ, Kromhout D, Nedeljkovic S, Nissinen A & et al. 1989. Seven Countries Study. First 20-year mortality data in 12 cohorts of six countries. *Annals of Medicine* 21:175-9.

Moorman RH. 1991. Relationship between organizational justice and organizational citizenship behaviors: do fairness perception influence employee citizenship? *Journal of Applied Psychology* 76:845-55.

O'Leary DH & Polak JF. 2002. Intima-media thickness: a tool for atherosclerosis imaging and event prediction. *American Journal of Cardiology* 90:18L-21L.

Porges SW. 1992. Vagal tone: a physiologic marker of stress vulnerability. *Pediatrics* 90:498-504.

Pulkki-Råback L, Puttonen S, Elovainio M, Raitakari OT, Juonala M & Keltikangas-Järvinen L. 2011. Adulthood EAS-temperament and carotid artery intima-media thickness: the Cardiovascular Risk in Young Finns study *Psychological Health* 26:61-75.

Puttonen S, Ravaja N & Keltikangas-Järvinen L. 2005. Cloninger's temperament dimensions and affective responses to different challenges. *Comprehensive Psychiatry* 46:128-34.

Räikkönen K, Hautanen A & Keltikangas-Järvinen L. 1996a. Feelings of exhaustion, emotional distress, and pituitary and adrenocortical hormones in borderline hypertension. *Journal of Hypertension* 14:713-8.

Räikkönen K, Keltikangas-Järvinen L, Adlercreutz H & Hautanen A. 1996b. Psychosocial stress and the insulin resistance syndrome. *Metabolism* 45:1533-8.

Räikkönen K, Keltikangas-Järvinen L, Hautanen A & Adlerkreutz H. 1997. Neuroendocrine mechanisms in chronic perceived stress: associations with the metabolic syndrome. *Endocrinology and Metabolism* 4:247-54.

Ravaja N, Keltikangas-Järvinen & Kettunen J. 2006. Cloninger's temperament dimensions and threat, stress, and performance appraisals during different challenges among young adults. *Journal of Personality* 74:287-310.

Reis MS & Saraiva PM. 2004. A comparative study of linear regression methods in noisy environments. *Journal of Chemometrics,* 18:526-36.

Repetti RL, Taylor SE & Seeman TE. 2002. Risky families: family social environments and the mental and physical health of offspring. *Psychological Bulletin* 128:330-66.

Rosenblum LA & Paully GS. 1984. The effects of varying environmental demands on maternal and infant behavior. *Child Development* 55:305-14.

Rosenström T, Hintsanen M, Kivimäki M, Jokela M, Juonala M, Viikari JS, Raitakari OT & Keltikangas-Järvinen L. 2011. Change in job strain and progression of atherosclerosis: The Cardiovascular Risk in Young Finns study. *Journal of Occupational Health Psychology* 16:139-50.

Rosipal R & Kramer N. 2006. Overview and recent advances in partial least squares. . *Lecture Notes in Computer Science* 3940:34-51.

Sapolsky RM. 1996. Stress, Glucocorticoids, and Damage to the Nervous System: The Current State of Confusion. *Stress* 1:1-19.

Sapolsky RM, Romero LM & Munck AU. 2000. How do glucocorticoids influence stress responses? Integrating permissive, suppressive, stimulatory, and preparative actions. *Endocrine Reviews* 21:55-89.

Selye H. 1973. The evolution of the stress concept. *American Scientist* 61:692-9.

Siegrist J, Starke D, Chandola T, Godin I, Marmot M, Niedhammer I & Peter R. 2004. The measurement of effort-reward imbalance at work: European comparisons. *Social Science & Medicine* 58:1483-99.

Stanton ME, Gutierrez YR & Levine S. 1988. Maternal deprivation potentiates pituitary-adrenal stress responses in infant rats. *Behavioral Neuroscience* 102:692-700.

Steelman LM, Assel MA, Swank PR, Smith KE & Landry SH. 2002. Early maternal warmth responsiveness as a predictor of child social skills: direct and indirect paths of influence over time. *Applied Developmental Psychology* 23:135-56.

Strelau J. 1998. *Temperament. A Psychological Perspective.* New York: Plenum Press

Tsuji H, Larson MG, Venditti FJ, Jr., Manders ES, Evans JC, Feldman CL & Levy D. 1996. Impact of reduced heart rate variability on risk for cardiac events. The Framingham Heart Study. *Circulation* 94:2850-5.

van Vegchel N, de Jonge J, Bosma H & Schaufeli W. 2005. Reviewing the effort-reward imbalance model: drawing up the balance of 45 empirical studies. *Social Science & Medicine* 60:1117-31.

Wasserman L. 2006. *All of nonparametric statistics. .* New York, USA: Springer-Verlag

Watanabe S. 2009. *Algebraic geometry and statistical learning theory.* New York, USA: Cambridge University Press

Watson D, Clark LA & Tellegen A. 1988. Development and validation of brief measures of positive and negative affect: the PANAS scales. *Journal of Personality and Social Psychology* 54:1063-70.

Åkerblom HK, Uhari M, Pesonen E, Dahl M, Kaprio EA & Nuutinen E. 1991. Cardiovascular risk in young Finns. *Annals of Medicine* 23:35-40.

# 3

# Pulse Pressure and Target Organ Damage

Adel Berbari and Abdo Jurjus
*American University of Beirut,*
*Lebanon*

## 1. Introduction

Hypertension remains the major risk for cardiovascular disease, stroke and end-stage nephropathy. Hypertension is traditionally defined in terms of elevated systolic and or diastolic blood pressure (BP). Recently, however, there has been increased recognition of the importance of high brachial pulse pressure (PP) as an important and independent predictor of increased cardiovascular morbidity and mortality, especially in senior subjects (Franklin et al., 2001). This paradigm shift is attributed to the aging of the population. The aging process is associated with an increased incidence of systolic hypertension, and in particular isolated systolic hypertension (ISH) (Franklin et al., 1999; Franklin et al. 2001; National High Blood Pressure Education Program Working Group, 1994). Both systolic and isolated systolic hypertension are characterized by wide (high) PP (Franklin et al. 2001 & National High Blood Pressure Education Program Working Group, 1994).

Increased pulse pressure (PP) defined as the difference between inappropriately elevated systolic blood pressure (SBP) and reduced diastolic blood pressure (DBP) at any value of mean arterial pressure (MAP) is a surrogate measure of increased arterial stiffness of central elastic arteries (aorta and its major branches) (Figure 1) (Dart & Kingwell, 2001; Safar et al., 2003). Arterial stiffness has emerged as an important independent predictor of adverse cardiorenal outcome in the general population (Figure 2) (Boutouyrie et al., 2002). Central PP is considered an accurate indicator of arterial stiffness (Boutouyrie et al., 2002). However, brachial PP is a widely accepted marker of arterial stiffness in the elderly and in some middle-aged individuals because central PP equalizes brachial PP during aging due to PP augmentation by early wave reflection (Dart & Kingwell, 2001).

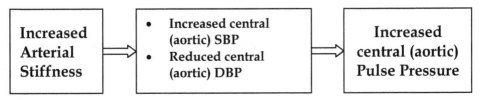

SBP= Systolic blood pressure, DBP= Diastolic blood pressure

Fig. 1. Determinants of Central Pulse Pressure

The relationship between PP and age is reported to be J-shaped, negative in subjects younger than 50 years and becoming positive after the age of 50 years. These findings suggest different pathophysiologic implications in younger versus older subjects. In subjects younger than 50 years of age, with preserved left ventricular dynamics, PP is related to a hyperdynamic cardiovascular state whereas, after the age of 60 years, arterial stiffening becomes a major determinant (Wilkinson et al., 2001). In fact, after the age of 60 years, the increase in PP results both from continuous elevation in SBP and a decrease in DBP (Franklin et al., 2001).

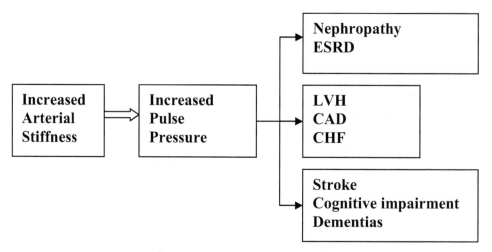

LVH= Left ventricular hypertrophy, CAD= Coronary artery disease, CHF= Congestive heart failure, ESRD= Endstage renal disease

Fig. 2. Relationship between increased arterial stiffness, increased pulse pressure and target organ disease

Several observational and clinical studies have indicated that, in both normotensive and hypertensive middle-aged and older subjects, wide PP is a better predictor of cardiovascular events and target organ disease than increased SBP and MAP adjusted for age, sex and other cardiovascular risk factors (Franklin et al., 2001). Further, a level of PP that predicts cardiovascular events in hypertensive patients appears to be equal or greater than 60-63mmHg (De Simone et al., 2005).

An increased brachial PP is an independent predictor of cardiovascular mortality not only in hypertensive men but also in normotensive men aged 40-69 years (Benetos et al., 1998). Thus, normotensive men with PP > 55mmHg were shown to have a 40% increased cardiovascular risk compared to normotensive men with same age but PP< 45mmHg (Benetos et al., 1998). Further, the predictive value of PP was observed even in well controlled hypertensive subjects (Benetos et al., 1998). Finally, the predictive power of PP has been demonstrated in subjects with evidence of other target organ involvement such as left ventricular dysfunction, endstage renal failure and in those with diabetes mellitus (Schram et al., 2002).

In contrast, in subjects younger than 50 years, brachial PP is not associated with a poor prognostic implication. In these subjects, the central arteries are more distensible and velocity of reflected pulse wave is low (Kotsis et al., 2011). As a result, SBP and PP increase significantly by about 12-14mmHg from central to peripheral arteries. This is known as the amplification phenomenon (Franklin et al., 2001 & Karamanoglu et al., 1993). Central and peripheral MAP and DBP, however, are not significantly different. Consequently, the peripheral (brachial) SBP and PP overestimate central (aortic) values (Franklin et al., 2001 & Karamanoglu et al., 1993). After the age of 55-60 years, as a result of arterial aging, central SBP and PP may increase even more than peripheral pressures. As a result, central SBP and PP become equal to or higher than peripheral (brachial) SBP and PP (Figure 3) (Franklin et al., 2001; Karamanoglu et al., 1993; Kotsis et al., 2011).

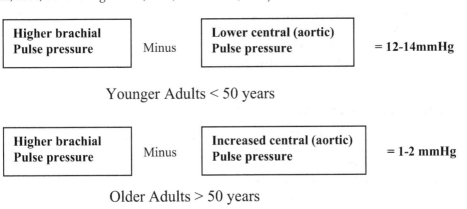

Fig. 3. Amplification phenomenon in younger and older adults

## 2. Genesis of the pulse pressure

The various BP components in the systemic circulation are the resultant of an interaction between left ventricular outflow (ejection) and properties of the large arterial system (aorta and its proximal major branches) (Benetos et al., 2010 & Van Bortel et al., 2001).

Ejection of blood from the left ventricle (LV) generates flow and pressure waves (Safar et al., 2003 & Wilkinson et al., 2001). The pressure wave generated by the LV travels down the arterial tree and is reflected back at any discontinuity of the arterial wall, namely at the multiple resistance arterioles and their bifurcation (Safar et al., 2003). The pressure waveform recorded at any site of the arterial tree is the sum of a forward traveling waveform, the incident pulse wave generated by left ventricular ejection and a back travelling wave, the reflected pulse wave (Safar et al., 2003 & Wilkinson et al., 2001).

### 2.1 Youth and early adulthood

In youth and early adulthood, the peak pressure recorded in the proximal aorta during LV ejection represents the SBP. Due to high distensibility of the system, the pressure wave form travels at low velocity (low pulse wave velocity- PWV) to the periphery and the reflected wave returns to the heart after closure of the aortic valve, so that it does not create an additional pressure load to the contracting LV (Safar et al., 2003). It does, however, increase the pressure during early diastole thereby enhancing DBP and improving coronary perfusion (Safar et al., 2003).

PP which represents pressure fluctuations resulting from episodic cardiac contraction is approximately 25mmHg in the aorta and is amplified to 40mmHg in the brachial and radial arteries.

## 2.2 Aging

In humans, the aging process is associated with structural and functional changes in the aorta and proximal elastic arteries. These vessels dilate and stiffen.

With increased arterial stiffness, the pulse wave travels faster, and reflected pulse wave merges earlier with the incident wave, augmenting aortic systolic blood pressure, rather than diastolic blood pressure (Safar et al., 2003 & Wilkinson et al., 2001). As a result, left ventricular load is increased and coronary perfusion is compromised (Safar et al., 2003 & Wilkinson et al., 2001).

## 3. Amplification phenomenon

BP amplification is defined as the elevation of PP from the central aorta towards the periphery and is mainly attributed to an increase in SBP (Benetos et al., 2011; McEniery et al., 2005). Pressure wave amplification can be explained by the reflection phenomenon of the oscillating BP wave (Benetos et al., 2011; McEniery et al., 2005). In the presence of compliant (i.e. low stiffness) central elastic arterial system as in young adults, PWV is low, the reflected pulse wave will attain the peripheral arteries (i.e. radial arteries) during systole due to their proximity to the reflecting sites, and the central arteries during the diastolic period (Benetos et al., 2011). This mechanism explains PP phenomenon namely why the peripheral (brachial, radial) is higher than the central (aortic) PP. The ratio of brachial / central PP varies from 70% in subjects younger than 20 years to 20% in those older than 80 years (McEniery et al., 2005). When expressed in absolute change in mmHg, the difference between brachial and central PP varies from 20 to 7 mmHg (Benetos et al., 2011; McEniery et al., 2005). Loss of PP amplification, associated with an increase in central PP and PWV have been shown to be significant predictors of all cause and cardiovascular mortality (Benetos et al., 2010).

### 3.1 Determinants of PP amplification

Several factors have been postulated to alter PP amplification including aging, gender, and traditional risk factors (McEniery et al., 2005).

In youth and early adulthood, PP increases significantly from central (aorta / proximal elastic arteries) to peripheral (brachial) arteries, leading to PP amplification. This phenomenon is attributed to higher SBP and slightly lower DBP in peripheral (brachial, radial) arteries. In contrast, MAP gradient between central and peripheral arteries is only 1-2mmHg.

In middle-aged and elderly subjects, the increasing stiffness of central elastic arterial system is associated with elevation of central SBP, reduction in DBP, widening of central PP and loss of PP amplification.

Females have a lower PP amplification than males of similar age which is attributed to:

i.   i) shorter arterial tree;
ii.  ii) additional gender related factors.

Subjects with hypertension, diabetes, dyslipidemia or established CV disease tend to have a low PP amplification independent of age, height or gender.

Age and gender remain the major determinants of PP amplification.

## 4. Kidney damage and pulse pressure

It is well established that hypertension and chronic kidney disease (CKD) are closely linked. Hypertension is the second most common primary diagnosis in patients with incident or prevalent endstage renal disease (ESRD). Further, most forms of CKD are etiologically related to hypertension (Udani et al., 2011). In addition, coexistent or superimposed hypertension is the major risk for progression of CKD (Hsu et al., 2005; Perry et al., 1995; Udani et al., 2011). The rates of CKD and ESRD in the USA attributed to hypertension have been steadily increasing partly attributed to the aging process (Udani et al., 2011).

Epidemiologic data and several clinical studies have documented a graded relationship between degree of BP elevation and renal functional impairment. Malignant hypertension, characterized by marked BP elevations (SBP/DBP ≥ 220/120mmHg) leads, if untreated, to severe renal damage and irreversible renal failure which is attributed to occlusive intra-renal arterial and arteriolar lesions (Bidani and Griffin, 2004). Conversely, data from several cohort studies provide strong support for nonmalignant hypertension as a causal risk for development of CKD and endstage renal failure (ESRD). In 12000 hypertensive patients from multiple Veterans Administration Centers followed up for 15 years, Perry et al. reported that uncontrolled hypertension was associated with a risk for development of CKD/ESRD(Perry et al., 1995). Specifically, the risk ratio for CKD was 2.8 for a pre-treatment SBP= 166-180mmHg, and 7.6 for a pre-treatment SBP>180mmHg (Perry et al., 1995).

Even modest BP elevation in the non-hypertensive range appears to confer increased risk of CKD. Compared to BP< 120/80mmHg, the adjusted risk ratio for developing ESRD was 1.62 for BP=120-129/80-84 mmHg and 1.98 for BP=130-139/84-89 mmHg in a cohort of 316675 adult members of the Kaiser Permanente of Northern California (Hsu et al., 2005).

### 4.1 Hypertensive nephropathy

### 4.1.1 Histopathologic patterns

Hypertension-induced kidney damage can be classified into two clinical and histopathologic patterns: 1) vascular, 2) glomerular.

The vascular pattern, often referred as nephrosclerosis can be further subdivided into two forms – namely benign and malignant nephrosclerosis (Bidani and Griffin, 2004). Benign nephrosclerosis, the most frequent form which occurs in the majority of patients with essential hypertension, is characterized by hyaline arteriosclerosis which is slowly progressive but does not compromise the vascular lumen (Bidani and Griffin, 2004). Accordingly, significant loss of nephrons and compromise of renal function are infrequent (Bidani and Griffin, 2004). In contrast, malignant hypertension is characterized by marked

BP elevation (SBP/DBP ≥ 220/120 mmHg) and occlusive arterial and arteriolar preglomerular lesions with prominent fibrinoid necrosis leading to ischemic glomerular injury (Bidani and Griffin, 2004). Rapid deterioration of renal function and irreversible renal failure can develop in the absence of adequate BP reduction (Bidani and Griffin, 2004). However, with the availability of effective modern antihypertensive therapy, malignant hypertension has become an uncommon cause of ESRD.

The glomerular pattern, characterized by an accelerated segmental or global glomerulosclerosis, is an increasingly recognized lesion of hypertension-induced kidney damage (Bidani and Griffin, 2002 & Bidani et al., 2009). It is often superimposed on the underlying primary nephropathy and occurs even with mild to moderate BP elevations. Further, these histopathologic renal changes are independent of presence of nephrosclerosis (Bidani and Griffin, 2002 & Bidani et al., 2009). In fact, vascular lesions are not prominent.

### 4.1.2 Mechanisms of hypertension-induced nephropathy (CKD)

The mechanisms of hypertension-induced renal injury and appearance of hypertensive nephropathy have not been completely elucidated. A growing body of evidence suggests a link between aortic stiffness and renal function (Mimran, 2006). Aortic stiffness causes increased SBP and wide (increased) PP, both factors associated with increased rates of decline in renal function and progression to renal impairment (Mimran, 2006).

### 4.2 Renal autoregulation

Disturbances in the mechanisms of renal autoregulation appear to play important roles in the appearance and progression of hypertensive nephropathy (Loutzenhiser et al., 2006).

One of most striking features of the renal circulation is the phenomenon of autoregulation by which the kidney maintains constant renal blood flow (RBF) and glomerular filtration rate (GFR) in the face of wide fluctuations of systemic BP (Loutzenhiser et al, 2002). This dual regulation of both RBF and GFR is achieved by proportionate changes in the tone of the preglomerular and postglomerular resistances (Loutzenhiser et al, 2002). This process is initiated by combination and integration of two mechanisms, the faster renal myogenic response and the slower tubuloglomerular feedback (TGF) system (Loutzenhiser et al, 2002). TGF involves a flow-dependent signal that is sensed at the macula densa and alters the tone of the adjacent preglomerular and postglomerular resistances (Loutzenhiser et al, 2002). The renal myogenic response involves a direct vasoconstriction of the afferent arteriole when this vessel is exposed to an increase in transmural pressure (Loutzenhiser et al, 2002, 2006).

By using the hydronephrotic rat kidney preparation, Loutzenhiser et al reported that the myogenic response is influenced only by the SBP, even when MAP is kept constant (Loutzenhiser et al, 2002, 2006).

Normally, increases in systemic BP, whether sustained or intermittent are prevented from fully reaching the renal microcirculation by proportionate vasoconstriction of the preglomerular afferent arterioles (Loutzenhiser et al, 2002, 2006). Systolic BP and PP appear to be the major determinants of the tone of the afferent arterioles, independent of MAP and DBP (Loutzenhiser et al, 2002, 2006). In fact, recent clinical studies indicate that hypertensive renal injury correlates most strongly with SBP and PP (Ford et al., 2010; Mimran, 2006; Safar, 2004; Verhave et al., 2005).

In contrast to the microcirculation of other organs, the renal microcirculation presents two special features. First, glomerular MAP and pulsatile pressures are high, representing about 60% of the aortic pressures (Mitchell, 2004). Second, because the resistance is higher in the efferent arteriole than in the afferent arteriole, the pressure drop across the afferent arteriole is low (Mitchell, 2004). These hemodynamic characteristics allow the maintenance of glomerular filtration but expose the glomerular microcirculation to high pressure injury and biotrauma (Mitchell, 2010). Under normal conditions, the renal myogenic response prevents transmission of the elevated MAP and pulsatile pressure from reaching the glomerular capillaries (Loutzenhiser et al, 2002).

Renal autoregulation mediates hypertension-induced nephropathy (CKD) by 2 mechanisms: i) intact renal autoregulation associated with elevated systemic BP levels within or beyond the autoregulatory threshold; ii) impaired renal autoregulatory process.

### 4.2.1 Intact renal autoregulation

#### 4.2.1.1 Elevated systemic BP levels within the autoregulatory threshold

In mild to moderate uncomplicated essential hypertension, the renal autoregulatory mechanisms are intact and BP levels remain within the autoregulatory threshold (Bidani & Griffin, 2002, 2004). The elevated systemic BP enhances the myogenic tone of the afferent arteriole, preserving the relative constancy of the glomerular capillary hydrostatic pressures and insulating the renal microcirculation from biotrauma (Bidani & Griffin, 2002, 2004). Renal functional impairment is minimal and development of CKD and ESRD is infrequent (Bidani & Griffin, 2002, 2004). However, prolonged exposure of the renal circulation to elevated systemic BP levels may initiate the pattern of benign nephrosclerosis in the afferent arterioles which is characterized by vascular lesions of nonspecific hyaline arteriosclerosis (Bidani & Griffin, 2002, 2004).

#### 4.2.1.2 Elevated systemic BP beyond the autoregulatory threshold

In contrast, in malignant hypertension, although the autoregulatory process is still preserved, the markedly elevated MAP levels, which exceed the upper threshold of the process, may cause severe renal vascular and glomerular disruptive lesions, resulting in severe renal functional impairment (Bidani & Griffin, 2002, 2004). However, with the advent of renal vascular disease, renal autoregulatory responses may become secondarily impaired leading to amplification of the renal damage.

A sudden severe BP elevation is much more likely to exceed the autoregulatory threshold than a progressive rise in BP to the same levels. This is due to the protection afforded by the rightward shift of the upper and lower limits of autoregulation, a characteristic feature in chronic hypertension (Bidani & Griffin, 2004).

### 4.2.2 Impaired renal autoregulation

Impaired renal autoregulation is frequently reported in states such as diabetes and CKD (Bidani & Griffin, 2004). This hemodynamic alteration tends to be manifested as dilatation of the afferent arteriole, glomerular hypertrophy, hyperfiltration injury and subsequent extracellular matrix production and glomerulosclerosis with irreversible reduction in GFR (Bidani & Griffin, 2004). In addition, increased aortic stiffness may contribute directly to renal injury by favoring increased transmission of PP to the renal microcirculation (Bidani & Griffin, 2004). Unlike benign and malignant nephrosclerosis, the histological lesions are glomerular, being characterized by glomerulosclerosis (Bidani & Griffin, 2004).

## 4.3 Clinical studies – Relation between SBP/PP and renal vascular nephropathy

Several longitudinal and cross-sectional studies indicate a relation between an increase in arterial stiffness and its corollaries, increased SBP/PP, and injury to the renal microcirculation.

### 4.3.1 Essential hypertension

#### 4.3.1.1 Systolic blood pressure (SBP)

In the Systolic Hypertension in the Elderly Program (SHEP) conducted in subjects older than 65 years with ISH, SBP emerged as the best predictor of an increase in serum creatinine within a 5-year period (Young et al., 2002). Similarly in a cohort of 722 subjects with treated essential hypertension, the decrease in GFR, within a 7-year observation period, was preferentially associated with baseline SBP (Vupputuri et al., 2003).

#### 4.3.1.2 Pulse pressure (PP)

Other clinical investigations revealed an association between PP and decline in renal function in older subjects. Fesler et al reported that in 132 never treated essential hypertension patients at baseline followed on treatment for 6.5 years, the yearly change in GFR was strongly and inversely correlated with PP independent of baseline GFR, age, MAP, body mass index, and microalbuminuria (Fesler et al., 2007). Gosse et al reported similar findings (Gosse et al., 2009). Measured either on clinic examination or by ambulatory BP monitoring in 375 patients with uncomplicated essential hypertension without proteinuria over a mean follow-up period of 14 years, initial baseline PP was an independent determinant of decline in renal function, pointing to the role of BP pulsatility as a glomerular biotrauma (Gosse et al., 2009).

### 4.3.2 Chronic Kidney Disease (CKD)

Aortic stiffening has been shown to predict loss of renal function also in CKD. Ford et al evaluated the relation between arterial stiffness and changes in renal function in 120 patients with CKD stage 3 and 4 enrolled in the prospective ACADEMIC (Arterial Compliance and Oxidant Stress as Predictors of Loss of Renal Function, Morbidity and Mortality in Chronic Kidney Disease (CKD) study) cohort (Ford et al., 2010). These investigators noted that, compared to those with lower PWV (12.3 m/sec), patients with higher PWV (13.9 m/s) experienced a greater progression of CKD, as determined by a greater decrease in the reciprocal of serum creatinine and greater than 25% decline in estimated glomerular filtration rate during 1 year follow-up (Ford et al., 2010).

Conversely, decreasing renal function may promote risk of accelerated rate of aortic stiffening. In 1290 untreated normotensive and hypertensive subjects with a serum creatinine < 130 μmol/L (< 1.47 mg/dl), Mourad et al reported an inverse association between aortic PWV and creatinine clearance calculated by the Cockcroft-Gault formula (Mourad et al., 2001). However the aortic PWV was significantly enhanced only in subjects exhibiting a reduced creatinine clearance in the lower tertile of normal values particularly in younger than 55 years of age. Baseline serum creatinine was the only predictor of the changes in arterial function (Mourad et al., 2001).

Similar associations between reduction in GFR and an acceleration of PWV were reported in the CRIC study in which unadjusted analysis indicated that each 10ml/min/1.73m$^2$ decrease in estimated GFR was associated cross-sectionally with a 0.5 m/s increase in aortic PWV (Townsend et al., 2010).

In patients with ESRD (stage V) , increased aortic stiffening, as measured by PWV may be a contributor to further deterioration in renal structure and function. Several uremia related factors have been postulated to account for the disease of the large arterial system (Udani et al., 2011).

## 4.4 Aging

The aging process is often associated with reduced renal function (Mimran, 2006). In the Multiple Risk Factor Intervention Trial (MRFIT), a high risk of ESRD was reported in patients with isolated systolic hypertension (ISH) (Klag et al., 1996). In a cohort of 212 patients with ISH, an inverse relationship between PP and GFR and effective renal plasma flow (ERPF) was documented in subjects 60 years of age and older independent of age, MAP and known cardiovascular factors (Verhave et al., 2005). This inverse relationship, however, was observed in elderly subjects exhibiting the highest tertile of PP (Verhave et al., 2005).

## 4.5 Microalbuminuria and pulse pressure

Increased urinary albumin excretion (UAE) is a well recognized risk for cardiovascular morbidity and mortality and a predictor of renal involvement (Sarnak et al., 2003).

The pathophysiologic mechanisms causing increased UAE have not been fully elucidated. However a link between BP and UAE is well recognized. Although earlier studies emphasized an association between DBP/MAP and UAE, more recent studies report stronger relations between SBP/PP and UAE (Farasat et al., 2010). In a cross-sectional study that included 211 untreated controls, patients with essential hypertension or clinically stable cardiovascular disease, Pedrinelli et al found that PP was the best predictor of UAE, defined as UAE≥15 μg/min (Pedrinelli et al., 2000). Similarly in a longitudinal study of 450 normotensive and untreated hypertensive subjects drawn from the Baltimore Study of Aging, only longitudinal levels of SBP and PP, pulsatile BP components, were independent predictors of UAE in men (Pedrinelli et al., 2000).

## 4.6 Renal transplantation and pulse pressure

Increased PP, a sign of arterial stiffness, is frequently recorded in renal transplant recipients (Fernandez-Fresnedo et al., 2005).

Several studies have demonstrated a relationship between PP and renal allograft function and survival. In a cohort of 493 renal transplant recipients with a median follow-up of 6.3

years, increased PP, recorded 3 months post-transplant emerged as an early and strong marker of poor allograft outcome (Bahous et al., 2006; Vetromile et al., 2009).Further, recent data suggest that immunosuppressive regimens which include Calcineurin inhibitors may also mediate both an increased risk of arterial stiffness and allograft dysfunction (Seckinger et al., 2008). Adequate BP control and immunosuppressive therapy free of Calcineurin inhibitors have been recommended to improve allograft outcome and prevent nephrotoxicity (Seckinger et al., 2008 & Vetromile et al., 2009).

## 5. Cardiovascular disease and pulse pressure

Epidemiologic surveys and clinical observations have established a strong association between indices of arterial stiffness (peripheral PP, central PP, aortic PWV, pressure wave amplification) and cardiovascular events in hypertensive and older subjects.

### 5.1 Structural and functional changes in the cardiovascular system

Arterial stiffness is associated with structural and functional changes in the central elastic arteries (aorta and proximal elastic branches). These vessels dilate and stiffen (Lakatta, 2003). The primary cause of the stiffening is marked disorganization of the normal elastic pattern, increased deposition of less extensible collagen fibers, fibrosis, inflammation, medial smooth muscle necrosis, calcification and diffusion of macromolecules into the arterial wall (Lakatta, 2003). The repetitive cycles of distension of the arterial wall which occur with each heart beat lead to fatigue, fraying and fracture of the elastic fibers and subsequent extensive impairment of the medical elastin fiber network (Lakatta, 2003).

With increasing stiffness of the central elastic arteries, pulse wave velocity is faster, leading to summation of reflected and incident pulse waves in systole, enhancing central SBP, reducing DBP and widening central PP (Benetos et al., 2010). The elevation in central SBP increases myocardial oxygen demand, enhances left ventricular load, generates a heightened LV systolic pressure to sustain a constant blood flow and impairs ventricular ejection. Moreover, the contemporary reduction in DBP, the latter being a determinant of coronary blood supply, compromises coronary perfusion, predisposes to subendocardial ischemia, myocardial infarction and arrhythmias (Mosley et al., 2007). Both an elevated SBP and wide PP promote hypertrophy of the left ventricle, with impaired left ventricular relaxation and diastolic heart failure (Mosley et al., 2007). Finally, PP, an index of oscillatory hemodynamic forces, is a significant modulator of formation and rupture of atherosclerotic plaques (Mosley et al., 2007).

Endothelial dysfunction and reduced bioavailability of nitric oxide, frequently associated with arterial stiffness, impair and limit the vasoactive and antiatherosclerotic properties of the vascular endothelium (Mosley et al., 2007).

A cross-talk has been recently documented between the central elastic arterial system and microcirculation of target organ damage (O'Rourke and Safar, 2005). Arterial stiffness and PP have a negative impact on the microcirculation of the kidney and brain, predisposing to renal impairment and deterioration in neurocognitive function (O'Rourke and Safar, 2005).

## 5.2 Clinical studies

Recent prospective and retrospective epidemiologic and clinical studies have demonstrated that an elevated PP is independently related, in both middle aged and older subjects, to an increased risk of cardiovascular events. In two independent French untreated male cohorts, the IPC (Investigations Preventives et Cliniques) composed of 15561 men aged 20 to 82 years who had 2 visits spaced 4 to 10 years apart, and the Paris Prospective Study including 6246 men aged 42 to 53 years examined over a period of 4 years, Benetos et al reported that an increase in SBP combined with a reduction in DBP, a hemodynamic pattern characteristic of wide PP, was associated with a highest risk of cardiovascular mortality, independent of age, initial BP levels and other risk factors (Benetos et al., 2000). In a different study, these same investigators noted that in untreated subjects, a spontaneous evolution towards a pattern of combined increase in SBP and reduced DBP over an extended period was associated with a 2 fold increase in cardiovascular mortality compared to those without changes in SBP and DBP (Benetos et al., 2000).

The relationship between pulsatile BP components and risk of cardiovascular events was also explored in 1109 patients with coronary artery disease. Intra-aortic BP indices were recorded during coronary angiography in these patients (Jankowski et al., 2008). After a 4.5 year follow-up, the ascertained primary endpoints (cardiovascular death, myocardial infarction, stroke, cardiac arrest, cardiac transplantation or myocardial revascularization) occurred in 22% of the patients (Jankowski et al., 2008). Central pulsatility (defined as PP/MAP) and central PP emerged as the primary endpoints with ratios of 1.3 and 1.25 respectively suggesting that central pulsatile BP indices were more important determinants of risk of cardiovascular events than steady BP components in patients with coronary artery disease (Chirinos et al. & Jankowski et al., 2008).

Premature stiffening of the arterial tree is frequently reported in insulin resistance and diabetes (Kengne et al., 2009 & Stehouwer et al., 2008). In the recent ADVANCE (Action in Diabetes and Vascular Disease: Preterax and Diamicron- Modified Release Controlled Evaluation Study) a clinical trial which enrolled 1140 subjects with type 2 diabetes, older than 55 years and one additional cardiovascular risk factor, the hazard ratio for cardiovascular events was 1.17 for SBP, 1.20 for PP, 1.12 for MAP and 1.04 for DBP. The investigators concluded that SBP and PP were the two best and DBP the least effective determinants of risk of major cardiovascular outcomes in relatively older diabetic patients (Kengne et al., 2009).

PP has been shown to be a predictor of heart failure especially in the elderly. In a sample of 2512 subjects aged $\geq$ 65 years, participants in the Established Population for Epidemiologic Study for the Elderly Program free of cardiovascular heart disease (CHD) and congestive heart failure (CHF) at baseline, a 10mmHg increment in PP was associated with an increased risk of CHD, CHF and overall mortality of 12%, 14% and 6% respectively both in normotensive subjects and in those with ISH (Vaccarino et al., 2000).

## 6. Cerebrovascular disease, stroke, neurocognitive dysfunction and pulse pressure

Several studies, in both population and patient-based cohorts have demonstrated a strong association between increased brachial PP and excess risk of stroke and neurocognitive dysfunction in both elderly and middle aged subjects (Hanon et al, 2005; Paultre & Mosca, 2005).

## 6.1 Mechanisms of cerebrovascular events

An increased arterial stiffness can enhance the risk of stroke through several mechanisms. An elevation in central PP enhances arterial remodeling both at the site of the extracranial and intracranial arteries, increasing carotid wall thickness, and predisposing to carotid stenosis, formation of atherosclerotic plaques and the likelihood of their rupture (Laurent et al., 2009). Central PP has been associated with increased prevalence and severity of cerebral white matter lesions (Kim et al., 2011 & Scuteri et al., 2011). A second mechanism relates to the specific features of the cerebral circulation. The torrential cerebral blood flow and low cerebrovascular resistance expose the cerebral microcirculation to high pressure fluctuations in the carotid and vertebral arteries which tend to increase three-to fourfold with age (O'Rourke & Safar, 2005). Finally, coronary heart disease and heart failure, often associated with arterial stiffness and high central PP, are also risk factors for stroke (Selvetella et al., 2003).

## 6.2 Clinical studies

Several epidemiologic surveys and clinical studies have documented that, in the elderly, high brachial PP was more predictive for stroke incidence and mortality than elevated SBP (>140mmHg). In the Boston Veterans Administration Study, PP was a stronger predictor for fatal cardiovascular outcome than were SBP and DBP among elderly subjects aged 60-85 years (Waldstein et al., 2008). Similar observations were reported in a prospective study of 5092 Chinese subjects. In this study, the incidence of total stroke, either ischemic or hemorrhagic, was related to PP (Zhang et al., 2004). In contrast, several other prospective studies identified SBP as a stronger predictor for incidence and mortality of stroke than PP (Miura et al., 2009).

Further, there is growing evidence that response of PP to antihypertensive therapy may also be relevant to outcome. In a post-hoc analysis of Systolic Hypertension in the Elderly Program (SHEP) trial data, an increase in PP (>10mmHg) on active drug treatment was associated with an increased risk of stroke (Vaccarino et al., 2001).. Another analysis of the same study revealed the enhanced risk of stroke resulted from excessive reduction in DBP with a threshold at about 60mmHg (Somes et al., 1999).

Elderly patients often have multiple comorbid conditions. These subjects are at increased postoperative complications when undergoing major surgical procedures. In a recent prospective study, a high brachial PP (>72mmHg) was reported to be associated with an increased risk of stroke during the postoperative period (Benjo et al., 2007).

In contrast to the well established relationship between brachial PP and risk of stroke in the elderly, data in middle aged subjects are controversial. A meta-analysis of prospective cohort studies reported that PP was not an independent risk factor for stroke. However, in a recent large cohort Japanese study which included 33372 participants free of cardiovascular disease at baseline and followed for 12 years, the JPHC study, PP was an independent stroke predictor among middle aged subjects with SBP<140mmHg, but not among those with higher SBP (Okada et al., 2011). Among persons of SBP<140mmHg, a 10mmHg higher PP at baseline was associated with 8.31mmHg higher SBP and 1.69mmHg lower DBP at baseline (Okada et al., 2011). These data suggest that, in middle aged subjects with SBP<140mmHg, it is the low DBP rather than the non hypertensive SBP which impacts the excess stroke risk (Okada et al., 2011).

Increased brachial PP is also a risk predictor for neurocognitive dysfunction in healthy elderly and middle aged normotensive and hypertensive individuals (Robbins et al., 2005). Impairment of cognitive function and memory loss are frequent in the aging population, especially among the elderly subjects (Henskens et al., 2008). Alzheimer's disease and vascular dementia are the most devastating manifestations of these neurocognitive disorders. Several longitudinal studies have emphasized an association between these dementias with increased PWV and a wide brachial PP, both indices of increased arterial stiffness (Qiu et al., 2003). In a community based cohort of 1270 elderly subjects (mean age ≥ 75 years) free of dementia at baseline, higher brachial PP (> 84 versus 70-84mmHg) was associated with increased risks of both Alzheimer's disease and vascular dementia (adjusted relative risks of 1.9 and 1.7 respectively) (Qiu et al., 2003). The association was particularly pronounced among women.

## 7. Therapeutic approaches

It is well established that reduction in BP and or improvement in arterial stiffness are associated with a reduction in risk of cardiovascular events (Dart & Kingwell, 2001). However it is often difficult to separate the effects of antihypertensive therapy on BP reduction alone from their direct effects on vascular wall properties. In fact, interventions that reduce BP and improve cardiovascular outcome are often associated with improvement in indices of arterial stiffness (PWV, PP) (Laurent et al., 2006; Laurent & Boutouyrie, 2007; Van Bortel et al., 2001).

Therapeutic mechanisms include both lifestyle issues and pharmacologic treatment.

### 7.1 Lifestyle measures

A large number of lifestyle measures have been postulated to reduce both BP and arterial stiffening. These include body weight reduction, exercise, lowering salt intake, smoking cessation and moderation of alcohol consumption.

#### 7.1.1 Weight reduction

Intentional weight reduction in obese hypertensive subjects is associated with significant fall in BP. Several clinical studies have shown that obese subjects whether normotensive or hypertensive exhibit increased arterial stiffness with its associated hemodynamic indices (increased PWV and PP) (Orr et al., 2008). In these subjects, weight loss with a hypocaloric diet improved arterial stiffness and reduced PWV and PP (Dengo et al., 2010). In some studies, an improvement in endothelial function was also reported (Miyaki et al., 2009).

#### 7.1.2 Dietary supplement

Several dietary supplements appear to improve functional characteristics of the elastic arterial system. Supplementation with n-3 polyunsaturated fatty acids reduces arterial stiffness in dyslipidemic subjects, probably by decreasing serum triglycerides (Nestel et al., 2002). A high dietary intake of isoflavones, the non-steroidal plant derived compounds rich in soy beans, and administration of red clover isoflavones reduce PWV (Van Der Schouw et al., 2002). These effects have been attributed to the affinity of isoflavones to human estrogen receptors.

Recent reports have demonstrated that cocoa use ameliorated endothelial function, as evidenced by improved endothelial flow mediated vasorelaxation (Ferri, 2006). Changes were more striking in older subjects. The amelioration in endothelial function has been attributed to the flavanols, a subclass of flavanoids, present in large quantities in cocoa beans (Ferri, 2006). Controlled experiments conducted with beverages rich in flavanoids (wine, fruit, vegetable, tea, purple grape juice) have documented similar endothelial benefits (Ferri, 2006).

The cocoa related improved endothelial functions have been linked to increased bioavailability of nitric oxide (Ferri, 2006). In clinical trials, cocoa supplementation has been associated with BP reduction in subjects with grade I hypertension, with ISH and in younger soccer players (Ferri, 2006; Taubert et al., 2003).

### 7.1.3 Salt intake

Salt is the most potent modulator of arterial stiffness (Zieman et al., 2005). High salt intake enhances the age-related changes in the vascular system (Zieman et al., 2005). High salt intake increases MAP and triggers structural and functional pressure-independent changes in the vascular wall. In experimental animals, exposure to high salt diet has been associated with alterations in the composition of the vascular wall that precede BP elevations by several weeks (Limas et al., 1980). In the human, short- and long-term salt restriction causes an improvement in arterial distensibility independent from the effect on BP levels (Aviolo et al., 1986). In a group of elderly subjects (mean age 64 ± 2 years) with isolated systolic hypertension, dietary salt restriction for 4 weeks was associated with fall in both supine resting SBP ($\approx$ 6mmHg), ambulatory SBP ($\approx$ 3mmHg) and enhanced carotid artery compliance by 46% (Gates et al., 2004).

### 7.1.4 Alcohol consumption

An association between alcohol consumption and increased arterial stiffness has been reported in several studies (Sierksma et al., 2004; Zieman et al., 2005). Conversely, moderation of alcohol intake appears to reduce significantly PWV in both genders, independently of changes in BP levels (Sierksma et al., 2004; Zieman et al., 2005).

### 7.1.5 Physical exercise

The age related increase in arterial stiffness can be partly reversed by a program of physical training. In middle aged sedentary men, 3 months of aerobic training (walking or jogging 40 minutes daily at 70-75% of maximum heart rate) enhanced arterial compliance to levels observed in similarly aged endurance trained subjects (Tanaka et al., 2000). However, moderate exercise does not appear to improve arterial stiffening in elderly subjects with isolated systolic hypertension (Miyachi et al., 2003; Tanaka et al., 2000; Zieman et al., 2005).

In contrast, resistance training (weight lifting) has been reported to increase arterial stiffness and is associated with more severe increase in left ventricular mass compared to sedentary controls (Bertovic et al., 1999).

## 7.2 Pharmacologic approach

Although antihypertensive therapy has targeted brachial (peripheral) BP parameters, recent studies suggest that control of central hemodynamic indices (central SBP, PP, PWV) afford better cardiorenal protection (The CAFÉ Investigators, for the Anglo-Scandinavian Cardiac Outcomes Trial (ASCOT) Investigators, 2006).

The therapeutic benefits of antihypertensive drugs are influenced by two major effects: i) the effect due to BP reduction; ii) the direct effect of the drug on the vessel wall (Weber et al., 2005). Drug therapy that favorably influences blood vessel function appears to directly enhance the mechanical properties of arterial wall, independent of BP changes. In a therapeutic trial on patients with endstage renal failure, a population at very high cardiovascular risk, longer survival was strongly related to the drug-induced reversibility of aortic stiffness measured by PWV independently of BP evaluation (Guerin et al., 2001).

Although all classes of antihypertensive drugs reduce BP effectively, they do not exert similar benefits on arterial structure and function (Van Bortel et al., 2001). Antihypertensive therapy should focus on modulating high PP, the latter parameter contributing to major risk of cardiorenal events in older hypertensive subjects (Van Bortel et al., 2001). In these subjects who frequently exhibit ISH or a disproportionate increase in SBP over DBP, causing a selective widening in PP, the goal of treatment should aim at decreasing SBP with maintenance or even enhancing DBP. These targets may be attained by an active improvement in arterial stiffness, change in wave reflection and reduction in left ventricular ejection (Van Bortel et al., 2001).

Inhibitors of the renin-angiotensin-aldosterone system (RAAS), calcium channel antagonists, nitrosovasodialtors, diuretics and 3-methylglutaryl-coenzyme A inhibitors (statins) appear to modulate arterial stiffness (Staessen and Birkenhager, 2005).

The RAAS inhibitors reduce arterial stiffness by inhibition of the vasoconstrictive action of angiotensin II and improvement in endothelial function (Van Bortel et al., 2001). In a substudy of the RENAAL clinical trial, administration of Losartan to diabetic patients with baseline PP≥90mmHg led to 53.5% risk reduction for ESRD alone and 35.5% risk reduction for ESRD or death (Bakris et al., 2003). A similar mode of action has been postulated for the aldosterone antagonists (Van Bortel et al., 2001). Calcium channel blockers, by exerting direct relaxing effects on vascular smooth muscle cells, appear to also achieve a reduction in arterial stiffness and wave reflection. Nitrosovasodialtors effectively reduce central SBP and PP, especially in patients with stiff arteries and enhanced wave reflections. The benefits provided by nitrates and phosphodiesterase type-5 inhibitors have been attributed to the increase in cyclic guanosine monophosphate in vascular smooth muscles (Weber et al., 2005). Diuretics reduce arterial stiffness by decreasing systemic BP (Cushman et al., 2001 & Weber et al., 2005).

In contrast, in clinical trials, atenolol or pure beta-blockade based-therapy did not provide cardiovascular protection compared to that afforded by newer classes of BP lowering agent, despite similar brachial BP levels (Conduit Artery Function Evaluation [CAFÉ] Study – Anglo Scandinavian Cardiac Outcomes Trial [ASCOT], 2006).

Administration of statins to overweight and obese subjects was associated with an improvement in arterial stiffness as evidenced by a significant reduction in PWV, independent of baseline cardiometabolic risk factors (Orr et al., 2009).

## 8. Conclusion

Increased PP, defined as the difference between inappropriately elevated SBP and reduced DBP at any value of MAP has recently emerged as an important and independent predictor of enhanced cardiovascular morbidity and mortality, especially in senior subjects. Central PP represents a surrogate measure of increased arterial stiffness of the central elastic arteries. However, brachial PP is a widely accepted marker of arterial stiffness in older subjects due to loss of amplification phenomenon and equalization with central PP.

In the general population, PP and age are positively correlated after the age of 50 years, whereas a negative correlation between these 2 parameters is found in adults younger than 50 years.

Interaction between left ventricular outflow and elastic properties of the central arteries creates incident forward propagating and reflected backward traveling pulse waves which summate either in diastole or systole. In young adults, due to high arterial distensibility, both pulse waves summate in diastole boosting central DBP, whereas in older subjects, due to increased arterial stiffness, summation occurs in late systole, generating a high SBP and loss of peripheral amplification.

Epidemiologic surveys and clinical studies have demonstrated, in the elderly, a close relationship between increased brachial PP and cardiovascular events, stroke, impairment in neurocognitive function and dementia, and vascular nephropathy and progression of CKD.

Therapeutic regimens include lifestyle modifications and pharmacologic medications. Therapeutic benefits have been reported when BP reduction has been associated with improved arterial function and reduced arterial stiffness.

## 9. References

Aviolo, AP., Clyde, KM., Beard, TC., Cooke, HM., Ho, KK., O'Rourke, MF. (1986). Improved Arterial Distensibility in Normotensive Subjects on a Low Salt Diet. *Arteriosclerosis*, Vol.6, pp. 166-169

Bahous, SA., Stephan, A., Blacher, J. & Safar, ME. (2006). Aortic Stiffness, Living Donors and Renal Transplantation. *Hypertension*, Vol. 47, pp. 216-221

Bakris, GL., Weir, MR., Shanifar, S., Zhang, Z., Douglas, J., Van Dijk, DJ., Brenner, BM., for the RENAAL Study Group. (2003). Effects of Blood Pressure level on Progression of Diabetic Nephropathy: Results from the RENAAL Study. *Archives of Internal Medicine*, Vol. 163, pp. 1555-1565

Benetos, A., Rudnichi, A., Safar, M. & Guize, L., (1998). Pulse Pressure and Cardiovascular Mortality in Normotensive and Hypertensive Subjects. *Hypertension*, Vol. 32, pp. 560-564

Benetos, A., Zureik, M., Morcet, J., Thomas, F., Bean, K., Safar, M., Ducimetiere, P., & Guize, L. (2000). A Decrease in Diastolic Blood Pressure Combined with an Increase in Systolic Blood Pressure Is Associated with a Higher Cardiovascular Mortality in Men *Journal of the American College of Cardiology*, Vol. 35, pp. 673-680

Benetos, A., Thomas, F., Joly, L., Blacher, J., Pannier, B., Labat, C., Salvi, P., Smulyan, H. & Safar, ME. (2010). Pulse Pressure Amplification: a Mechanical Biomarker of Cardiovascular Risk. *Journal of the American College of Cardiology*, Vol. 55, pp. 1032-1037

Benetos, A., Salvi, P. & Lacolley, P. (2011). Blood Pressure Regulation during the Aging Process: the End of the "Hypertension Era"? *Journal of Hypertension*, Vol. 29, pp. 646-652

Benjo, A., Thompson, RE., Fine, D., Hogue, CH., Alejo, D., Kaw, A., Gerstenblith, G., Shah, A., Berkowitz, DE. & Nyhan, D. (2007). Pulse Pressure is an Independent Predictor of Stroke Development after Cardiac Surgery. *Hypertension*, Vol. 50, pp. 630-635

Bertovic, DA., Waddell, TK., Gatzka, CD., Cameron, JD., Dart, AM. & Kingwell, BA. (1999). Muscular Strength Training is Associated with Low Arterial Compliance and High Pulse Pressure. *Hypertension*, Vol. 33, pp. 1385-1391

Bidani, AK. & Griffin, KA. (2002). Long-Term Renal Consequences of Hypertension for Normal and Diseased Kidneys. *Current Opinion in Nephrology and Hypertension*, Vol. 11, pp. 73-80

Bidani, AK. & Griffin, KA. (2004). Pathophysiology of Hypertensive Renal Damage-Implications for Therapy. *Hypertension*, Vol. 44, pp. 595-601

Bidani, AK., Griffin, AK., Williamson, G., Wang, X. & Loutzenhiser, R. (2009). Protective Importance of the Myogenic Response in the Renal Circulation. *Hypertension*, Vol. 54, pp. 393-398

Boutouyrie, P., Tropeano, AI., Asmar, R., Gautier, I., Benetos, A., Lacolley, P. & Laurent, S. (2002). Aortic Stiffness is an Independent Predictor of Primary Coronary Events in Hypertensive Patients – A Longitudinal Study. *Hypertension*, Vol. 39, pp. 10-15

Chirinos, JA., Zambrano, JP., Chakko, S., Veerani, A., Schob, A., Willens, HJ., Perez, G. & Mendez, AJ. (2005). Aortic Pressure Augmentation Predicts Adverse Cardiovascular Events in Patients with Established Coronary Artery Disease. *Hypertension*, Vol.45, pp. 980-985

CAFÉ Investigators for the Anglo-Scandinavian Cardiac Outcomes Trial (ASCOT) Investigators, CAFÉ Steering Committee and Writing Committee, Williams, B., Lacy, PS., Thom, SM., Cruickshank, K., Stanton, A., Collier, D., Hughes, AD., Thurston, H. & O'Rourke, M. (2006). Differential Impact of Blood Pressure-Lowering Drugs on Central Aortic Pressure and Clinical Outcomes: Principal Results of the Conduit Artery Function Evaluation (CAFÉ) Study. *Circulation*, Vol. 113, pp. 1213-1225

Cushman, WC., Materson, BJ., Williams, DW., Reda, DJ & for the Veterans Affairs Cooperative Study Group on Antihypertensive Agents. (2001). Pulse Pressure Changes with Six Classes of Antihypertensive Agents in a Randomized Controlled Trial. *Hypertension*,Vol. 38, pp. 953-957

Dart, AM. & Kingwell, BA. (2001). Pulse Pressure – A Review of Mechanisms and Clinical Relevance. *Journal of the American College of Cardiology*, Vol. 37, pp. 975-984

Dengo, AL., Dennis, EA., Orr JS., Marinik, EL., Ehrlich, E., Davy, B. & Davy KJ. (2010). Arterial Destiffening with Weight Loss in Overweight and Obese Middle-Aged and Older Subjects. *Hypertension*, Vol. 55, pp. 855-861

De Simone, G., Roman MJ., Alderman, MH., Galderisi, M., De Divitiis, O. & Devereux, RB. (2005). Is High Pulse Pressure a Marker of Preclinical Cardiovascular Disease. *Hypertension*, Vol. 45, pp. 575-579

Farasat, SM., Valdes, C., Shetty, V., Muller, DC., Egan, JM., Metter, EJ., Ferrucci, L. & Najjar, SS. (2010). Is Longitudinal Pulse Pressure a Better Predictor of 24-Hour Urinary Albumin Excretion than Other Indices of Blood Pressure. *Hypertension*, Vol. 55, pp. 415-421

Fernandez-Fresnedo, G., Escallada, R., Martin de Francisco, AL., Ruiz, JC., Sanz de Castro, S., Gonzalez Cotorruelo, J. & Arias, M. (2005). Association between Pulse Pressure and Cardiovascular Disease in Renal Transplant Patients. *American Journal of Transplantation*, Vol. 5, pp. 394-398

Ferri, C., Grassi, D. & Grassi, G. (2006). Cocoa Beans, Endothelial Function and Aging: an Unexpected Friendship. *Journal of Hypertension*, Vol. 24, pp. 1471-1474

Fesler, P., Safar, ME., Du Cailar, G., Ribstein, J. & Mimran, A. (2007). Pulse Pressure is an Independent Determinant of Renal Function During Treatment of Essential Hypertension. *Journal of Hypertension*, Vol. 25, pp. 1915-1920

Ford, ML., Tomlinson, LA., Chapman, TP., Rajkumar, C. & Holt, SG. (2010). Aortic Stiffness is Independently Associated with Rate of Renal Function Decline in Chronic Kidney Disease Stages 3 and 4. *Hypertension*, Vol. 55, pp. 1110-1115

Franklin, SS., Khan SA., Wong ND., Larson, MG. & Levy, D. (1999). Is Pulse Pressure Useful in Predicting Risk for Coronary Heart Disease? The Framingham Heart Study. *Circulation*, Vol. 100, pp. 354-360

Franklin, SS., Jacobs, MJ., Wong, ND., L'Italien, GJ. & Lapuerta, P. (2001). Predominance of Isolated Systolic Hypertension among Middle-Aged and Elderly US Hypertensives: Analysis Based on National Health and Nutrition Survey (NHANES) III. *Hypertension*, Vol. 37, pp. 869-874

Franklin, SS., Larson, MG., Khan, AS., Wong, ND., Leip EP., Kannel, WK. & Levy, D. (2001). Does the Relation of Blood Pressure to Coronary Heart Disease Risk Change with Aging? The Framingham Heart Study. *Circulation*, Vol. 103, pp. 1245-1249

Gates, PE., Tanaka, H., Hiatt, WR. & Seals, DR. (2004). Dietary Sodium Restriction Rapidly Improves Large Artery Elastic Compliance in Older Adults with Systolic Hypertension. *Hypertension*, Vol. 44, pp. 35-41

Guerin, AP., Blacher, J., Pannier, B., Marchais, SJ., Safar, ME. & London, GM. (2001). Impact of Aortic Stiffness Attenuation on Survival of Patients in End-Stage Renal Failure. *Circulation*, Vol. 103, pp. 987-992

Gosse, P., Coulon, P., Papaioannou, G., Litalien, J. & Lemetayer, P. (2009). Long-Term Decline in Renal Function is Linked to Initial Pulse Pressure in the Essential Hypertensive. *Journal of Hypertension*, Vol. 27, pp. 1303-1308

Hanon, O., Haulton, S., Lenoir, H., Seux, ML., Rigaud, AS., Safar, M., Girerd, X. & Forette, F. (2005). Relationship Between Arterial Stiffness and Cognitive Function in Elderly Subjects with Complaints of Memory Loss. *Stroke*, Vol. 36, pp. 2193-2197

Henskens, LHG., Kroon, AA., Van Oostenbrugge, RJ., Gronenschild, EHBM., Fuss-Lejeune, MMJJ., Hofman, PAM., Lodder, J. & De Leeuw, PW. (2008). Increased Pulse Wave Velocity is Associated With Silent Cerebral Small-Vessel Disease in Hypertensive Patients. *Hypertension*, Vol. 52, pp. 1120-1126

Hsu, C-Y., McCulloch, CE., Darbinian, J., Go, AS. & Iribarren, C. (2005). Elevated Blood Pressure and Risk of End-Stage Renal Disease in Subjects Without Baseline Kidney Disease. *Archives of Internal Medicine*, Vol. 165, pp. 923-928

Jankowski, P., Kawecka-Jaszcz, K., Czarnecka, D., Brzozowska-Kiszka, M., Styczkiewicz, K., Loster, M., Kloch-Badelek, M., Wilinski, J., Curylo, AM. & Dudek, D. on behalf of the Aortic Blood Pressure and Survival Study Group. (2008). Pulsatile but Not Steady Component of Blood Pressure Predicts Cardiovascular Events in Coronary Patients. *Hypertension*, Vol. 51, pp. 1-8

Karamanoglu, M., O'Rourke, MF., Avolio, AP. & Kelly, RP. (1993). An Analysis of the Relationship Between Central Aortic and Peripheral Upper Limb Pressure Waves in Man. *European Heart Journal*, Vol. 14, pp. 160-167

Kengne, AP., Czernichow, S., Huxley, R., Grobbee, D., Woodward, M., Neal, B., Zoungas, S., Cooper, M., Glasziou, P., Hamet, P., Harrap, SB., Mancia, G., Poulter, N., Williams, B. & Chalmers, J. on behalf of the ADVANCE Collaborative Group. (2009). Blood Pressure Variables and Cardiovascular Risk: New Findings from ADVANCE. *Hypertension*, Vol. 54, pp. 399-404

Kim, CK., Lee, SH., Kim, BJ., Ryu, WS. & Yoon, BW. (2011). Age-Independent Association of Pulse Pressure with Cerebral White Matter Lesions in Asymptomatic Elderly Individuals. *Journal of Hypertension*, Vol. 29, pp. 325-329

Klag, MJ., Whelton, PK., Randall, BL., Neaton, JD., Brancati, FL., Ford, CE., Shulman, NB. & Stamler, J. (1996). Blood Pressure and End-Stage Renal Disease in Men. *New England Journal of Medicine*, Vol. 334, pp. 13-18

Kotsis, V., Stabouli, S., Karafillis, I. & Nilsson, P. (2011). Early Vascular Aging and the Role of Central Blood Pressure. *Journal of Hypertension*, Vol., 29, pp. 1847-1853

Lakatta, EG. (2003). Arterial and Cardiac Aging: Major Shareholders in Cardiovascular Disease Enterprises. Part III: Cellular and Molecular Clues to Heart and Arterial Aging. *Circulation*, Vol. 107, pp. 490-497

Laurent, S., Tropeano, A-I. & Boutouyrie, P. (2006). Pulse Pressure Reduction and Cardiovascular Protection. *Journal of Hypertension*, Vol. 24 (Suppl 3), pp. S13-S18

Laurent, S. & Boutouyrie, P. (2007). Recent Advances in Arterial Stiffness and Wave reflection in Human Hypertension. *Hypertension*, Vol. 49, pp. 1202-1206

Laurent, S., Briet, M. & Boutouyrie, P. (2009). Large and Small Artery Cross-Talk and Recent Morbidity-Mortality Trials in Hypertension. *Hypertension*, Vol. 54, pp. 388-392

Limas, C., Westrum, B., Limas, CJ. & Cohn, JN. (1980). Effect of Salt on the Vascular Lesions of Spontaneously Hypertensive Rats. *Hypertension*, Vol.2, pp. 477-489

Loutzenhiser, R., Bidani, A. & Chilton, L. (2002). Renal Myogenic Response-Kinetic Attributes and Physiologic Role. *Circulation Research*, Vol. 90, pp. 1316-1324

Loutzenhiser, R., Griffin, K., Williamson, G. & Bidani, A. (2006). Renal Autoregulation: New Perspectives Regarding the Protective and Regulatory Roles of the Underlying Mechanisms. *American Journal of Physiology-Regulatory, Integrative and Comparative Physiology*, Vol. 290, pp. R1153-R1167

McEniery, CM., Yasmin., Hall, IR., Qasem, A., Wilkinson, IB. & Cockroft, JR. on behalf of the ACCT Investigators. (2005). Normal Vascular Aging: Differential Effects on Wave Reflection and Aortic Pulse Wave Velocity: the Anglo-Cardiff Collaborative Trial (ACCT). *Journal of the American College of Cardiology*, Vol. 46, pp. 1753-1760

Mimran, A. (2006). Consequence of Elevated Pulse Pressure on Renal Function. *Journal of Hypertension*, Vol. 24 (Suppl.3), pp. S3-S7

Mitchell, G. (2004). Increased Aortic Stiffness: an Unfavorable Cardiorenal Connection. *Hypertension*, Vol. 43, pp. 151-153

Mitchell, GF., Hwang, S-J., Vasan, RS., Larson, MG., Pencina, MJ., Hamburg, NM., Vita, JA., Levy, D. & Benjamin, EJ. (2010). Arterial Stiffness and Cardiovascular Events. The Framingham Heart Study. *Circulation*, Vol. 121, pp. 505-511

Miura, K., Nakagawa, H., Ohashi, Y., Harada, A., Taguri, M., Kushiro, T., Takahashi, A., Nishinaga, M., Soejima, H. & Ueshima, H. for the Japan Arteriosclerosis Longitudinal Study (JALS) Group. (2009).Four Blood Pressure Indexes and the Risk of Stroke and Myocardial Infarction in Japanese Men and Women: A Meta-Analysis of 16 Cohort Studies. Circulation, Vol. 119, pp. 1892-1898

Miyachi, M., Donato, AJ., Yamamoto, K., Takahashi, K., Gates, PE., Moreau, KL. & Tanaka, H. (2003). Greater Age-Related Reductions in Central Arterial Compliance in Resistance-Trained Men. *Hypertension*, Vol. 41, pp. 130-135

Miyaki, A., Maeda, S., Yoshizawa, M., Misono, M., Saito, Y., Sasai, H., Endo, T., Nakata, Y., Tanaka, K. & Ajisaka, R. (2009). Effect of Weight Reduction with Dietary Intervention on Arterial Distensibility and Endothelial Function in Obese Men. *Angiology*, Vol. 60, pp. 351-357

Mosley II, WJ., Greenland, P., Garside, DB. & Lloyd, Jones. (2007). Predicitve Utility of Pulse Pressure and Other Blood Pressure Measures for Cardiovascular Outcomes. *Hypertension*, Vol. 49, pp. 1256-1264

Mourad, JJ., Pannier, B., Blacher, J., Rudnichi, A., Benetos, A., London, GM. & Safar, ME. (2001). Creatinine Clearance, Pulse Wave Velocity, Carotid Compliance and Essential Hypertension. *Kidney International*, Vol. 59, pp. 1834-1841

National High Blood Pressure Program Working Group. (1994). National High Blood Pressure Program Working Group Report on Hypertension in the Elderly. Hypertension, Vol. 23, pp. 275-285

Nestel, P., Shige, H., Pomeroy, S., Cehun, M., Abbey, M., & Raederstorff D., (2002). The n-3 Fatty Acids Eicosapentaenoic and Docosahexaenoic Acid Increase Systemic Arterial Compliance in Humans. *The American Journal of Clinical Nutrition*. Vol. 76, pp.326-330

Okada, K., Iso, H., Cui, R., Inove, M. & Tsugane, S. (2011). Pulse Pressure is an Independent Risk Factor for Stroke among Middle-Aged Japanese with Normal Systolic Blood Pressure: the JPHC Study. *Journal of Hypertension*, Vol. 29, pp. 319-324

O'Rourke, MF. & Safar, ME. (2005). Relationship between Aortic Stiffening and Microvascular Disease in Brain and Kidney: Cause and Logic of Therapy. *Hypertension*, Vol. 46, pp. 200-204

Orr, JS., Gentile, CL., Davy, BM. & Davy, KP. (2008). Large Artery Stiffening with Weight Gain in Humans: Roll of Visceral fat Accumulation. *Hypertension*, Vol. 51, pp. 1519-1524

Orr, JS., Dengo, L., Rivero, JM., & Davy, KP. (2009). Arterial Destiffening with Atorvastatin in Overweight and Obese Middle-Aged and Older Adults. *Hypertension*, Vol. 54, pp. 763-768

Paultre, F. & Mosca, L. (2005). Association of Blood Pressure Indices and Stroke Mortality in Isolated Systolic Hypertension. *Stroke*, Vol. 36, pp. 1288-1290

Pedrinelli, R., Dell'omo, G., Penno, G., Bandinelli, S., Bertini, A., Di Bello, V. and Mariani, M. (2000). Microalbuminuria and Pulse Pressure in Hypertensive and Atherosclerotic Men. *Hypertension,* Vol. 35, pp. 48-54

Perry, HMJr., Miller, JP., Fornoff, JR., Baty, JD., Sambhi, MP., Rutan, G., Moskowitz, DW. & Carmody, SE. (1995). Early Predictors of 15-Year End Stage Renal Disease in Hypertensive Patients. *Hypertension*, Vol. 25, pp. 587-594

Qiu, C., Winblad, B., Viitanen, M. & Fratiglioni, L. (2003). Pulse Pressure and Risk of Alzheimer Disease in Persons Aged 75 Years and Older: A Community-Based, Longitudinal Study. *Stroke*, Vol. 34, pp. 594-599

Robbins, MA., Elias, MF., Elias, PK. & Buoge, MM. (2005). Blood Pressure and Cognitive Function in an African-American and Caucasian-American Sample: the Maine-Syracuse Study. *Psychosomatic Medicine*, Vol. 67, pp. 707-714

Safar, ME., Levy, BI. & Struitjker-Boudier, H. (2003). Current Perspectives on Arterial Stiffness and Pulse Pressure in Hypertension and Cardiovascular Diseases. *Circulation*, Vol. 107, pp. 2864-2869

Safar, ME. (2004). Peripheral Pulse Pressure, Large Arteries and Microvessels. *Hypertension*, Vol. 44, pp. 121-122

Sarnak, MJ., Levey, AS., School Werth, AC., Coresh, J., Culleton, B., Hamm, LL., McCullough, PA., Kasike, BL., Kelepouris, E., Klag, MJ., Parfrey, P., Pfeffer, M., Raij, L., Spinosa, DJ. & Wilson PW. (2003). Kidney Disease as a Risk Factor for Development of Cardiovascular Diseases: a Statement from the American Heart Association Councils on Kidney in Cardiovascular Disease, High Blood Pressure Research, Clinical Cardiology, and Epidemiology and Prevention. *Circulation*, Vol. 108, pp. 2154-2169

Schram, MT., Kostense, PJ., Van Dijk, R.A.J.M., Dekker, JM., Nijpels, G., Bouter, LM., Heine RJ. & Stehouwer, C.D.A. (2002). Diabetes, Pulse Pressure and Cardiovascular Mortality: the Hoorn Study. *Journal of Hypertension*, Vol. 20, pp. 1743-1751

Scuteri, A., Nilsson, PM., Tzourio, C., Redon, J. & Laurent, S. (2011). Microvascular Brain Damage with Aging and Hypertension: Pathophysiological Consideration and Clinical Implications. *Journal of Hypertension*, Vol. 29, pp. 1469-1477

Seckinger, J., Sommerer, C., Hinkel, U-P., Hoffmann, O., Zeier, M., Schwenger, V. (2008). Switch of Immunosuppression from Cyclosporine A to Everolimus: Impact on Pulse Wave Velocity in Stable De Novo Renal Allograft Recipients. *Journal of Hypertension*, Vol. 26, pp. 2213-2219

Selvetella, G., Notte, A., Maffei, A., Calistri, V., Scamardella, V., Frati, G., Trimarco, B.,Colonnese, C. & Lembo, G. (2003). Left Ventricular Hypertrophy is Associated with Asymptomatic Cerebral Damage in Hypertensive Patients. *Stroke*, Vol. 34, pp. 1766-1770

Sierksma, A., Muller, M., Van Der Schouw, YT., Grobbee, DE., Hendriks, HF. & Bots, ML. (2004). Alcohol Consumption and Arterial Stiffeness in Men. *Journal of Hypertension*, Vol. 22, pp. 357-362

Somes, GW., Pahor, M., Shorr, RI., Cushman, WC. & Applegate, WB. (1999). The Role of Diastolic Blood Pressure When Treating Isolated Systolic Hypertension. *Annals of Internal Medicine*, Vol. 159, pp. 2004-2009

Staessen, JA. & Birkenhäger, WH. (2005). Evidence that New Antihypertensives are Superior to Older Drugs. *Lancet*, Vol. 366, issue 9489, pp. 869-871

Stehouwer, CD., Henry, RM. & Ferreira, I. (2008). Arterial Stiffness in Diabetes and the Metabolic Syndrome: a Pathway to Cardiovascular Disease. *Diabetologia*, Vol. 51, pp. 527-539

Tanaka, H., Dinenno, FA., Monahan, KD., Clevenger, CM., Desouza, CA. & Seals, DR. (2000). Aging Habitual Exercise and Dynamic Arterial Compliance. *Circulation*, Vol. 102, pp. 1270-1275

Taubert, D., Berkels, R., Roesen, R. & Klaus, W. (2003). Chocolate and Blood Pressure in Elderly Individuals with Isolated Systolic Hypertension. *Journal of the American Medical Association*, Vol. 290, pp. 1029-1030

Townsend, RR., Wimmer, NJ. & Chirinos, JA. (2010). Aortic PWV in Chronic Kidney Disease: a CRIC Ancillary Study. *American Journal of Hypertension*, Vol. 23, pp. 282-289

Udani, S., Lazich, I. & Bakris, GL. (2011). Epidemiology of Hypertensive Kidney Disease. *Nature Reviews of Nephrology*, Vol. 7, pp. 11-21

Vaccarino, V., Holford, TR. & Krumholz, HM. (2000). Pulse Pressure and Risk for Myocardial Infarction and Heart Failure in the Elderly. *Journal of the American College of Cardiology*, Vol. 36, pp. 130-138

Vaccarino, V., Berger, AK., Abramson, J., Black, HR., Setaro, JF., Davey, JA. & Krumholz, HM. (2001). Pulse Pressure and Risk of Cardiovascular Events in the Systolic Hypertension in the Elderly Program. *American Journal of Cardiology*, Vol. 88, pp. 980-986

Van Bortel, LMAB., Struitjker-Boudier, HAJ. & Safar, ME. (2001). Pulse Pressure, Arterial Stiffness and Drug Treatment of Hypertension. *Hypertension*, Vol. 38, pp. 914-921

Van Der Schouw, YT., Pijpe, A., Lebrun, CEI., Bots, ML., Peeters, PHM., Van Staveren, WA., Lamberts, SWJ. & Grobbee, DE. (2002). Higher Usual Dietary Intake of Phytoestrogens Is Associated with Lower Aortic Stiffness in Postmenopausal Women. *Arteriosclerosis, Thrombosis and Vascular Biology*, Vol. 22, pp. 1316-1322

Verhave, JC., Fesler, P., Du Cailar, G., Ribstein, J., Safar, ME. & Mimran, A.(2005). Elevated Pulse Pressure Is Associated with Low Renal Function in Elderly Patients with Isolated Systolic Hypertension. *Hypertension*, Vol. 45, pp. 586-591

Vetromile, F., Szwarc, I., Garrigue, V., Delmas, S., Fesler, P., Mimran, A., Ribstein, J. & Mourad, G. (2009). Early High Pulse Pressure is Associated with Graft Dysfunction and Predicts Poor Kidney Allograft Survival. *Transplantation*, Vol. 88, pp. 1088-1094

Vupputuri, S., Batuman V., Muntner, P., Bazzano, LA., Lefante, JJ., Whelton, PK. & He, J. (2003). Effect of Blood Pressure on Early Decline in Kidney Function among Hypertensive Men. *Hypertension*, Vol. 42, pp. 1144-1149

Waldstein, SR., Rice, SC., Thayer, JF., Najjar, SS., Scuteri, A. & Zonderman, AB. (2008). Pulse Pressure and Pulse Wave Velocity are Related to Cognitive Decline in the Baltimore Longitudinal Study of Aging. *Hypertension*, Vol. 51, pp. 99-104

Weber, T., Auer, J., O'Rourke, MF., Kvas, E., Lassnig, E., Lamm, G., Stark, N., Rammer, M. & Eber, B. (2005). Increased Arterial Wave Reflections Predict Severe Cardiovascular Events in Patients Undergoing Percutaneous Coronary Interventions. *European Heart Journal*, Vol. 26, pp. 2657-2663

Wilkinson, IB., Franklin, SS., Hall, IR., Tyrrell, S. & Cockroft, JR. (2001). Pressure Amplification Explains why Pulse Pressure is Unrelated to Risk in Young Subjects. *Hypertension*, Vol. 38, pp. 1461-1466

Young, JH., Klag, MJ., Muntner, P., Whyte, JL., Pahor, M. & Coresh, J. (2002). Blood Pressure and Decline in Kidney Function: Findings from the Systolic Hypertension in the Elderly Program (SHEP). *Journal of the American Society of Nephrology*, Vol. 13, pp. 2776-2782

Zhang, XF., Attia, J., D'Este, C. & Yu, XH. (2004). Prevalence and Magnitude of Classical Risk Factors for Stroke in a Cohort of 5092 Chinese Steelworkers over 13.5 Years of Follow-Up. *Stroke*, Vol. 35, pp. 1052-1056

Zieman, SJ., Melenovsky, V., & Kass, DA. (2005). Mechanisms, Pathophysiology and Therapy of Arterial Stiffness. *Arteriosclerosis, Thrombosis, Vascular Biology*, Vol. 25, pp. 932-934

# 4

# An Anti-Inflammatory Approach in the Therapeutic Choices for the Prevention of Atherosclerotic Events

Aldo Pende and Andrea Denegri
*Clinic of Internal Medicine 1, Department of Internal Medicine,*
*University of Genoa School of Medicine, Genoa,*
*Italy*

## 1. Introduction

Atherosclerosis, with its dramatic events, represents a heavy burden in terms of morbidity and mortality throughout the entire world (Gibbons et al., 2008). Although the risk factors are very well known and addressed by every physician (genetic background, physical inactivity, hypertension, dyslipidemia, diabetes mellitus, obesity and metabolic syndrome, smoking), the precise mechanisms of the plaque formation and rupture are not completely clarified. These limitations are confirmed by the difficulties in obtaining better results in both primary and secondary prevention of cardiovascular events: recent results of completed clinical trials (such as NAVIGATOR, ACCORD, ROADMAP) suggest that we have reached a limit in terms of reducing events by simply addressing common risk factors appropriately (Zanchetti, 2009). As a matter of fact, at the present time we cannot prevent 70% of clinical events, also with administration of all well established anti-atherosclerotic therapeutics. In addition at least 10% of coronary events can occur in apparently healthy subjects in the absence of traditional risk factors (Baigent et al., 2005; Greenland et al., 2003).

The inflammatory paradigm has represented an important achievement in the understanding of the atherosclerotic process: abundant laboratory and clinical evidence accumulated over the last twenty years, also from our research group (Montecucco et al. 2010), confirming the hypothesis that inflammation exerts a major role through the different stages of atherosclerosis (Ross, 1999; Hansson, 2005; Hansson & Libby, 2006; Libby et al., 2009). Therefore it would be interesting to evaluate how the therapeutic choices exerted by physicians can modulate the inflammatory activation (the so called pleiotropic effects): in other terms do the drugs we use in the attempt of counteracting atherosclerosis (such as anti-hypertensive drugs, statins, fibrates, aspirin, anti-diabetic drugs) exert their protective effects through their main site of action (decrease of blood pressure, cholesterol, triglycerides, and glucose, anti-platelets actions) or can an additional anti-inflammatory effect be proposed, at least for some of them? This is the reason why recently Ridker proposed a clinical trial with low-dose methotrexate, a powerful anti-inflammatory drug extensively used in the treatment of auto-immune disease (suc as rheumatoid arthritis), in post-myocardial infarction (MI) patients (Ridker, 2009); another testable drug could be canakinumab, a human monoclonal antibody targeted against interleukin-1β (Libby et al., 2011).

In theory these approaches have a great appeal because their main target is represented by the basic mechanism of the atherosclerotic process, i.e. the inflammatory activation, but the risk of untoward effects can overcome the expected benefits: particularly in primary prevention the possible depression of the immune system and defense against cancer may be too dangerous in a substantially healthy population. In addition the involvement of the immune system, and consequently the inflammatory activation, is not completely elucidated because the entire network is particularly complex with many pathways, both redundant and with opposite effects, and many cells (Libby et al., 2011). Another reason for our difficulties is represented by the realization of the incomplete concordance between atherosclerosis in human vessels and the possible animal models (Bentzon & Falk, 2010): the hypotheses generated by the experimental research frequently do not find a confirmation in a clinical scenario.

The road of the anti-inflammatory approach in the treatment of atherosclerosis is paved by many defeats: table 1 tries to summarize the possible explanations.

| Possible explanations | Example |
|---|---|
| Important side effects | NSAIDs, Corticosteroids, Torcetrapib |
| Activation of dangerous pathways | COX-2 inhibitors |
| Secondary target | Fibrates |
| Unfavourable effects on lipid profile | Rosiglitazone |
| Marked differences *in vitro* vs. *in vivo* conditions | Anti-oxidant agents |
| Too late and too shy treatment | All the possible options? |

Table 1. Possible reasons of negative or partly successful trials for atherosclerosis

A new and theoretically safer way to modulate the inflammatory activation could involve new lipid anti-inflammatory mediators, such as lipoxins, resolvins, protectins, and maresins: these molecules derive from the transformation of both the ω-6 fatty acid arachidonic acid and the ω-3 fatty acids eicosapentaenoic acid and docosahexaenoic acid via actions of lipoxygenase, cyclooxygenase-2 and aspirin-acetylated COX-2 enzymes (Hersberger, 2010; Maskrey et al., 2011). These mediators exert significant effects favoring the resolution of the inflammatory process through the activation of a specific program, characterized by apoptosis and subsequent clearance of inflammatory cells. Again anti-inflammatory mediators are tightly linked, in terms of chemical structure and synthetic pathways, to pro-inflammatory molecules, such as leukotrienes. At the present time, among available drugs, aspirin and statins seem to be able to activate these pathways significantly (Spite & Serhan, 2010): the theoretical advantage would be represented by targeting inflammation without precipitating sustained immunosuppression.

Another important preliminary consideration is related to the ongoing debate about the appropriate timing of the beginning in anti-atherosclerotic treatments (Steinberg, 2010; Pletcher & Hulley, 2010). Although we need to never forget the fundamental role of healthy lifestyle choices, we know that some people are at potential high risk of vascular damage and consequently in this subset a more aggressive pharmacological approach can be advisable. The two opposite points of view are represented by physicians who support an aggressive therapy (at least with statins and antihypertensives, when indicated) at young age, i.e. at the beginning of the atherosclerotic process, and physicians who underline the risk of the creation of a "pseudodisease" (Lauer, 2011).

Directly linked to this topic is the role of biomarkers and vascular imaging in supporting treatment decisions: if we identify subclinical markers of atherosclerotic damage, we can use them in the prognostic stratification and consequently in rational therapeutic strategies. This consideration is an implicit criticism to the Framingham Risk Score (and other related risk calculators), a simple, relatively inexpensive, and useful way to predict cardiovascular events in the general population (Shah, 2010; Forrester, 2010). Limitations of the Framingham Risk Score include a substantial underestimation of lifetime risk and misclassification of some subgroups of subjects; in addition it does not incorporate family history and some components of the metabolic syndrome, important risk factors for coronary heart disease, and more importantly does not take into consideration the possible help of the noninvasive detection of subclinical atherosclerosis. Therefore we can reasonably affirm that Framingham Risk Score is very useful at the population level, but it remains suboptimal for individual subjects.

Subclinical atherosclerosis always begins with fatty streak lesions, which are already extensively diffuse by 30 years of age (Shah, 2010; Lauer, 2010): although we know that fatty streaks are reversible, we are also aware that this lesion is certainly the precursor of the stenotic plaque. Do we have validated imaging tools for subclinical atherosclerosis? Essentially, we can rely on coronary calcium score, obtained by computed tomography without contrast, and on carotid intima-media thickness, evaluated by B-mode ultrasonography (US). With some limitations (Shah, 2010; U.S. Preventive Services Task Force, 2009) they represent a useful aid in better classification of risk categories in human subjects: some years ago the SHAPE (Screening for Heart Attack Prevention and Education) Task Force recommended noninvasive atherosclerosis imaging of all asymptomatic men (age 45 – 75 years) and women (age 55 – 75 years), except those at very low risk, to augment conventional cardiovascular risk assessment algorithms (Naghavi et al., 2006): recently these guidelines were positively evaluated in the Dallas Heart Study, with significant bidirectional reclassification of eligibility for lipid-lowering therapy in the participants (See et al., 2008).

About serum biomarkers the role of high-sensitivity C-reactive protein (hsCRP) is well established and will be evaluated in depth for statins. Recently 30 biomarkers for atherosclerosis, or more in general cardiovascular diseases, were studied in two large cohorts totalling more than 9,000 subjects (Blankenberg et al., 2010): a consistent association with incident cardiovascular events was observed for hsCRP, B-type natriuretic peptide and cardiac troponin I. These observations allowed the development of a biomarker score which was positively validated in a cohort of male subjects.

The present article will present updated information about the anti-inflammatory effects of different classes of drugs and the possible therapeutic advantages obtained with this approach. Before starting the evaluation we need to never forget the fundamental protective role exerted by a healthy lifestyle: very recently we extensively reviewed these choices and their great social value (Pende & Dallegri, 2011). However we know that their implementation and long-term compliance is very low: a possible help is the potentiation of population-based strategies, such as smoking bans and food legislation against trans-fats and high amount of salt.

Table 2 gives some information about the clinical trials discussed in the review with full definition of the names.

| Clinical trial acronym | Clinical trial name | Drugs tested |
|---|---|---|
| ACCORD-Lipid | Action to Control Cardiovascular Risk in Diabetes | Simvastatin, fenofibrate |
| AFCAPS/TexCAPS | Air Force/Texas Coronary Atherosclerosis Prevention Study | Statins |
| ARBITER 6-HALTS | Arterial Biology for the Investigation of the Treatment Effects of Reducing Cholesterol 6 - HDL and LDL Treatment Strategies in Atherosclerosis | Ezetimibe, niacin |
| ARIC | Atherosclerosis Risk in Communities | Multiple drugs |
| ARISE | Aggressive Reduction of Inflammation Stops Events | Succinobucol |
| A-to-Z | Aggrastat to Zocor | Simvastatin |
| CAMELOT | Comparison of Amlodipine vs Enalapril to Limit Occurrences of Thrombosis | Amlodipine, enalapril |
| CARE | Cholesterol and Recurrent Events | Pravastatin |
| DEFINE | Determining the Efficacy and Tolerability of CETP Inhibition with Anacetrapib. | Anacetrapib |
| HPS2-THRIVE | Treatment of High density lipoprotein to Reduce the Incidence of Vascular Events | Niacin/laropiprant |
| ILLUMINATE | Investigation of Lipid Level Management to Understand its Impact in Atherosclerotic Events | Torcetrapib |
| JUPITER | Justification for the Use of Statin in Prevention: an Intervention Trial Evaluating Rosuvastatin | Rosuvastatin |
| MIRACL | Myocardial Ischemia Reduction with Aggressive Cholesterol Lowering | Atorvastatin |
| NAVIGATOR | Nateglinide and Valsartan in Impaired Glucose Tolerance Outcomes Research | Nateglinide, valsartan |
| PLASMA | Phospholipase Levels And Serological Markers of Atherosclerosis | Varepladib |
| PROactive | Prospective Pioglitazone Clinical Trial in Macrovascular Events | Pioglitazone |
| PROVE IT-TIMI 22 | Pravastatin or Atorvastatin Evaluation and Infection Therapy Thrombolysis in Myocardial Infarction 22 | Pravastatin, atorvastatin |
| REVERSAL | Reversing Atherosclerosis with Aggressive Lipid Lowering | Pravastatin, atorvastatin |
| ROADMAP | Randomised Olmesartan and Diabetes Microalbuminuria Prevention | Olmesartan |
| SOLID-TIMI 52 | Stabilization of Plaques Using Darapladib — Thrombolysis in Myocardial Infarction 52 | Darapladib |
| STABILITY | Stabilization of Atherosclerotic Plaque by Initiation of Darapladib Therapy | Darapladib |
| VISTA-16 | Vascular Inflammation Suppression to Treat Acute Coronary Syndrome for 16 Weeks | Varespladib |

Table 2. Acronyms of clinical trials discussed in this review

## 2. HMG-CoA reductase inhibitors (statins)

Although the main mechanism of action of this class of drugs is the inhibition of the cholesterol synthesis, since the end of the last century a significant anti-inflammatory effect appeared to be present as additional explanation of the results in randomized controlled trials. The specific biomarker for inflammation was CRP and this molecule maintained its role in many different trials until present time.

Although the association between CRP and coronary artery disease was first observed more than two decades ago (Berk et al., 1990), researchers are still debating about the precise position of CRP in clinical and experimental atherosclerosis (Ridker, 2007; Schunkert & Samani, 2008; Casas et al., 2008; Nordestgaard, 2009; Anand & Yusuf, 2010; Boekholdt & Kastelein, 2010; Després, 2011; Keavney, 2011): some authors think that CRP exerts a fundamental role in the beginning of the vascular inflammatory process (for example through the activation of the classical complement pathway and enhancement of the innate immune response), instead a more conservative opinion regards CRP no more than a useful but unspecific biomarker of inflammation (an innocent bystander). In practical terms, its long half-life (about 19 h), its limited cost and possibility of replication of the assay in the follow-up without health issues for the patients represent good features. In addition CRP seems to meet most of the American Heart Association (AHA) statement criteria for use of a novel cardiovascular risk marker (proof of concept, prospective validation, incremental value beyond other risk factors, and clinical utility) (Hlatky et al., 2009). For these reasons Ridker et al. proposed and validated a new clinical risk algorithm, Reynolds risk score for both women (Ridker at al., 2007) and men (Ridker et al., 2008a), which incorporates information on both inflammation (hsCRP) and genetics (parental history of premature MI). The utility of hsCRP for risk reclassification was confirmed also in the Framingham Heart Study (Wilson et al., 2008).

Statins can exert their anti-inflammatory role through different effects: the combined actions are called pleiotropic effects and are abundantly reviewed in the literature (C.Y. Wang et al., 2007; Ludman et al., 2009). The main mechanism seems to be always related to the inhibition of HMG-CoA reductase enzyme, involved in the rate-limiting step in cholesterol biosynthesis, but also in the production of isoprenoid intermediates, such as farnesyl-pyrophosphate and geranyl-geranyl-pyrophosphate: these molecules are important for the post-translational modification of small GTP-binding proteins Ras, Rac, and Rho, which are known to modulate vascular smooth muscle cell proliferation, platelet aggregation, and plaque stability.

Returning to statin trials, CARE study of secondary prevention was able to demonstrate, in a post hoc analysis, that pravastatin decreased CRP levels significantly in comparison to placebo; this decrease did not correlate with the reduction in cholesterol levels (Ridker et al., 1999). Few years later similar results were obtained in a primary prevention study, the AFCAPS/TexCAPS trial (Ridker et al., 2001): an interesting observation was the absence of clinical benefits in subjects with low density lipoprotein (LDL)-cholesterol <150 mg/dl and hsCRP levels <2 mg/l, instead a significant benefit was found in those with LDL-cholesterol levels <150 mg/dl and hsCRP >2 mg/l. Further studies, such as MIRACL (Kinlay et al., 2003), REVERSAL (Nissen et al., 2005), A to Z (Morrow et al., 2006), and PROVE IT-TIMI 22(Ridker et al., 2005), demonstrated effects of statins on CRP. Again in all these studies the statin-induced reductions of CRP and LDL-cholesterol levels were only weakly correlated, whereas the decrease in CRP was correlated with slowed atherosclerosis progression, in an independent way with respect to LDL-cholesterol decrease. In PROVE IT-TIMI 22 and in A to Z trials the best outcomes were observed in individuals who reached both LDL-cholesterol levels <70 mg/dl and hsCRP <2.0 mg/l. Therefore the concept of a "dual target" for statin therapy (LDL-cholesterol and CRP) was introduced.

A step forward was represented by the JUPITER trial (Ridker et al., 2008b). JUPITER was a large, double-blind, placebo-controlled trial, multinational, primary prevention trial, which recruited 17,802 apparently healthy subjects with entry criteria of less than 130 mg/dl for LDL-cholesterol levels and hs-CRP levels of 2.0 mg/dl or higher. Subjects were randomly assigned to 20 mg/d of rosuvastatin or placebo and continued their usual standard care; the primary end point was a combination of MI, stroke, arterial revascularization, hospitalization for unstable angina, or death from cardiovascular causes.

The trial was terminated prematurely, after a mean of only 1.9 years of follow-up by an indipendent data and safety monitoring board. The absolute risk reduction was 1.2%, with the primary endpoint occurring in 2.8% of subjects in the placebo arm versus 1.6% of subjects in the rosuvastatin arm. The active treatment reduced the risk for first MI by 55%, the risk for venous thromboembolism by 52%, the need for coronary artery bypass grafting (CABG) or percutaneous coronary intervention (PCI) by 47%, and total mortality by 20%. On the basis of the Kaplan-Meier estimates and with a forward projection of the results, about 25 subjects would have to be treated for 5 years to prevent one primary endpoint. This estimate is very favourable, compared to trials evaluating statins in hyperlipidemic patients, where the 5-year number needed to treat patients was between 44 and 65; more strikingly in hypertension treatment the 5-year number needed to treat patients ranged between 86 and 140. The treatment with rosuvastatin was well tolerated even at very low attained levels of LDL-cholesterol (less than 50 mg/dl) with consequent lower risk of cardiovascular events (Hsia et al., 2011). Moreover the study demonstrated a 43% reduction in venous thrombosis. Another limited but important finding was the increase in the rate of diabetes mellitus as well as a small, significant increase in the median value of glycated hemoglobin: this observation was confirmed in a recent meta-analysis of 13 statin trials which showed a 9% increased risk of development of diabetes associated with statin therapy (Sattar et al., 2010).

The publication of the JUPITER trial spurred intense debate, sometimes with harsh criticisms to the authors (de Lorgeril et al., 2010; Kaul et al., 2010): the main points were the too early termination (with possible overestimation of the results), unprecise definitions of the endpoints (in particular about mortality), the undertreatment for the usual care of the involved patients, the increased health costs of this preventive approach, the excessive role of the pharmaceutical company. The trial however survived to the critics and convinced the United States Food and Drug Administration to approve the indication of rosuvastatin for reduction of acute MI, stroke, CABG, and PCI in men >50 years of age and women >60 years of age with hsCRP levels ≥2 mg/l who also have 1 additional cardiovascular risk factor. In addition in 2009 Canadian Cardiovascular Society guidelines included the results of the JUPITER trial recommending that also subjects at intermediate risk, defined as 10 – 20% risk at 10 years by Framingham criteria, should be treated with a statin when hsCRP is >2 mg/l.

JUPITER conclusions were similar to the results subsequently obtained in the ARIC study (Yang et al., 2009), again showing that, starting with individuals at highest risk, the relative cardiovascular event rates are high LDL-cholesterol + high CRP > high CRP + low LDL-cholesterol > high LDL-cholesterol + low CRP > low LDL-cholesterol + low CRP.

Another cholesterol-lowering drug, frequently administered with a statin, is ezetimibe, an inhibitor of the intestinal cholesterol transporter Niemann-Pick C1-like protein (NPC1L1): this drug can reduce LDL-cholesterol levels by almost 20% in individuals already taking a statin. However no clinical trial results have so far demonstrated that this combination will reduce cardiovascular events in comparison with statins only. In terms of anti-inflammatory effects ezetimibe per se did not reduce CRP levels, but it was able to help statin in decreasing CRP more deeply (Al Badarin et al., 2009).

## 3. High Density Lipoprotein (HDL)-modulating agents

Main focus of anti-atherosclerotic therapy is correctly the decrease in LDL-cholesterol levels. Although the success in terms of cardiovascular prevention was outstanding, we know that it is limited: as already stated, no more than 25-30% relative risk reduction was observed in statin monotherapy trials with a large amount of individuals in the active arm still suffering a cardiovascular event. This can be related to the different levels attained for LDL-cholesterol in the trials with progressive updates of the international guidelines for atherosclerosis with the motto "lower for LDL-cholesterol is always better" (Grundy, 2008), but undoubtedly a residual risk is still present: "lower LDL-cholesterol is better but it is not enough" (Superko & King III, 2008).

Another related observation, based on arteriographic findings, is the positive significant effect of statins on the decrease in the rate of atherosclerotic progression but the absent effect on any regression, something demonstrated on the contrary with a combined treatment (LDL-cholesterol reduction + HDL-cholesterol increase) (Superko & King III, 2008). This was confirmed recently by the conclusions of the ARBITER 6-Halts study which compared the effects of ezetimibe, an inhibitor of cholesterol absorption, and extended-release niacin in high risk patients already with statin therapy: the primary end point was the change in the intima-media thickness of common carotid artery (Taylor et al., 2009). Niacin was significantly superior to ezetimibe in the primary end point, suggesting again that the addition of a HDL-cholesterol raising drug to a statin is superior to a further LDL-cholesterol decreasing strategy.

Although a recent meta-analysis has suggested that increasing HDL-cholesterol does not reduce the risk of cardiovascular events in human subjects (Briel et al., 2009), animal studies have provided strong evidence that HDL-cholesterol is protective (Haas & Mooradian, 2011). HDL exerts a key role in the reverse cholesterol transport, whereby cholesterol is transported from peripheral cells to the liver and consequently fostering the removal of this molecule from the lipid-laden macrophages at the vascular level. In addition HDL particles have been shown to be involved in direct anti-oxidative, anti-apoptotic, anti-thrombotic, and also anti-inflammatory functions (Tabet & Rye, 2009), suggesting further protection against the atherosclerotic process. However we need to be aware that, during the inflammatory activation, HDL particles can shift to a "dysfunctional" setting, showing on the contrary pro-inflammatory properties (Säemann et al., 2010): therefore the functional properties of HDL reflect its role more appropriately than mere serum concentrations.

At the present time, among HDL-cholesterol-increasing drugs, niacin (nicotinic acid) is the most effective agent, raising HDL-cholesterol by 20-30% (Farmer, 2009) with an important side effect (flushing), which can be attenuated by both an extended-release formulation (Knopp et al., 1998) and a combination with a prostaglandin D2 receptor 1 antagonist, laropiprant (Perry, 2009). The results of the HPS2-THRIVE ongoing study will give us important information about the therapeutic role of this combination in the prevention of cardiovascular events. In the meantime we already know that niacin exerts direct anti-inflammatory effects, in particular an anti-oxidant and a CRP-decreasing activity (Sanyal et al., 2007; Thoenes et al., 2007).

The most effective way to increase HDL-cholesterol was thought to be the inhibition of the cholesteryl ester transfer protein (CETP), the enzyme responsible for the transfer of cholesteryl esters from HDL particles to very low-density lipoproteins and LDLs (Barter & Kastelein, 2006). The first developed CETP-inhibitor was torcetrapib, which was evaluated in the ILLUMINATE trial (Barter et al., 2007): in this study patients at high cardiovascular risk were randomly assigned to receive either torcetrapib + atorvastatin or placebo + atorvastatin. Despite the very favourable lipid changes obtained in the torcetrapib arm (a 72% increase in HDL-cholesterol and a 25% decrease in LDL-cholesterol), the rate of major cardiovascular events was increased by 25% and the deaths from cardiovascular causes by 40%; all-cause mortality was increased by 58% and an increase in blood pressure and aldosterone levels, therefore unrelated to CETP inhibition, was also observed in the active arm. Whereas the pressor and aldosterone-stimulating effects could explain the cardiovascular results, it was harder to understand the increased rate of deaths from noncardiovascular causes induced by torcetrapib: the increase was due to more deaths from cancers and infections. Since CETP inhibition alters the size and the composition of the HDL particles (Barter & Kastelein, 2006), these qualitative changes could predispose to an increased susceptibility to neoplasms and infections.

These negative results did not stop the development of other drugs of the same class: very recently the safety of anacetrapib was positively evaluated in the DEFINE study (Cannon et al., 2010) and the increased HDL particles exhibited a strong ability to suppress macrophage toll-like receptor 4-mediated inflammatory responses (Yvan-Charlet et al., 2010). A more direct way to stimulate the reverse cholesterol transport is the infusion of reconstituted HDL or Apo A-I mimetic peptides: with both therapeutic approaches a potent anti-inflammatory effect was observed (Natarajan et al., 2010).

## 4. Anti-platelet agents

Atherosclerotic thrombotic events are always characterized by an important inflammatory activation which is a consequence of the release of chemokines and cytokines from the platelets (Gurbel et al., 2009); however platelets are also involved in the initiation and the early progression of atherosclerosis mediating leukocyte recruitment and adhesion to the vascular wall (Antoniades et al., 2010). Many markers of platelet activation are currently investigated: in this context prospective studies and meta-analysis suggest a correlation between an increase in mean platelet volume and the risk of thrombosis (Gasparyan et al., 2011); in addition the soluble form of CD40 ligand has been studied in sera of human subjects and seems to have a prognostic role in atherothrombosis (Antoniades et al., 2010).

The most used anti-platelet drug, aspirin, is able to decrease serum CRP and patients with the highest baseline CRP levels derives the greatest benefit from this drug.

Trials of cardiovascular prevention with aspirin do not always confirm the positive effects of an anti-thrombotic approach, at least in the primary setting: also recently updated guidelines suggest judicious use of anti-platelet drug (Bell et al., 2011). The limited protective effects of aspirin have led to the concept of aspirin resistance (Gasparyan et al., 2008).

## 5. Phospholipase A$_2$ and ACAT inhibitors

In atherosclerosis the interactions between lipoprotein metabolism and inflammation are modulated by the complex phospholipase A$_2$ (PLA$_2$) superfamily. This family comprises five types of enzymes, of which the secretory PLA$_2$ (sPLA$_2$) and the lipoprotein-associated PLA$_2$ (Lp-PLA$_2$) have been associated with atherogenesis (Garcia-Garcia & Serruys, 2009). These enzymes catalyze the hydrolysis of the centre (sn-2) ester bond of phospholipids to produce non-esterified fatty acids (in particular arachidonic acid) and lysophospholipids (lysophosphatidylcholine): the atherogenic consequences are the formation of smaller and denser HDL and LDL particles, the formation of vascular LDL aggregates, the increased LDL oxidation, the synthesis of potent inflammatory lipid mediators such as prostaglandins and leukotrienes (Rosenson, 2009). Therefore inhibitors of the types of PLA$_2$ have been developed and have reached the phase III clinical evaluation, one for LpPLA2 (darapladib) and one for sPLA2 (varespladib).

In human studies darapladib induced a small but significant decrease in the inflammatory markers hsCRP and interleukin-6 with no changes in plasma lipid levels. In the IBIS-2 trial after 12 months the drug did not affect the primary end point, coronary plaque volume evaluated by intravascular ultrasound (IVUS); however necrotic core size remained unchanged in the active arm but increased in those treated with placebo (Boekholdt et al., 2008). Darapladib is now being evaluated in two large placebo-controlled cardiovascular outcome studies – STABILITY and SOLID-TIMI 52. As for varespladib, in the PLASMA Phase II the drug was demonstrated to induce a decrease in both oxidized LDL and CRP; an ongoing Phase III cardiovascular outcome study (VISTA-16) have recruited high risk patients.

Another important enzyme involved in the cellular cholesterol metabolism is acyl-coenzyme A:cholesterol acyltransferase (ACAT): this protein is able to catalyse cholesteryl ester formation by transfer of fatty acyl chain from acyl-coenzyme A to cholesterol. Two isozymes are present, one expressed in macrophages in atherosclerotic lesions (ACAT-1) and the other mainly expressed in small intestine (ACAT-2): therefore nonselective pharmacological inhibition of ACAT was expected to exert a double favourable effect, suppressing both foam cell formation in arterial walls and cholesterol intestinal absorption. Unfortunately results of the studies in human subjects were disappointing: avasimibe and pactimibe, the two nonselective ACAT inhibitors developed for clinical use, gave null or negative results (Fazio & Linton, 2006). Very recently a potent and selective ACAT-1 inhibitor, K-604, with significant anti-atherosclerotic effects *in vitro* and in experimental animals, entered a Phase II trial (Yoshinaka et al., 2010).

## 6. Leukotriene pathway inhibitors

Leukotrienes (LTs) belong to the family of eicosanoids and exert potent pro-inflammatory smooth muscle constrictive actions. It is well known their involvement in many inflammatory and allergic diseases, such as rheumatoid arthritis, inflammatory bowel disease, and bronchial asthma. Initially a leukotriene receptor blocker, i.e. montelukast, was administered to acute coronary syndrome patients to evaluate the endothelial function in brachial artery (clinicaltrials.gov NCT00351364, data unpublished). Subsequently inhibitors of both 5-lipoxygenase (5-LO) (atreleuton) and 5-lipoxygenase activating protein (FLAP) (veliflapon) were studied in human subjects. Atreleuton, a potent 5-LO inhibitor, was administered in acute coronary syndrome patients for 24 weeks and was able to reduce both the appearance of new coronary plaques and the volume of noncalcified plaques in comparison with placebo; these effects were paralleled by a 66% reduction of hsCRP (Tardif et al., 2010). Instead veliflapon, a weak FLAP inhibitor, induced a decrease in LTB4 production and myeloperoxidase activity with a nonsignificant reduction in CRP (Hakonarson et al., 2005).

## 7. CCR2 blockade

One of the main players in the inflammatory cascade induced by the atherosclerotic changes is chemokine CC motif ligand 2 (CCL2), also known as monocyte chemoattractant protein-1: this chemokine, through the interaction with its receptor chemokine receptor 2 (CCR2), efficiently induces the recruitment of circulating blood monocytes to become plaque macrophages. Very recently MLN1202, a highly specific humanized monoclonal antibody that recognizes CCR2 and inhibits CCL2 binding, was evaluated in a randomized, double-blind, placebo-controlled trial: the main aim was to measure possible decrease in hsCRP with the active treatment in cardiovascular high-risk patients (Gilbert et al., 2011). The results of this preliminary study confirmed a significant 26% reduction in the inflammatory marker, but obviously we need to perform outcome studies in order to establish a role of this new therapeutic approach in the treatment of atherosclerosis.

## 8. Peroxisome Proliferator-Activated Receptor (PPAR) agonists and Polyunsaturated Fatty Acids (PUFAs)

PPARs are ligand-activated transcription factors belonging to the nuclear receptor superfamily (Oyekan, 2011). Through cellular mechanisms called transactivation, binding of PPAR/nuclear retinoid receptor (RXR) heterodimers to PPAR response elements (PPREs) in the promoter region of target genes, and transrepression, interference with transcription factors such as nuclear factor-kB (NF-kB) and activator protein-1 (AP-1), these transcription factors exert multiple and complex effects involving the regulation of the vascular tone, inflammation and metabolism. The PPAR family consists of three isoforms, α, γ, and β/δ, which possess distinct functions, with corresponding agonists.

PPAR-α agonists (fibric acid derivatives = fibrates) have demonstrated potentially very favourable effects on serum lipids with a significant decrease in triglyceride levels and more modest effects on LDL-cholesterol (a decrease) and HDL-cholesterol (an increase); in addition LDL size is modified with a decrease of more atherogenic small dense particles. All these positive changes are theoretically complementary to those induced by statins

(Abourbih et al., 2009) and are paralleled by a significant anti-inflammatory modulation, as demonstrated both *in vitro* and *in vivo* (Adameova et al., 2009). Despite these considerations and the long time of clinical evaluation (more than 30 years in Europe), considerable controversy still remains about therapeutic efficacy, also after recent reevaluation (Jun et al., 2010; Goldfine et al., 2011).

The same negative results were observed in the ACCORD-Lipid substudy which compared a statin monotherapy with a combination therapy with a statin + a fibrate in type 2 diabetic patients, who are the population with the theoretical maximal advantage from the combination (Ginsberg et al., 2010). However a prespecified analysis showed a 31% reduction in the primary end point (nonfatal MI, nonfatal stroke, or death from cardiovascular causes) in the subgroup of patients with the most negative metabolic profile (baseline triglyceride levels >204 mg/dl and HDL-cholesterol levels <34 mg/dl).

PPAR-γ agonists (thiazolidinediones = glitazones) was known as anti-inflammatory agents for a long time (Duan et al., 2009): two molecules are available for administration in humans, pioglitazone and rosiglitazone. They have a specific therapeutic indication for type 2 diabetes mellitus due to their improvement in insulin sensitivity, supporting the interpretation of type 2 diabetes mellitus as an auto-inflammatory disease (Dinarello, 2010; N. Wang et al., 2011). *In vitro*, in human blood monocytes, pioglitazone reduces synthesis of IL-1β, tumor necrosis factor (TNF)-α, IL-6, MCP-1, Toll-like receptors (TLRs) (Dasu et al., 2009). Also *in vivo*, in human subjects, pioglitazone exerts potent anti-inflammatory effects with a significant decrease in hsCRP levels in both diabetic and nondiabetic individuals (Pfützner et al., 2010).

Like fibrates, cardiovascular end points evaluated in large randomized studies with glitazones gave disappointing results. The only published outcome trial with this group of drugs is the PROactive trial (Dormandy et al., 2005): in this study pioglitazone induced a nonsignificant reduction in the primary end point (a composite of death, nonfatal MI, stroke, major leg amputation, acute coronary syndrome, and coronary or leg revascularization); however the principal secondary end point (a composite of all-cause death, nonfatal MI, and stroke) was significantly reduced by 16%. On the contrary in different trials rosiglitazone gave some suspicions about detrimental effects on cardiovascular events: a large meta-analysis concluded that this drug may increase the risk of cardiovascular events (MI, death) (Nissen & Wolski, 2007), possibly through a more favourable effect of pioglitazone on the lipid profile (Goldberg et al., 2005). A possible step forward in the development of PPARs is the evaluation of a dual α/γ agonist: after the withdrawal of muraglitazar and tesaglitazar for important toxicities, aleglitazar is currently being investigated in type 2 diabetic patients (Paras et al., 2010).

Other drugs which are able to decrease triglyceride levels are omega-3 fatty acids: the attempt to copy Eskimo diet was successful in the secondary prevention of cardiovascular diseases with important complex anti-inflammatory effects, which probably involve the above mentioned mediators resolvins (De Caterina, 2011).

## 9. Succinobucol and fasudil

Another possible target for atherosclerosis treatment is represented by the blockade of the oxidative stress, and in particular of the oxidation of lipoproteins (Libby et al., 2011): this was the reason why anti-oxidant vitamins (vitamin C and E) were evaluated in randomized controlled trials, unfortunately with no success (Kris-Etherton et al., 2004). Two drugs exert similar potent *in vitro* anti-oxidant effects and have been studied in atherosclerotic patients: succinobucol and fasudil. Succinobucol is a derivative of probucol, previously withdrawn at Phase III evaluation for safety concerns, with well-demonstrated anti-inflammatory and anti-oxidant effects in endothelial and blood mononuclear cells (Kunsch et al., 2004). The ARISE trial recently examined the effects of succinobucol on cardiovascular events in patients with a recent acute coronary syndrome: there was no significant difference in the primary end point (cardiovascular death, resuscitated cardiac arrest, MI, stroke, unstable angina, or coronary revascularization); the composite secondary end point of cardiovascular death, MI, cardiac arrest and stroke was 19% lower in the succinobucol arm compared to placebo and reached statistical significance (Tardif et al., 2008). Another interesting observation of the study, tertiary end point, was the 63% relative reduction in the onset of new diabetes, related to a reduction in glycosilated haemoglobin in diabetic patients.

Fasudil is an inhibitor of Rho-kinase, an important downstream effector of the small GTP-binding protein RhoA (Satoh et al., 2011). It has been demonstrated that the RhoA/Rho-kinase pathway exerts a specific role in the pathogenesis of vasospasm, atherosclerosis, ischemia-reperfusion injury, hypertension, stroke, and heart failure. Fasudil is already marketed in Japan for the acute treatment of cerebral vasospasm but the possible additional indications in human subjects are not completely established (Zhou et al., 2011).

## 10. Anti-hypertensive drugs

Despite intensive research the pathogenesis of hypertension, the leading risk factor of death in the entire world (Ezzati et al., 2002), remains elusive. The hypothesis of a low-grade inflammatory activation could explain many aspects of the hypertensive process and therefore is actively investigated (Harrison et al., 2011; Leibowitz & Schiffrin, 2011; Montecucco et al., 2011). If we can translate these observation to the clinical ground, the therapeutic strategies should keep account of possible anti-inflammatory modulations of the hypotensive drugs adding more fuel to the controversy about the protective role exerted by the blood pressure reduction *per se* or the presence of additional pleiotropic actions of some classes of drugs with respect to others: "outcomes beyond blood pressure control?" (Sever et al., 2006; Staessen et al., 2010). In this context the renin-angiotensin system inhibitors (angiotensin-converting enzyme inhibitors, angiotensin II receptor blockers, renin inhibitors) could be the best choice since the fundamental role of this system in the activation of the vascular inflammation is widely demonstrated (Marchesi et al., 2008): this is confirmed by the *in vivo* demonstration of a significant decrease of various inflammatory markers induced by these drugs (reviewed in Montecucco et al., 2009).

However, the most comprehensive guidelines for the treatment of hypertension do not consider an inflammation-based approach: on the contrary the updated versions of the European Society of Hypertension/European Society of Cardiology guidelines did not confirm the role of CRP as a cardiovascular risk factor for the prognostic stratification, as proposed in the first edition (Mancia et al., 2007). All the hypertension guidelines emphasize the control of blood pressure levels as the main target for the therapeutic choices, without a classification of the different available drugs and suggesting that frequently we need to prefer a drug combination to improve effectiveness and limit side effects. In terms of the atherosclerotic process a partial confirmation of this approach comes from the IVUS substudy of the CAMELOT trial which demonstrated a significant slowing in the progression of the atheroma volume with a calcium-antagonist (amlodipine, a potent and possibly more effective hypotensive drug) compared to an angiotensin-converting enzyme inhibitor (enalapril) (Nissen et al., 2004).

## 11. Immunosuppressive agents

In this section we will discuss the anti-atherosclerotic effects of drugs developed for immunosuppression and therefore without a primary metabolic action. In terms of immunosuppression nothing is more powerful and studied than corticosteroids (Rhen & Cidlowski, 2005). 35 years ago corticosteroid administration was shown to exert deleterious effects in patients with MI (Roberts et al., 1976); however very recently oral prednisone was used successfully to prevent restenosis after PCI with bare metal stents in comparison with bare metal stents alone(better event-free survival) and drug-eluting stents (similar outcome) (Ribichini et al., 2011).

As discussed in the introduction, a proof-of-concept for the role of inflammation in the atherosclerotic process would be a clinical trial with well tolerated anti-inflammatory drugs, devoid of metabolic effects: methotrexate and canakinumab could be good choices and have been proposed recently.

For other drugs the tolerability in uncomplicated atherosclerotic subjects could be more problematic with a disadvantageous risk-benefit ratio, but their potentially positive cardiovascular effects in patients with a specific immunosuppressive indication can be carefully monitored in clinical trials for post hoc analysis (Westlake et al., 2010). Another possible application is the administration of these drugs for a limited period of time (e.g. for a few days after PCI).

TNF-α antagonists are extensively used in autoimmune diseases with a significant cardiovascular protection (Tracey et al., 2008), possibly related to the pivotal role of this cytokine in vascular dysfunction: recently, in a population of subjects who underwent carotid endarterectomy for a significant stenosis, we found an increase in TNF-α plasma levels in symptomatic patients for an ischemic cerebrovascular event with respect to asymptomatic patients (Montecucco et al., 2010). TNF-α antagonists have been evaluated in vascular disorders accompanying chronic disordes (Crohn' s disease and rheumatoid arthritis) with the demonstration of improvement in endothelial function (Schinzari et al., 2008; Hürlimann et al., 2002). In addition to the anti-inflammatory effects, these drugs also induce a favourable lipid profile with an increase in HDL-cholesterol and apolipoprotein A-I (van Eijk et al., 2009).

IL-1 seems to exert a central role in the intense inflammatory response which follows a MI. Using a recombinant form of the naturally occurring antagonist (anakinra), a pilot study was recently performed to test the safety and effects of this drug on post-MI left ventricular remodelling and CRP serum levels (Abbate et al., 2010). Anakinra was able to mitigate significantly left ventricular remodelling, evaluated  with both cardiac magnetic resonance and echocardiography, and the changes in CRP levels correlated with the changes in cardiac anatomy.

Another new important inflammatory pathway involves p38 mitogen-activated protein kinase (MAPK). This phosphorylation cascade can be activated by a vascular injury, such as coronary stenting with subsequent neointimal proliferation and in-stent restenosis (Schieven, 2005), and represents an important intracellular switch for the production of key inflammatory cytokines (IL-1$\beta$, TNF-$\alpha$, and IL-6), inflammatory enzyme cyclooxygenase-2 and matrix metalloproteases. Recently a p38 MAPK inhibitor (dilmapimod, SB-681323) has been shown to significantly attenuate the inflammatory activation induced by a PCI procedure with positive consequences in post-procedural outcomes (Sarov-Blat et al., 2010).

Interesting observations came from the administration of the immunosuppressive drug mycophenolate mofetil in atherosclerotic patients for a limited period of time: the drug, devoid of effects on both serum lipids and blood pressure, was able to attenuate cellular and biochemical inflammatory activation in the unstable carotid plaques of patients who subsequently underwent endarterectomy for advanced stenosis (van Leuven et al., 2006; Van Leuven et al., 2010). At the very beginning of the clinical evaluation are the inhibitors of Toll-like receptors, involved in the innate immune response (Hennessy et al., 2010; Cole & Monaco, 2010).

## 12. Conclusion

Recently the title of an editorial in Circulation was "Could direct inhibition of inflammation be the *next big thing* in treating atherosclerosis?" (Natarajan & Cannon, 2010). This is certainly a fascinating strategy because it tries to exert a fully pathogenetic approach, though we need not to forget the frustrations, caused by so many disappointing results. In this context we know that it is not always wise to found our evaluation on surrogate end points: only randomized controlled trials with cardiovascular hard end points can give the final answer.

---

**Take-home messages**
- Lifestyle choices are an essential part of the cardiovascular prevention and physicians must exert every effort to obtain a good compliance from patients
- In terms of therapeutic control of the different risk factors physicians must reach better results
- At the present time physicians have to focus at the single risk factors with the awareness that the inflammatory activation is important for the atherosclerotic process
- hsCRP represents a useful marker of inflammation and an excellent support for the prognostic stratification
- Additional help can derive from carotid US and coronary calcium score
- In the context of blockade of the inflammatory activation statins and RAS-inhibitors offer good choices in terms of safety and effectiveness
- Specific ant-inflammatory drugs need to be carefully evaluated with appropriate trials
- At the present time these drugs may be useful for a limited period of time (e.g.: after a PCI)
- Intense investigation on this topic will certainly suggest new therapeutic targets and strategies

---

In this review we tried to give an update of the experimental and clinical data with already marketed drugs or with Phase III therapeutic principles but we did not discuss the possible use of an immunomodulating (not immunosuppressive) approach: expansion of regulatory

T cells, a subset of T lymphocytes with a well demonstrated anti-inflammatory role, and atherosclerosis-specific immunization are thought as promising therapeutic opportunities and are actively investigated (Klingerberg & Hansson, 2009; van Puijvelde et al., 2008).

Although at the present time the physicians are confident with the use of drugs developed for particular aspects of the atherosclerotic spectrum (decrease of blood pressure, decrease in LDL-cholesterol, increase in HDL-cholesterol, decrease in glucose, etc.), the "unfinished business" of cardiovascular prevention (Libby, 2005) drives our efforts to find new targets and strategies against the pernicious activation of inflammation in atherosclerosis.

## 13. Acknowledgments

This work was supported by grant n. 2008.0812-132 from Fondazione Carige.

The authors declare that they have no conflicts of interest.

## 14. References

Abbate A., Kontos M., Grizzard J.D., Biondi-Zoccai G.G.L., Van Tassel B.W., Robati R., Roach L.M., Arena R.A., Roberts C.S., Varma A., Gelwix C.C., Salloum F.N., Hastillo A., Dinarello C.A., & Vetrovec G.W. (2010). Interleukin-1 blockade with anakinra to prevent adverse cardiac remodeling after acute myocardial infarction (Virginia Commonwealth University Anakinra Remodeling Trial [VCU-ART] Pilot Sudy). *American Journal of Cardiology*, Vol.105, No.10, (May 2010), pp. 1371-1377, ISSN 1879-1913

Abourbih S., Filion K.B., Joseph L., Schiffrin E.L., Rinfret S., Poirier P., Pilote L., Genest J., & Eisenberg M.J. (2009). Effect of fibrates on lipid profiles and cardiovascular outcomes: a systematic review. *American Journal of Medicine*, Vol.122, No.10, (August 2009), pp. 962e1-962e8, ISSN 1555-7162

Adameova A., Xu Y.J., Duhamel T.A., Tappia P.S., Shan L., & Dhalla N.S. (2009). Anti-atherosclerotic molecules targeting oxidative stress and inflammation. *Current Pharmaceutical Design*, Vol.15, No.27, (2009), pp. 3094-3107, ISSN 1381-6128

Al Badarin F.J., Kullo I.J., Kopecky S.L., & Thomas R.J. (2009). Impact of ezetimibe on atherosclerosis: is the jury still out? *Mayo Clinic Proceedings*, Vol.84, No.4, (April 2009), pp. 353-361, ISSN 1942-5546

Anand S.S., & Yusuf S. (2010). C-reactive protein is a bystander of cardiovascular disease. *European Heart Journal*, Vol.31, No.17, (July 2010), pp. 2092-2097, ISSN 1522-9645

Antoniades C., Bakogiannis C., Tousoulis D., Demosthenous M., Marinou K., & Stefanadis C. (2010). Platelet activation in atherogenesis associated with low-grade inflammation. Inflammation and Allergy Drug Targets, Vol.9, No.5, (December 2010), pp. 334-345, ISSN 1871-5281

Baigent C., Keech A., Kearney P.M., Blackwell L., Buck G., Pollicino C., Kirby A., Sourjina T., Peto R., Collins R., & Simes R. (2005). Efficacy and safety of cholesterol-lowering treatment: prospective meta-analysis of data from 90,056 participants in 14 randomised trials of statins. *Lancet*, Vol.366, No.9494, (June 2005), pp. 1267-1278, ISSN 1474-547X

Barter P.J., & Kastelein J.J.P. (2006). Targeting cholesteryl ester transfer protein for the prevention and management of cardiovascular disease. *Journal of the American College of Cardiology*, Vol.47, No.3, (February 2006), pp. 492-499, ISSN 1558-3597

Barter P.J., Caulfield M., Eriksson M., Grundy S.M., Kastelein J.J.P., Komajda M., Lopez-Sendon J., Mosca L., Tardif J.C., Waters D.D., Shear C.L., Revkin J.H., Buhr K.A., Fisher M., Tall A.R., & Brewer B. (2007). Effects of torcetrapib in patients at high risk for coronary events. *New England Journal of Medicine*, Vol.357, No.21, (November 2007), pp. 2109-2122, ISSN 1533-4406

Bell A.D., Roussin A., Cartier R., Chan W.S., Douketis J.D., Gupta A., Kraw M.E., Lindsay T.F., Love M.P., Pannu N., Rabasa-Lhoret R., Shuaib A., Teal P., Theroux P., Turpie A.G., Welsh R.C., & Tanguay J.F. (2011). The use of antiplatelet therapy in the outpatient setting: Canadian Cardiovascular Society guidelines executive summary. *Canadian Journal of Cardiology*, Vol.27, No.2, (March 2011), pp. 208-221, ISSN 1916-7075

Bentzon J.F., & Falk E. (2010). Atherosclerotic lesions in mouse and man: is it the same disease? *Current Opinion in Lipidology*, Vol.21, No.5, (October 2010), pp. 434-440, ISSN 1473-6535

Berk B.C., Weintraub, W.S., & Alexander R.W. (1990). Elevation of C-reactive protein in "active" coronary artery disease. *American Journal of Cardiology*, Vol.65, No.3, (January 1990), pp. 168-172, ISSN 1879-1913

Blankenberg S., Zeller T., Saarela O., Havulinna A.S., Kee F., Tunstall-Pedoe H., Kuulasmaa K., Yarnell J., Schnabel R.B., Wild P.S., Münzel T.F., Lackner K.J., Tiret L., Evans A., & Salomaa V. (2010). Contribution of 30 biomarkers to 10-year cardiovascular risk estimation in 2 population cohorts: the MONICA, risk, genetics, archiving, and monograph (MORGAM) biomarker project. *Circulation*, Vol.121, No.22, (June 2010), pp. 2388-2397, ISSN 1524-4539

Boekholdt S.M., de Winter R.J., & Kastelein J.J.P. (2008). Inhibition of lipoprotein-associated phospholipase activity by darapladib. Shifting gears in cardiovascular drug development: are anti-inflammatory drugs the next frontier? *Circulation*, Vol.118, No.11, (September 2008), pp. 1120-1122, ISSN 1524-4539

Boekholdt S.M., & Kastelein J.J.P. (2010). C-reactive protein and cardiovascular risk: more fuel to the fire. *Lancet*, Vol.375, No.9709, (January 2010), pp. 95-96, ISSN 1474-547X

Briel M., Ferreira-Gonzalez I., You J.J., Karanicolas P.J., Akl E.A., Wu P., Blechacz B., Bassler D., Wei X., Sharman A., Whitt I., Alves da Silva S., Khalid Z., Nordmann A.J., Zhou Q., Walter S.D., Vale N., Bhatnagar N., O'Regan C., Mills E.J., Bucher H.C., Montori V.M., & Guyatt G.H. (2009). Association between change in high density lipoprotein cholesterol and cardiovascular disease morbidity and mortality: systematic review and meta-regression analysis. *British Medical Journal*, Vol.338, No.92, (February 2009), doi:10.1136/bmj.b92, ISSN 1468-5833

Cannon C.P., Shah S., Dansky H.M., Davidson M., Brinton E.A., Gotto A.M., Stepanavage M., Liu S.X., Gibbons P., Ashraf T.B., Zafarino J., Mitchel Y., & Barter P. (2010). Safety of anacetrapib in patients with or at high risk of coronary heart disease. *New England Journal of Medicine*, Vol.363, No.25, (December 2010), pp. 2406-2415, ISSN 1533-4406

Casas J.P., Shah T., Hingorani A.D., Danesh J., & Pepys M.B. (2008). C-reactive protein and coronary heart disease: a critical review. *Journal of Internal Medicine*, Vol.264, No.4, (October 2008), pp. 295-314, ISSN 1365-2796

Cole J.E., & Monaco C. (2010). Treating atherosclerosis: the potential of Toll-like receptors as therapeutic target. *Expert Review of Cardiovascular Therapy*, Vol.8, No.11, (November 2010), pp. 1619-1635, ISSN 1477-9072

Dasu M., Park S., Devaraj S., & Jialal I. (2009). Pioglitazone inhibits Toll-like receptor expression and activity in human monocytes and db/db mice. *Endocrinology*, Vol.150, No.8, (August 2009), pp. 3457-3464, ISSN 1945-7170

De Caterina R. (2011). n-3 fatty acids in cardiovascular disease. *New England Journal of Medicine*, Vol.364, No.25, (June 2011), pp. 2439-2450, ISSN 1533-4406

de Lorgeril M., Salen P., Abramson J., Dodin S., Hamazaki T., Kostucki W., Okuyama H., Pavy B., & Rabacus M. (2010). Cholesterol lowering, cardiovascular diseases, and the rosuvastatin-jupiter controversy: a critical reappraisal. *Archives of Internal Medicine*, Vol.170, No.12, (June 2010), pp. 1032-1036, ISSN 1538-3679

Després J.P. (2011). CRP: star trekking the galaxy of risk markers. *Lancet*, Vol.377, No.9764, (February 2011), pp. 441-442, ISSN 1474-547X

Dinarello C.A. (2010). Anti-inflammatory agents: present and future. *Cell*, Vol.140, No.6, (March 2010), pp. 935-950, ISSN 1097-4172

Dormandy J.A., Charbonnel B., Eckland D.J.A., Erdmann E., Masi-Benedetti M., Moules I.K., Skene A.M., Tan, M.H., Lefebre P.J., Murray G.D., Standl E., Wilcox R.G., Mokan M., Norkus A., Pirags V., Podar T., Scheen A., Scherbaum W., Scherntaner G., Schmitz O., Skrha J., Smith U., & Taton J. (2005). Secondary prevention of macrovascular events in patients with type 2 diabetes in the PROactive Study (PROspective pioglitAzone Clinical Trial In macroVascular Events): a randomised controlled trial. *Lancet*, Vol.366, No.9493, (October 2005), pp. 1279-1289, ISSN 1474-547X

Duan S.Z., Usher M.G., & Mortensen R.M. (2009). PPARs: the vasculature, inflammation and hypertension. *Current Opinion in Nephrology and Hypertension*, Vol.18, No.2, (March 2009), pp. 128-133, ISSN 1473-6543

Ezzati M., Lopez A.D., Rodgers A., Vander Hoorn S., & Murray C.J.L. (2002). Selected major risk factors and global and regional burden of disease. *Lancet*, Vol.360, No.9343, (November 2002), pp. 1347-1360, ISSN 1474-547X

Farmer J.A. (2009). Nicotinic acid: a new look at an old drug. *Current Atherosclerosis Reports*, Vol.11, No.2, (March 2009), pp. 87-92, ISSN 1523-3804

Fazio S., & Linton M. (2006). Failure of ACAT inhibition to retard atherosclerosis. *New England Journal of Medicine*, Vol.354, No.12, (March 2006), pp. 1307-1309, ISSN 1533-4406

Forrester J.S. (2010). Redifining normal low-density lipoprotein cholesterol: a strategy to unseat coronary disease as the nation's leading killer. *Journal of the American College of Cardiology*, Vol.56, No.8, (August 2010), pp. 630-636, ISSN 1558-3597

Garcia-Garcia H.M., & Serruys P.W. (2009). Phospholipase $A_2$ inhibitors. *Current Opinion in Lipidology*, Vol.20, No.4, (August 2009), pp. 327-332, ISSN 1473-6535

Gasparyan A.Y., Watson T., & Lip G.Y. (2008). The role of aspirin in cardiovascular prevention: implications of aspirin resistance. *Journal of the American College of Cardiology*, Vol.51, No.19, (May 2008), pp. 1829-1843, ISSN 1558-3597

Gasparyan A.Y., Ayvazyan L., Mikhailidis D.P., & Kitas G.D. (2011). Mean platelet volume: a link between thrombosis and inflammation?. *Current Pharmaceutical Design*, Vol.17, No.1, (2011), pp. 47-58, ISSN 1873-4286

Gibbons R.J., Jones D.W., Gardner T.J., Goldstein L.B., Moller J.H., & Yancy C.W. (2008). The American Heart Association' s 2008 statement of principles for healthcare reform. *Circulation*, Vol.118, No.21, (November 2008), pp. 2209-2218, ISSN 1524-4539

Gilbert J., Lekstrom-Himes J., Donaldson D., Lee Y., Hu M., Xu J., Wyant T., & Davidson M. (2011). Effect of CC chemokine receptor 2 CCR2 blockade on serum C-reactive protein in individuals at atherosclerotic risk and with a single nucleotide polymorphism of the monocyte chemoattractant protein-1 promoter region. *American Journal of Cardiology*, Vol.107, No.6, (March 2011), pp. 906-911, ISSN 1879-1913

Ginsberg H.N., Elam M.B., Lovato L.C., Crouse III J.R., Leiter L.A., Linz P., Friedewald W.T., Buse J.B., Gerstein H.C., Probstfield J., Grimm R.H., Ismail-Beigi F., Bigger J.T., Goff Jr. D.C., Cushman W.C., Simons-Morton D.G., & Byington R.P. (2010). Effects of combination lipid therapy in type 2 diabetes mellitus: the ACCORD study group. *New England Journal of Medicine*, Vol.362, No.17, (April 2010), pp. 1563-1574, ISSN 1533-4406

Goldberg R.B., Kendall D.M., Deeg M.A., Buse J.B., Zagar A.J., Pinaire J.A., Tan M.H., Khan M.A., Perez A.T., & Jacober S.J. (2005). A comparison of lipid and glycemic effects of pioglitazone and rosiglitazone in patients with type 2 diabetes and dyslipidemia. *Diabetes Care*, Vol.28, No.7, (July 2005), pp. 1547-1554, ISSN 1935-5548

Goldfine A.B., Kaul S., & Hiatt W.R. (2011). Fibrates in the treatment of dyslipidemias – time for a reassessment. *New England Journal of Medicine*, Vol. 365, No.6, (August 2011), pp. 481-484, ISSN 1533-4406

Grundy S.M. (2008). Promise of low-density lipoprotein-lowering therapy for primary and secondary prevention. *Circulation*, Vol.117, No.4, (January 2008), pp. 569-573, ISSN 1524-4539

Greenland P., Knoll M.D., Stamler J., Neaton J.D., Dyer A.R., Garside D.B., & Wilson P.W. (2003). Major risk factors as antecedents of fatal and nonfatal coronary heart disease events. *Journal of the American Medical Association*, Vol.290, No.7, (August 2003), pp. 891-897, ISSN1538-3598

Gurbel P.A., Bliden K.P., Kreutz R.P., Dichiara J., Antonino M.J., & Tantry U.S. (2009). The link between heightened thrombogenicity and inflammation: pre-procedure characterization of the patient at high risk for recurrent events after stenting. *Platelets*, Vol.20, No.2, (March 2009), pp. 97-104, ISSN 1369-1635

Haas M.J., & Mooradian A.D. (2011). Inflammation, high-density lipoprotein and cardiovascular dysfunction. *Current Opinion in Infectious Diseases*, Vol.24, No.3, (June 2011), pp. 265-272, ISSN 1535-3877

Hakonarson H., Thorvaldsson S., Helgadottir A., Gudbjartsson D., Zink F., Andresdottir M., Manolescu A., Arnar D.O., Andersen K., Sigurdsson A., Thorgeirsson G., Jonsson A., Agnarsson U., Bjornsdottir H., Gottskalksson G., Einarsson A., Gudmundsdottir H., Adalsteinsdottir A.E., Gudmundsson K., Kristjansson K., Hardarson T., Kristinsson A., Topol E.J., Gulcher J., Kong A., Gurney M., Thorgeirsson G., & Stefansson K. (2005). Effects of a 5-lipoxygenase-activating protein inhibitor on biomarkers associated with risk of myocardial infarction: a randomized trial.

*Journal of the American Medical Association*, Vol.293, No.18, (May 2005), pp. 2245-2256, ISSN 1538-3598

Hansson G.K. (2005). Inflammation, atherosclerosis, and coronary artery disease. *New England Journal of Medicine*, Vol.352, No.16, (April 2005), pp. 1685-1695, ISSN 1533-4406

Hansson G.K., & Libby P. (2006). The immune response in atherosclerosis: a double-edged sword. *Nature Reviews Immunology*, Vol.6, No.7, (July 2006), pp. 508-519, ISSN 1474-1733

Harrison D.G., Guzik T.J., Lob H.E., Madhur M.S., Marvar P.J., Thabet S.R., Vinh A., & Weyand C.M. (2011). Inflammation, immunity, and hypertension. *Hypertension*, Vol.57, No.2, (February 2011), pp. 132-140, ISSN 1524-4563

Hennessy E.H., Parker A.E., & O'Neill L.A.J. (2010). Targeting Toll-like receptors: emerging therapeutics. *Nature Reviews Drug Discovery*, Vol.9, No.4, (April 2010), pp. 293-307, ISSN 1474-1784

Hersberger M. (2010). Potential role of the lipoxygenase derived lipid mediators in atherosclerosis: leukotrienes, lipoxins and resolvins. *Clinical Chemistry and Laboratory Medicine*, Vol.48, No.8, (August 2010), pp. 1063-1073, ISSN 1434-6621

Hlatky M.A., Greenland P., Arnett D.K., Ballantyne C.M., Criqui M.H., Elkind M.S.V., Go A.S., Harrell Jr. F.E., Hong Y., Howard B.V., Howard V.J., Hsue P.Y., Kramer C.M., McConnell J.P., Normand S.L.T., O'Donnell C.J., Smith S.C., & Wilson P.W.F. (2009). Criteria for evaluation of novel markers of cardiovascular risk: a scientific statement from the American Heart Association. *Circulation*, Vol.119, No.17, (May 2009), pp. 2408-2416, ISSN 1524-4539

Hsia J., MacFayden J.G., Monyak J., & Ridker P.M. (2011). Cardiovascular event reduction and adverse events among subjects attaining low-density lipoprotein cholesterol <50 mg/dl with rosuvastatin. The Jupiter Trial (Justification for the Use of Statins in Prevention: an Intervention Trial Evaluating Rosuvastatin). *Journal of the American College of Cardiology*, Vol.57, No.16, (April 2011), pp. 1666-1675, ISSN 1558-3597

Hürlimann D., Forster A., Noll G., Enseleit F., Chenevard R., Distler O., Béchir M., Spieker L.E., Neidhart M., Michel B.A., Gay R.E., Lüscher T.F., Gay S., & Ruschitzka F. (2004). Anti-tumor necrosis factor-α treatment improves endothelial function in patients with rheumatoid arthritis. *Circulation*, Vol.106, No.17, (October 2004), pp. 2184-2187, ISSN 1524-4539

Jun M., Foote C., Lv J., Neal B., Patel A., Nicholls S.J., Grobbee D.E., Cass A., Chalmers J., & Perkovic V. (2010). Effects of fibrates on cardiovascular outcomes: a systematic review and meta-analysis. *Lancet*, Vol.375, No.9729, (May 2010), pp. 1875-1884, ISSN 1474-547X

Kaul S., Morrissey R.P., & Diamond G.A. (2010). By Jove! What is a clinician to make of JUPITER? *Archives of Internal Medicine*, Vol.170, No.12, (June 2010), pp. 1073-1077, ISSN 1538-3679

Keavney B. (2011). C reactive protein and the risk of cardiovascular disease: are clearly linked but a causal associatiuon is unlikely. *British Medical Journal*, Vol.342, (February 2011), pp. 393-394, ISSN 1468-5833

Kinlay S., Schwartz G.G., Olsson A.G., Rifai N., Leslie S.J., Sasiela W.J., Szarek M., Libby P., & Ganz P. (2003). High-dose atorvastatin enhances the decline in inflammatory markers in patients with acute coronary syndromes in the MIRACL study. *Circulation*, Vol.108, No.13, (September 2003), pp. 1560-1566, ISSN 1524-4539

Klingenberg R., & Hansson G.K. (2009). Treating inflammation in atherosclerotic cardiovascular disease: emerging therapies. *European Heart Journal*, Vol.30, No.23, (December 2009), pp. 2838-2844, ISSN 1522-9645

Knopp R.H., Alagona P., Davidson M., Goldberg A.C., Kafonek S.D., Kashyap M., Sprecher D., Superko H.R., Jenkins S., & Marcovina S. (1998). Equivalent efficacy of a time-release form of niacin (Niaspan) given once-a-night versus plain niacin in the management of hyperlipidemia. *Metabolism*, Vol.47, No.9, (September 1998), pp. 1097-1104, ISSN 0026-0495

Kris-Etherton P.M., Lichtenstein A.H., Howard B.V., Steinberg D., & Witztum R. (2004). Antioxidant vitamin supplements and cardiovascular disease. *Circulation*, Vol.110, No.5, (August 2004), pp. 1726-1728, ISSN 1524-4539

Kunsch C., Luchoomun J., Grey J.Y., Olliff L.K., Saint L.B., Arrendale R.F., Wasserman M.A., Saxena U., & Medford R.M. (2004). Selective inhibition of endothelial and monocyte redox-sensitive genes by AGI-1067: a novel antioxidant and anti-inflammatory agent. *Journal of Pharmacology and Experimental Therapeutics*, Vol.308, No.3, (March 2004), pp. 820-829, ISSN 1521-0103

Lauer M.S. (2010). Screening asymptomatic subjects for subclinical atherosclerosis: not so obvious. *Journal of the American College of Cardiology*, Vol.56, No.2, (July 2010), pp. 106-108, ISSN 1558-3597

Lauer M.S. (2011). Pseudodisease, the next great epidemic in coronary atherosclerosis. *Archives of Internal Medicine*, Vol.171, No.14, (July 2011), pp. 1268-1269, ISSN 1538-3679

Leibowitz A, & Schiffrin E.L. (2011). Immune mechanisms in hypertension. *Current Hypertension Reports*, Epub. Ahead of Print, (August 2011), ISSN 1534-3111

Libby P. (2005). The forgotten majority: unfinished business in cardiovascular risk reduction. *Journal of the American College of Cardiology*, Vol.46, No.7, (October 2005), pp. 1225-1228, ISSN 1558-3597

Libby P., Ridker P.M., & Hansson G.K. (2009). Inflammation in atherosclerosis: from pathophysiology to practice. *Journal of the American College of Cardiology*, Vol.54, No.23, (December 2009), pp. 2129-2138, ISSN 1558-3597

Libby P., Ridker P.M., & Hansson G.K. (2011). Progress and challenges in translating the biology of atherosclerosis. *Nature*, Vol.473, No.7347, (May 2011), pp. 317-325, ISSN 1476-4687

Ludman A., Venugopal V., Yellon D.M., & Hausenloy D.J. (2009). Statins and cardioprotection – more than just lipid lowering ? *Pharmacology and Therapeutics*, Vol.122, No.1, (April 2009), pp. 30-43, ISSN 1879-016X

Mancia G., De Backer G., Dominiczak A., Cifkova R., Fagard R., Germanò G., Grassi G., Heagerty A.M., Kjeldsen S.E., Laurent S., Narkiewicz K., Ruilope L., Rynkiewicz A., Schmieder R.E., Struijker Boudier H.A.J., & Zanchetti A. (2007). 2007 guidelines for the management of arterial hypertension. *Journal of Hypertension*, Vol.25, No.9, pp. 1105-1187, ISSN 1473-5598

Marchesi C., Paradis P., & Schiffrin E.L. (2008). Role of the renin-angiotensin system in vascular inflammation. *Trends in Pharmacological Sciences*, Vol. 29, No.7, (July 2008), pp. 367-374, ISSN 0165-6147

Maskrey B.H., Megson I.L., Whitfield P.D., & Rossi A.G. (2011). Mechanisms of resolution of inflammation: a focus on cardiovascular disease. *Arteriosclerosis Thrombosis and Vascular Biology*, Vol.31, No.5, (May 2011), pp. 1001-1006, ISSN 1524-4636

Montecucco F., Pende A., & Mach F. (2009). The renin-angiotensin system modulates inflammatory processes in atherosclerosis: evidence from basic research and clinical studies. *Mediators of Inflammation*, Vol.2009, 752406, ISSN 1466-1861

Montecucco F., Lenglet S., Bertolotto M., Pelli G., Gayet-Ageron A., Palombo D., Pane B., Spinella G., Steffens S., Raffaghello L., Pistoia V., Ottonello L., Pende A., Dallegri F., & Mach F. (2010). Systemic and intraplaque mediators of inflammation are increased in patients symptomatic for ischemic stroke. *Stroke*, Vol.41, No.7, (July 2010), pp. 1394-1404, ISSN 1524-4628

Montecucco F., Pende A., Quercioli A., & Mach F. (2011). Inflammation in the pathophysiology of essential hypertension. *Journal of Nephrology*, Vol.24, No.1, (January-February 2011), pp. 23-34, ISSN 1724-6059

Morrow D.A., de Lemos J.A., Sabatine M.S., Wiviott S.D., Blazing M.A., Shui A., Rifai N., Califf R.M., & Braunwald E. (2006). Clinical relevance of C-reactive protein during follow-up of patients with acute coronary syndromes in the Aggrastat-to-Zocor Trial. *Circulation*, Vol.114, No.4, (July 2006), pp. 281-288, ISSN 1524-4539

Naghavi M., Falk E., Hecht H.S., & Shah P.K. (2006). The first SHAPE (Screening for Heart Attack Prevention and Education) guideline. *Critical Pathways in Cardiology*, Vol.5, No.4, (December 2006), pp. 187-190, ISSN 1535-2811

Natarajan P., & Cannon C.P. (2010). Could direct inhibition of inflammation be the "next big thing" in treating atherosclerosis. *Arteriosclerosis Thrombosis and Vascular Biology*, Vol.30, No.11, (November 2010), pp. 2081-2083, ISSN 1524-4636

Natarajan P., Ray K.K., & Cannon C.P. (2010). High-density lipoprotein and coronary heart disease: current and future therapies. *Journal of the American College of Cardiology*, Vol.55, No.13, (March 2010), pp. 1283-1299, ISSN 1558-3597

Nissen S.E., Tuczu E.M., Libby P., Thompson P.D., Ghali M., Garza D., Berman L., Shi H., Buebendorf E., & Topol E.J. (2004). Effect of antihypertensive agents on cardiovascular events in patients with coronary disease and normal blood pressure. The CAMELOT study: a randomized controlled trial. *Journal of the American Medical Association*, Vol.292, No.18, (November 2004), pp. 2217-2226, ISSN 1538-3598

Nissen S.E., Tuczu E.M., Schoenhagen P., Crowe T., Sasiela W.J., Tsai J., Orazem J., Magorien R.D., O'Shaughnessy C., & Ganz P. (2005). Statin therapy, LDL cholesterol, C-reactive protein, and coronary artey disease. *New England Journal of Medicine*, Vol.352, No.1, (January 2005), pp. 29-38, ISSN 1533-4406

Nissen S.E., & Wolski K. (2010). Rosiglitazone revisited: an updated meta-analysis of risk for myocardial infarction and cardiovascular mortality. *Archives of Internal Medicine*, Vol.170, No.14, (July 2010), pp. 1191-1201, ISSN 1538-3679

Nordestgaard B.G. (2009). Does elevated C-reactive protein cause human atherothrombosis? Novel insights from genetics, intervention trials, and elsewhere. *Current Opinion in Lipidology*, Vol.20, No.5, (October 2009), pp. 393-401, ISSN 1473-6535

Oyekan A. (2011). PPARs and their effects on their cardiovascular system. *Clinical and Experimental Hypertension*, Vol.33, No.5, (August 2011), pp. 287-293, ISSN 1525-6006

Paras C., Hussain M.M., & Rosenson R.S. (2010). Emerging drugs for hyperlipidemia. *Expert Opinion on Emerging Drugs*, Vol.15, No.3, (September 2010), pp. 433-451, ISSN 1744-7623

Pende A., & Dallegri F. (2011). Anti-inflammatory approaches to reduce acute cardiovascular events: Not only benefits. *Current Pharmaceutical Biotechnology*, Epub. Ahead of Print, (April 2011), ISSN 1389-2010

Perry C.M. (2009). Extended-release niacin (nicotinic acid)/laropiprant. *Drugs*, Vol.69, No.12, (August 2009), pp. 1665-1679, ISSN 012-6667

Pfützner A., Schöndorf T., Hanefeld M., & Forst T. (2010). High-sensitivity C-reactive protein predicts cardiovascular risk in diabetic and nondiabetic patients: effects of insulin-sensitizing treatment with pioglitazone. *Journal of Diabetes Science and Technology*, Vol.4, No.3, (May 2010), pp. 706-716, ISSN 1932-2968

Pletcher M., & Hulley S.B. (2010). Statin therapy in young adults: ready for prime time? *Journal of the American College of Cardiology*, Vol.56, No.8, (August 2010), pp. 637-640, ISSN 1558-3597

Ribichini F., Tomai F., De Luca G., Boccuzzi G., Presbitero P., Pesarini G., Ferrero V., Ghini A.S., Abukaresh R., Aurigemma C., De Luca L., Zavalloni D., Soregaroli D., Marino P., Garbo R., Zanolla L., & Vassanelli C. (2011). Immunosuppressive therapy with oral prednisone to prevent restenosis after PCI. A multicenter randomized trial. *American Journal of Medicine*, Vol.124, No.5, (May 2011), pp. 434-443, ISSN 1555-7162

Ridker P.M., Rifai N., Pfeffer M.A., Sacks F.M., & Braunwald E. (1999). Long-term effects of pravastatin on plasma concentration of C-reactive protein. The Cholesterol and Recurrent Events (CARE) investigators. *Circulation*, Vol.100, Vol.3, (July 1999), pp. 230-235, ISSN 1524-4539

Ridker P.M., Rifai N., Clearfield M., Downs J.R., Weis S.E., Miles J.S., & Gotto Jr., A.M. (2001). Measurement of C-reactive protein for the targeting of statin therapy in the primary prevention of acute coronary events. *New England Journal of Medicine*, Vol.344, No.26, (June 2001), pp. 1959-1965, ISSN 1533-4406

Ridker P.M., Cannon C.P., Morrow D., Rifai N., Rose L.M., McCabe C.H., Pfeffer M.A., & Braunwald E. (2005). C-reactive protein levels and outcomes after statin therapy. *New England Journal of Medicine*, Vol.352, No.1, (January 2005), pp. 20-28, ISSN 1533-4406

Ridker P.M. (2007). C-reactive protein and the prediction of cardiovascular events among those at intermediate risk: moving an inflammatory hypothesis toward consensus. *Journal of the American College of Cardiology*, Vol.49, No.21, (May 2007), pp. 2129-2138, ISSN 1558-3597

Ridker P.M., Buring J.E., Rifai N., & Cook N.R. (2007). Development and validation of improved algorithms for the assessment of global cardiovascular risk in women: the Reynolds Risk Score. *Journal of the American Medical Association*, Vol.297, No.6, (February 2007), pp. 611-619, ISSN 1538-3598

Ridker P.M., Paynter N.P., Rifai N., Gaziano J.M., & Cook N.R. (2008a). C-reactive protein and parental history improve global cardiovascular risk prediction: the Reynolds Risk Score for Men. *Circulation*, Vol.118, No.22, (November 2008), pp. 2243-2251, ISSN 1524-4539

Ridker P.M., Danielson E., Fonseca F.A., Genest J., Gotto Jr., A.M., Kastelein J.J., Koenig W., Libby P., Lorenzatti A.J., MacFadyen J.G., Nordestgaard B.G., Shepherd J.,

Willerson J.T., & Glynn R.J. (2008b). Rosuvastatin to prevent vascular events in men and women with elevated C-reactive protein. *New England Journal of Medicine*, Vol.359, No.21, (November 2008), pp. 2195-2207, ISSN 1533-4406

Ridker P.M. (2009). Testing the inflammatory hypothesis of atherothrombosis: scientific rationale for the cardiovascular inflammation reduction trial (CIRT). *Journal of Thrombosis and Haemostasis*, Vol.7, No.Suppl.1, (July 2009), pp. 332-339, ISSN 1538-7836

Roberts R., DeMello V., Sobel B.E. (1976). Deleterious effects of methylprednisolone in patients with myocardial infarction. *Circulation*, Vol.53, No.Suppl. 3, (March 1976), pp. 1204-1206, ISSN 1524-4539

Rosenson R.S. (2009). Future role for selective phospholipase $A_2$ inhibitors in the prevention of atherosclerotic cardiovascular disease. *Cardiovascular Drugs and Therapy*, Vol.23, No.1, (February 2009), pp. 93-101, ISSN 1573-7241

Ross R. (1999). Atherosclerosis – an inflammatory disease. *New England Journal of Medicine*, Vol.340, No.2, (January 1999), pp. 115-126, ISSN 1533-4406

Säemann M.D., Poglitsch M., Kopecky C., Haidinger M., Hörl W.H., & Weichhart T. (2010). The versatility of HDL: a crucial anti-inflammatory regulator. *European Journal of Clinical Investigation*, Vol.40,No.12, (December 2010), pp. 1131-1143, ISSN 1365-2362

Sanyal S., Karas R.H., Kuvin J.T. (2007). Present-day uses of niacin: effects on lipid and non-lipid parameters. *Expert Opinion in Pharmacotherapy*, Vol.8, No.11, (August 2007), pp.1711-1717, ISSN 1744-7666

Sarov-Blat L., Morgan J.M., Fernandez P., James R., Fang Z., Hurle M.R., Baidoo C., Willette R.N., Lepore J.J., Jensen S.E., & Sprecher D.L. (2010). Inhibition of p38 mitogen-activated protein kinase reduces inflammation following coronary vascular injury in humans. *Arteriosclerosis Thrombosis and Vascular Biology*, Vol.30, No.11, (November 2010), pp. 2256-2263, ISSN 1524-4636

Satoh K., Fukumoto Y., & Shimokawa H. (2011). Rho-kinase: important new therapeutic target in cardiovascular diseases. *American Journal of Physiology Heart and Circulatory Physiology* , Vol.301, No.2, (August 2011), pp. H287-H296, ISSN 1522-1539

Sattar N., Preiss D., Murray H.M., Welsh P., Buckley B.M., de Craen A.J., Seshasai S.R., McMurray J.J., Freeman D.J., Jukema J.W., Macfarlane P.W., Packard C.J., Stott D.J., Westendorp R.G., Shepherd J., Davis B.R., Pressel S.L., Marchioli R., Marfisi R.M., Maggioni A.P., Tavazzi L., Tognoni G., Kjekshus J., Pedersen T.R., Cook T.J., Gotto A.M., Clearfield M.B., Downs J.R., Nakamura H., Ohashi Y., Mizuno K., Ray K.K., & Ford I. (2010). Statins and risk of incident diabetes: a collaborative meta-analysis of randomised statin trials. *Lancet*, Vol.375, No.9716, (February 2010), pp. 735-742, ISSN 1474-547X

Schieven G.L. (2005). The biology of p38 kinase: a central role in inflammation. *Current Topics in Medicinal Chemistry*, Vol.5, No.10, (September 2005), pp. 921-928, ISSN 1568-0266

Schinzari F., Armuzzi A., De Pascalis B., Mores N., Tesauro M., Melina D., & Cardillo C. (2008). Tumor necrosis factor-α antagonism improves endothelial dysfunction in patients with Crohn's disease. *Clinical Pharmacology and Therapeutics*, Vol.83, No.1, (January 2008), pp. 70-76, ISSN 1532-6535

Schunkert H., & Samani N.J. (2008). Elevated C-reactive protein in atherosclerosis – chicken or egg? *New England Journal of Medicine*, Vol.359, No.18, (October 2008), pp. 1953-1955, ISSN 1533-4406

See R., Lindsey J.B., Patel M.J., Ayers C.R., Khera A., McGuire D.K., Grundy S.M., & de Lemos J.A. (2008). Application of the Screening for Heart Attack Prevention and Education Task Force recommendations to an urban population: observations from the Dallas Heart Study. *Archives of Internal Medicine*, Vol.168, No.10, (May 2008), pp. 1055-1062, ISSN 1538-3679

Sever P.S., Poulter N.R., Elliott W.J., Jonsson M.C., & Black H.R. (2006). Management of hypertension: is it the pressure or the drug? *Circulation*, Vol.113, No.23, (June 2006), pp. 2754-2774, ISSN 1524-4539

Shah P.K. (2010). Screening asymptomatic subjects for subclinical atherosclerosis: can we, does it matter, and should we? *Journal of the American College of Cardiology*, Vol.56, No.2, (July 2010), pp. 98-105, ISSN 1558-3597

Spite M, & Serhan C.N. (2010). Novel lipid mediators promote resolution of acute inflammation: impact of aspirin and statins. *Circulation Research*, Vol.107, No.10, (November 2010), pp. 1170-1184, ISSN 1524-4571

Staessen J.A., Richart T., Wang Z., Thijs, L. (2010). Implications of recently published trials of blood pressure-lowering drugs in hypertensive or high-risk patients. *Hypertension*, Vol.55, No.4, (April 2010), pp. 819-831, ISSN 1524-4563

Steinberg D. (2010). Earlier intervention in the management of hypercholesterolemia: what are we waiting for? *Journal of the American College of Cardiology*, Vol.56, No.8, (August 2010), pp. 627-629, ISSN 1558-3597

Superko H.R., & King III S. (2008). Lipid management to reduce cardiovascular risk: a new strategy is required. *Circulation*, Vol.117, No.4, (January 2008), pp. 560-568, ISSN 1524-4539

Tabet F., & Rye K.A. (2009). High-density lipoproteins, inflammation and oxidative stress. *Clinical Science*, Vol.116, No.2, (January 2009), pp. 87-98, ISSN 1470-8736

Tardif J.C., McMurray J.J., Klug E., Small R., Schumi J., Choi J., Cooper J., Scott R., Lewis E.F., L'Allier P.L., & Pfeffer M.A. (2008). Effects of succinobucol (AGI-1067) after an acute coronary syndrome: a randomised, double-blind, placebo-controlled trial. *Lancet*, Vol.371, No.9626, (May 2008), pp. 1761-1768, ISSN 1474-547X

Tardif J.C., L'Allier P.L., Ibrahim R., Grégoire J.C., Nozza A., Cossette M., Kouz S., Lavoie M.A., Paquin J., Brotz T.M., Taub R., & Pressacco J. (2010). Treatment with 5-lipoxygenase inhibitor VIA-2291 (atreleuton) in patients with recent acute coronary syndrome. *Circulation Cardiovascular Imaging*, Vol.3, No.3, (May 2010), pp. 298-307, ISSN 1942-0080

Taylor A.J., Villines T.C., Stanek E.J., Devine P.J., Griffen L., Miller M., Weissman N.J., & Turco M. (2009). Extended-release niacin or ezetimibe and carotid intima-media thickness. *New England Journal of Medicine*, Vol.361, No.22, (November 2009), pp. 2113-2122, ISSN 1533-4406

Thoenes M., Oguchi A., Nagamia S., Vaccari C.S., Hammoud R., Umpierrez G.E., & Khan B.V. (2007). The effects of extended-release niacin on carotid intimal media thickness, endothelial function and inflammatory markers in patients with the metabolic syndrome. *International Journal of Clinical Practice*, Vol.61, No.11, (November 2007), pp. 1942-1948, ISSN 1368-5031

Tracey D., Klareskog L., Sasso E.H., Salfeld J.G., & Tak P.P. (2008). Tumor necrosis factor antagonist mechanisms of action: a comprehensive review. *Pharmacology and Therapeutics*, Vol.117, No.2, (February 2008), pp. 244-279, ISSN 0163-7258

U.S. Preventive Services Task Force (2009). Using nontraditional risk factors in coronary heart disease risk asessment: U.S. Preventive Services Task Force recommendation statement. *Annals of Internal Medicine*, Vol.151, No.7, (October 2009), pp. 474-482, ISSN 1539-3704

van Eijk I.C., de Vries M.K., Levels J.H., Peters M.J., Huizer E.E., Dijkmans B.A., van der Horst-Bruinsma I.E., Hazenberg B.P., van de Stadt R.J., Wolbink G.J., & Nurmohamed M.T. (2009). Improvement of lipid profile is accompanied by atheroprotective alterations in high-density lipoprotein composition upon tumor necrosis factor blockade: a prospective cohort study in ankylosing spondylitis. *Arthritis and Rheumatism*, Vol.60, No.5, (May 2009), pp. 1324-1330, ISSN 0004-3591

van Leuven S.I., Kastelein J.J., Allison A.C., Hayden M.R., & Stroes E.S. (2006). Mycophenolate mofetil (MMF): firing at the atherosclerotic plaque from different angles? *Cardiovascular Research*, Vol.69, No.2, (February 2006), pp. 341-347, ISSN 0008-6363

van Leuven S.I., van Wijk D.F., Volger O.L., de Vries J.P., van der Loos C.M., de Kleijn D.V., Horrevoets A.J., Tak P.P., van der Wal A.C., de Boer O.J., Pasterkamp G., Hayden M.R., Kastelein J.J., & Stroes E.S. (2010). Mycophenolate mofetil attenuates plaque inflammation in patients with symptomatic carotid artery stenosis. *Atherosclerosis*, Vol.211, No.1, (July 2010), pp. 231-236, ISSN 1879-1484

van Puijvelde G.H.M., van Es T., Habets K.L.L., Hauer A.D., van Berkel T.J.C., & Kuiper J. (2008). A vaccine against atherosclerosis: myth or reality? *Future Cardiology*, Vol.4, No.2, (March 2008), pp. 125-133, ISSN 1744-8298

Wang C.Y., Liu P.Y., & Liao J.K. (2008). Pleiotropic effects of statin therapy: molecular mechanisms and clinical results. *Trends in Molecular Medicine*, Vol.14, No.1, (January 2008), pp. 37-44, ISSN 1471-4914

Wang N., Yin R., Liu Y., Mao G., & Xi F. (2011). Role of peroxisome proliferator-activated receptor-γ in atherosclerosis: an update. *Circulation Journal*, Vol.75, No.3, (March 2011), pp. 528-535, ISSN 1346-9843

Westlake S.L., Colebatch A.N., Baird J., Kiely P., Quinn M., Choy E., Ostor A.J., & Edwards C.J. (2010). The effect of methotrexate on cardiovascular disease in patients with rheumatoid arthritis: a systematic literature review. *Rheumatology*, Vol.49, No.2, (February 2010), pp. 295-307, ISSN 1462-0332

Wilson P.W., Pencina M., Jacques P., Selhub J., D'Agostino Sr. R., & O'Donnell C.J. (2008). C-reactive protein and reclassification of cardiovascular risk in the Framingham Heart Study. *Circulation Cardiovascular Quality and Outcomes*, Vol.1, No.2, (November 2008), pp. 92-97, ISSN 1941-7705

Yang E.Y., Nambi V., Tang Z., Virani S.S., Boerwinkle E., Hoogeveen R.C., Astor B.C., Mosley T.H., Coresh J., Chambless L., & Ballantyne C.M. (2009). Clinical implications of JUPITER (Justification fo the Use of statins in Prevention: an Intervention Trial Evaluating Rosuvastatin) in a U.S. population. *Journal of the American College of Cardiology*, Vol.54, No.25, (December 2009), pp. 2388-2395, ISSN 1558-3597

Yoshinaka Y., Shibata H., Kobayashi H., Kuriyama H., Shibuya K., Tanabe S., Watanabe T., & Miyazaki A. (2010). *Atherosclerosis*, Vol.213, N.1, (November 2010), pp. 85-91, ISSN 1879-1484

Yvan-Charvet L., Kling J., Pagler T., Li H., Hubbard B., Fisher T., Sparrow C.P., Taggart A.K., & Tall A.R. (2010). Cholesterol efflux potential and antiinflammatory properties of high-density lipoprotein after treatment with niacin or anacetrapib. *Arteriosclerosis Thrombosis and Vascular Biology*, Vol.30, No.7, (July 2010), pp.1430-1438, ISSN 1524-4636

Zanchetti A. (2009). Bottom blood pressure or bottom cardiovascular risk? How far can cardiovascular risk be reduced? *Journal of Hypertension*, Vol.27, No.8, (August 2009), pp. 1509-1520, ISSN 1473-5598

Zhou Q., Gensch C., & Liao J.K. (2011). Rho-associated coiled-coil-forming kinases (ROCKs): potential targets for the treatment of atherosclerosis and vascular disease. *Trends in Pharmacological Sciences*, Vol.32, No.3, (March 2011), pp. 167-173, ISSN 1873-3735

# 5

# Gender-Specific Aspects in the Clinical Presentation of Cardiovascular Disease

Chiara Leuzzi, Raffaella Marzullo,
Emma Tarabini Castellani and Maria Grazia Modena*
*Department of Cardiovascular Disease, Women's Clinic*
*University of Modena and Reggio Emilia,*
*Italy*

## 1. Introduction

In the industrialized countries, the cardiovascular disease (CVD) is the leading cause of mortality and morbidity in women after of 50 years. Genetic, hormonal and metabolic influences are involved in gender differences, including the epidemiology, symptoms, diagnosis, progression, prognosis and management of these pathologies.

Recent advances in the field of cardiovascular medicine have not led to significant drops in case fatality rates for women, compared to the dramatic reductions achieved for men. Such gender-specific difference in cardiovascular disease mortality are probably related to a knowledge gap about CVD in women. Thus, much of the evidence supporting contemporary recommendations for testing, prevention, and treatment of CVD in women is extrapolated from studies conducted predominantly on middle-aged men. For example pharmacological therapy is hampered by defective evidence.

Only recently, significant sex-related differences in prevalence, presentation, management and outcomes of CVD, have been evaluated and discovered.

The ability of knowing and recognizing gender differences in CVD may facilitate a rapid identification of cardiac signs and symptoms of warning and may avoid significant delays in diagnosis and treatment in women. This compendium will briefly summarize gender-related differences in several manifestations of CVD, with a special focus also on arrhythmias and heart failure.

## 2. Risk factors

Traditionally, guidelines classify women as being at high, intermediate or low risk on risk profile, based on Framingham risk scores. Despite major traditional risk factors are the same in both sexes, gender-specific differences are noted, and these differences are related to different outcome. For this reason, a new approach in evaluation of cardiovascular risk in

---

* Corresponding Author

women considers a multifactorial model that includes a complex interaction between sex hormones and traditional risk factors.

## 2.1 Traditional risk factors

There is also substantial gender-related differences in the prevalence and outcome in traditional risk factors. For example, overall rates of hypertension and smoking are higher in men, but their presence is associated with a worse outcome in women. The prevalence of hypertension is lower in pre-menopausal women than men, whereas in post-menopausal women it is higher than in men. In fact about 50% of post-menopausal women experience of moderate to severe hypertension or take antihypertensive therapy.

Several studies have clearly demonstrated a strong relationship between level of blood pressure and risk for cardiovascular events. In this setting, hypertension is one of the most risk factors for stroke, myocardial infarction, heart failure, aortic disease and chronic renal failure. Mechanisms responsible for the increase in blood pressure in post-menopausal women are complex and multifactorial, including loss of estrogen, oxidative stress, endothelial dysfunction, modification in renin-angiotensin system and sympathetic activation.

Hypertension may appears as an isolated disease, more typical of elderly women, or as part of the metabolic syndromes (MS), more frequently in early postmenopausal women. MS is a constellation of interrelated risk factors that promote the development of CVD. The presence of MS worsens the severity of hypertension and reduces the response to treatment. Than, MS is considered a unfavourable prognostic factor in hypertension post-menopausal women. On the other hand hypertension tends to associate with other metabolic risk factors and about one-half patients with essential hypertension are insulin resistant. In addition women with MS have chronic subclinical inflammation and systemic endothelial dysfunction. Endothelial dysfunction is common after the menopause and its detection may precede overt disease such as hypertension and diabetes.

Data derived from population studies demonstrate that total cholesterol measurements are higher in men until the fifth decade of life but, beyond this age, women have greater values. Examining the lipoprotein subclassis, women have less LDL particles than men and have about two-fold higher concentration of HDL particles then men. Particularly, HDL cholesterol inversely correlates with coronary artery disease (CAD) in young men and in women of all ages. Women typically experience a relatively mild decline in HDL cholesterol at the time of menopause.

Hypertriglyceridemia is also a more potent independent risk factor for CAD in women as compared with men. In fact, in presence of hypertriglyceridemia, the risk of CVD is twice in women.

Another strong risk factors in women is diabetes. Diabetic women have significantly higher cardiovascular mortality when compared with diabetic men, because diabetes eliminates the 'female advantage' of a lower CAD prevalence and outcome risk that exists for the female in general population. Furthermore diabetes is an independent predictor of 'atypical' presentation of acute myocardial infarction in women.

At the onset of diabetes-related cardiovascular complications, women have higher out-of-hospital mortality than men, and those who reach hospital are more likely to die from an initial cardiac event and are also at high risk of post-event complications.

## 2.2 Gender-specific risk factors

Other factors are unique to the female: menopause, which affects especially if early and hypothalamic-hypoestrogenism occurring in fertile women.

Menopause is a physiological condition associated with endothelial dysfunction, due to lack of estrogens. Than, the deficiency of female gonadal hormones may represent a major risk factor for menopausal hypertension, due to related modifications of blood vessel structure and the elicit response to a vasoactive substances.

Furthermore, dysfunction of the endotelium causes reduction or abolition of vasoprotective factors, inducing a proinflammatory, proliferative and procoagulatory milieu. These changes favour the development of cardiovascular risk factors, as hypertension.

Gender-specific opportunities for identifying women's risk (e.g., prior preeclampsia) also deserve further exploration.

Preeclampsia is a disorder of pregnancy diagnosed by gestational hypertension and proteinuria. Abnormal placentation resulting in preeclampsia and intrauterine growth restriction is a major cause of both maternal and perinatal morbidity and mortality.

Prior preeclampsia is associated with increased risk of CVD, including myocardial infarction, ischemic heart disease, stroke and endstage renal disease. Particularly, the increased risk for future vascular disease is more pronounced in women with early-onset preeclampsia. Although the symptoms of preeclampsia resolve over a number of weeks after delivery, maternal vascular dysfunction may persist for years.

Endothelial dysfunction, however, is considered a central component of the pathophysiology of preeclampsia and known to contribute to the pathogenesis of hypertension and cardiovascular sequelae. Several factors contribute to the endothelial dysfunction in the post-partum state. Abnormal placenta, for example, release antiangiogenic factors, harmful to the vascular endothelium. Often, women with a history of peeclampsia or intrauterine growth restriction have high cholesterol levels, high blood pressure and insulin resistance.

Frequently, preeclamptic women are obese, and obesity associated with insulin resistance, may reduce endothelial dependent blood flow response.

Behavioral factors also, such as chronic stress, lack of social support, and family demands, as well as biological processes, including genetics, may contribute to the development of CVD in this setting.

Similarly, women with a history of polycystic ovary syndrome have a increased risk of CVD and have a greater frequency of multiple risk factors including central obesity, insulin resistance, and a greater prevalence of the metabolic syndrome and diabetes.

## 2.3 Inflammatory risk factors

Beside the traditional and female specific risk factors, novel risk markers such as inflammatory markers are being studied.

Women are at increased risk of inflammatory and autoimmune disease. The risk of mortality and morbidity from CVD is very high in autoimmune diseases, as systemic lupus erythematosus or rheumatoid arthritis. Various possible mechanisms have been proposed to explain the excess rate of cardiovascular mortality in patients with autoimmune disease.

A combination of traditional (dyslipidemia, hypertension, diabetes, and smoking) and nontraditional risk factors, including high inflammation, antiphospholipid antibodies and lipid oxidation, contribute to CVD in autoimmune diseases. Inflammation is a key component in the development of atherosclerosis in this setting. In fact, inflammation leads to the activation of endothelial cells, which, through an increase in the expression of leukocyte adhesion molecules, promotes a pro-atherosclerotic environment. Expression of proinflammatory cytokines and inflammatory mediators influences all stages of atherosclerosis development, from early atheroma formation to thrombus development responsible for events such as myocardial infarction. Proinflammatory cytokines may promote both traditional (e.g., dyslipidemia, insulin resistance) and nontraditional (e.g., oxidative stress) systemic cardiovascular risk factors.

Than in these patients, is commonly found a presence of endothelial dysfunction, a loss of arterial compliance and dysfunction in the microvascolature, resulting in myocardial flow heterogeneity.

Others factors contribute to poor prognosis: undertreatment of cardiovascular comorbidity may contribute to increased cardiovascular mortality in these patients. However, some drugs, largely used in this setting, may worsen cardiovascular profile: e.g. corticosteroids promote hypertension, dyslipidemia, and diabetes.

Then, novel risk stratification, including inflammatory markers and reproductive hormones, is developing to assess global cardiovascular risk in women.

## 3. Coronary heart disease

Coronary heart disease (CHD) is the most common cause of death amongst women, who experience more complications after acute myocardial infarction (AMI) than men.

It has been demonstrated that the epidemiology, the clinical manifestation and the progression of CHD are different in both sexes. The women developed CHD about 10-20 years later than men, in part by the influence of hormones and in part by the genetic sex.

Particularly, at the time of first experience of AMI, women are more likely to have diabetes mellitus or heart failure (HF) than men.

In addition, the prevalence of obstructive coronary disease is particularly low in premenopausal women, whilst increases dramatically for a woman after age 50.

The most common initial presentation of CHD is a AMI or sudden cardiac death and up to half of all women presenting with an acute myocardial infarction report no prior chest pain symptoms. There would appear to be an interaction effect of symptom presentation with age, in that older women often present in a similar way to men.

Several studies have indicated that women have "atypical" symptoms such as back pain, dyspnea, indigestion, nausea/vomiting and weakness. Frequently women reported pain in the jaw and neck and describe their symptoms as more anguished and frightening (emotional component) compared with men. Furthermore, prodromal symptoms are described up to 1 month before the onset of AMI such unusual fatigue (70.7%), sleep disturbance (47.8%) and shortness of breath (42.1%). The atypical presentation may explain the rate of under-diagnosed AMI, the under treatment of acute coronary syndromes and the worse outcomes characterized by increased hospital morbidity, higher mortality and fewer evidence-based therapies in women.

In the postmenopausal women, the plaque rupture is the main mechanism of acute coronary syndromes like as in the men. The higher mortality noted for younger women when compared with age-matched men is due the higher frequency of plaque erosion (Fig. 1). In an autopsy series, women also had a greater frequency of distal microvascular embolization in the setting of a fatal epicardial thrombosis when compared to men, independently of the type of thrombus or presence of necrosis. AMI and sudden death in women can occur also in spontaneous coronary artery dissection. This event is more frequent in the peri-partum period and can involve all coronary tree, but more frequently affects the left anterior descending artery. The dissection can involve every coronary, but in women frequently involves the left anterior descending coronary artery, whereas in man the right coronary artery is more frequently involved.

Many as 50% of patients undergoing coronary angiography for typical or atypical chest pain do not have obstructive CAD. An alternative mechanism of pain in women may be a coronary microvascular dysfunction, known as syndrome X. Most of these patients have an 'abnormal' exercise stress test, myocardial perfusion defects on gated Single-photon emission computed tomography or stress-induced wall motion abnormalities on echocardiography, but normal coronary angiography.

However, differentiation between these mechanisms of chest pain is important, because 'noncardiac' chest pain is not associated with cardiovascular sequelae and may require further medical evaluation and treatment. By contrast, syndrome X, which is thought to be caused by microvascular dysfunction, is associated with inducible metabolic ischaemia and can be treated by improving microvascular vasomotor tone with oral L-arginine, a precursor to vascular nitric oxide, and oestrogen.

Despite the absence of CAD and low risk for adverse cardiac events, a majority of those patients continue to have symptoms that contribute to a poor quality of life and consumption of large amounts of health care resources because of repeated evaluations and hospitalizations. Recently, Han et al. studied patients with obstructive CAD who underwent simultaneous intravascular ultrasound and coronary reactivity assessment and demonstrated that men have a greater atheroma burden and more diffuse epicardial endothelial dysfunction while women have more disease of the microcirculation. The coronary micro-vascular dysfunction, the smaller coronary artery lumens, the less collateral circulation than men and more prominent positive remodeling support the higher rate of angina, and acute coronary syndromes in the absence of obstructive CAD particularly during exertion or stress.

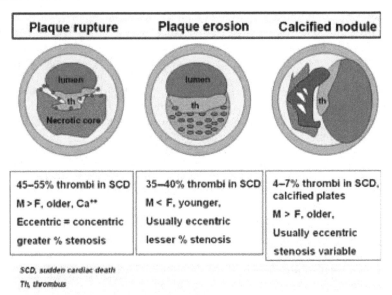

SCD, sudden cardiac death; Th, thrombus

Fig. 1. Gender differences in plaque morphologic features in an autoptic series of patients who died for sudden cardiac death, modified from reference 13.

## 4. Heart failure

The lifetime risk of developing HF is about 20% for both men and women. There are differences between men and women in clinical presentation, aetiology, treatment and outcome in HF, and these differences lead to different outcome.

The women are older than men and present more frequent hypertension and diabetes.

Diabetes mellitus is one of the strongest additional risk factors for the development of HF in women with CAD.

The systolic function is usually better preserved and the prevalence of ischemic etiology is lower respect to hypertension and valvular diseases. Another cause of HF includes cardiac toxicity from chemotherapeutic agents used to treat breast malignancy.

Mullens et al. show that the survival rate in women with non-ischemic cardiomyopathy was better than men, irrespective of baseline characteristics, while there was no advantage in presence of ischemic cause. The reason of different outcome remains unclear but might in part be related to sex differences in etiology.

The diagnosis of HF is a clinical diagnosis based on a constellation of symptoms and signs. Women with impaired systolic left ventricular function are more likely than men to have dependent edema, jugular venous distension, and an S3 gallop.

Furthermore, normal brain natriuretic peptide value, a biomarker used to identify patients with symptoms of HF, are higher in women versus men.

Current guidelines for HF therapy also are not sex specific due to under-representation of women and lack of sex-specific, prospective, randomized clinical trials. Indeed, women receive less life-prolonging treatment (ACE-I, beta-blockers and spironolactone) than men, in the presence of normal left ventricular function, while there no difference if etiology of HF is CAD.

Cardiac resynchronization therapy, an important therapy for HF, is beneficial for both women and men. Data suggest CRT is preferable to medical therapy alone in women for the combined end point of total mortality and hospital stay for major cardiovascular events.

A peculiar type of left ventricular dysfunction and HF typical in women is Takotsubo cardiomyopathy. This disease is typically observed in post-menopausal women and the highest frequency of occurrence is between the seventh and eighth decade of life.

The reason for the much more common occurrence in postmenopausal women is unclear.

It is characterized by a left ventricular dysfunction, electrocardiographic changes like an acute myocardial infarction and release of cardiac biomarkers, in the absence of obstructive coronary disease. The emotionally or physical stress are usually the triggers. The catecholamine-mediated cardio-toxicity, multi-vessels coronary vasospasm and abnormalities in coronary micro-vascular function have been postulated as pathophysiologic mechanisms.

The left ventricular dysfunction is reversible within weeks, despite a dramatic clinical presentation (similar to acute myocardial infarction but in the absence of obstructive coronary disease) and substantial risk of complications in the acute setting.

Another cause of left ventricular dysfunction and HF typical in women is peripartum cardiomyopathy (PPCM). This disease develops in the last month of pregnancy or within 5 months post-partum with no pre-existing cardiac disease or identifiable cause. The incidence is very low (<1%) and varies on the basis of the population studied. Risk factors include advanced maternal age, African descent, twin pregnancy, usage of tocolytics, and poverty.

The etiology remains unknown, but potential causes include abnormal immune response to pregnancy, increased myocyte apoptosis, genetic predisposition. Only 20% may worsen up to the death or transplantation, while one-half of PPCM patients recover normal systolic function within 6 months.

## 5. Arrhythmias

It is been demonstrated that women had a higher resting heart rate than did men (3 to 5 beats faster for minute). These finding may be explained by differences in exercise tolerance, autonomic modulation and intrinsic properties of the sinus node, influencing in part by hormonal influences. Burke et al. reported an higher average heart rate during the follicular or luteal phases of the menstrual cycle, although the response to double autonomic blockade was identical regardless of phase.

Several authors demonstrated differences in QT interval between men and women. Women have a longer corrected QT interval and the difference becomes more pronounced at lower heart rates. Rautaharju et al. reported that this difference was due to a drop in the corrected QT that occurred in males after puberty (when androgen levels are highest). Then, the interval in men gradually increased with age until 50 years, at which point it paralleled that of women. The actions of hormonal influences in QT differences was confirmed in families with genotipically characterized long QT syndrome. In addition, the torsades de pointes correlated to both congenital and acquired long QT Syndrome was more frequent in women.

There are many differences in incidence, prevalence, presentation and clinical course of many arrhythmias. Inappropriate sinus tachycardia is more common in women. Rodigruez et al. reported in patients undergoing invasive electrophysiologic testing for various tachycardias that the atrio-ventricular node reentrant tachycardia (AVNRT) was twice times more common in women, whereas atrial tachycardia affected both sexes equally. In addition, the atrio-ventricular reentrant (circus-movement) tachycardia (AVRT), atrial fibrillation (AF), and ventricular fibrillation (VF) occurred more often in men. These trends for supra-ventricular tachycardias (SVTs), AF, VF, were confirmed in the Framingham cohort. Myerburg and associates found that the inducing SVT during electrophysiologic testing was greatest at the onset of menses or during the premenstrual phase. Rossano et al. confirmed that the SVT prone state is hindered by estrogen and facilitated by progesterone.

The SVTs new- onset or exacerbation are most common arrhythmia during pregnancy and the postpartum period in absence o f structural heart disease. The mechanisms for increase in this situation may be related to progesteronerich gravid state, increased intravascular volume and autonomic tone.

The Atrial Fibrillation (AF) is the most prevalent in men, although its incidence increases with age both in men and women. Women with AF are more symptomatic, older and have lower quality of life and more co-morbidities than men. Also they present more likely a higher heart rate, longer episodes and increase incidence of embolic strokes compared to men. Data from the Euro Heart Survey on Atrial Fibrillation demonstrated that women are usually treated less aggressively, with fewer cardioversions and catheter ablations. In this study, albeit both genders received anticoagulation therapy, women experienced a significantly higher rate of stroke and major bleeding events.

## 6. References

[1] Leuzzi C, Sangiorgi GM and Modena MG (2010) Gender-specific aspects in the clinical presentation of cardiovascular disease Fundam Clin Pharmacol. N. 24(6):711-7
[2] Athyros VG, Ganotakis E, Kolovou GD et al (2011). Assessing The Treatment Effect in Metabolic Syndrome without Perceptible Diabetes (ATTEMPT): A Prospective-Randomized Study in Middle Aged Men and Women. Curr Vasc Pharmacol Apr 11. [Epub ahead of print].
[3] Leuzzi C, Modena MG (2011). Hypertension in postmenopausal women: pathophysiology and treatment. High Blood Press Cardiovasc Prev. N. 18;13-8.
[4] Shaw LJ, Bugiardini R, and Bairey Merz CN (2009) Women and Ischemic Heart Disease: Evolving Knowledge J. Am. Coll. Cardiol. N: 54;1561-1575
[5] Bairey Merz CN et al.(2006) Insights from the NHLBI-Sponsored Women's Ischemia Syndrome Evaluation (WISE) Study: Part II: gender differences in presentation,

diagnosis, and outcome with regard to gender-based pathophysiology of atherosclerosis and macrovascular and microvascular coronary disease. J. Am. Coll. Cardiol. N:47 S21-S29

[6] Vitale C, Miceli M, Rosano GM.(2007) Gender-specific characteristics of atherosclerosis in menopausal women: risk factors, clinical course and strategies for prevention. Climacteric. 2007 N.10; 16-20

[7] Association A.H.. Heart Disease and Stroke Statistics: 2004 Update. available at: http://americanheart.org/downloadable/heart/1072969766940HSStats2004Update.pdf

[8] Yinon Y, Kingdom JCP, Odutayo A (2010). Vascular Risk Vascular Dysfunction in Women With a History of Preeclampsia and Intrauterine Growth Restriction : Insights Into Future. Circulation N. 122, 1846-1853

[9] Bairey Merz N et al.(2004) Women's Ischemic Syndrome Evaluation: current status and future research directions: report of the National Heart, Lung and Blood Institute workshop: October 2-4, 2002: executive summary. Circulation N:109, 805-807

[10] Bugiardini R, Estrada JL, Nikus K et al. (2010) Gender bias in acute coronary sindromes. Curr Vasc Pharmacol. N.8;276-84

[11] Vaccarino V et al.(1999) Sex-based differences in early mortality after myocardial infarction. National Registry of Myocardial Infarction 2 Participants. N. Engl. J. Med. N:341 217-225

[12] Nabel EG et al.(2002) Women's Ischemic Syndrome Evaluation: current status and future research directions: report of the National Heart, Lung and Blood Institute workshop: October 2-4, 2002: Section 3: diagnosis and treatment of acute cardiac ischemia: gender issues. Circulation N: 109 e50-e52. 25

[13] Kolodgie FD et al. (2004) Pathologic assessment of the vulnerable human coronary plaque. Heart N: 90 1385-1391. 26

[14] Farb A et al. (2003) Pathological mechanisms of fatal late coronary stent thrombosis in humans. Circulation N:108, 1701-1706

[15] Shaver PJ, Carrig TF and Baker WP (1978)Postpartum coronary artery dissection. Br. Heart J. N: 40 83-86

[16] Basso C, Morgagni G.L., Thiene G.(1996) Spontaneous coronary artery dissection: a neglected cause of acute myocardial ischaemia and sudden death. Heart N: 75, 451-454

[17] Han SH et al.(2008)Sex differences in atheroma burden and endothelial function in patients with early coronary atherosclerosis. Eur Heart J N: 29, 1359-69

[18] Lloyd-Jones DM.(2001) The risk of congestive heart failure: sobering lessons from the Framingham Heart Study. Curr. Cardiol. Rep. N:3, 184-190

[19] O'Meara E et al.(2007) Sex differences in clinical characteristics and prognosis in a broad spectrum of patients with heart failure: results of the Candesartan in Heart failure: Assessment of Reduction in Mortality and morbidity (CHARM) program. Circulation N: 115 3111- 3120

[20] Hsich EM and Pina IL. (2009) Heart failure in women: a need for prospective data. J. Am. Coll. Cardiol. N: 54 491-498

[21] Mullens W et al. (2008) Gender differences in patients admitted with advanced decompensated heart failure. Am. J. Cardiol. N:102, 454-458

[22] Komajda M et al. (2003) The EuroHeart Failure Survey programme – a survey on the quality of care among patients with heart failure in Europe. Part 2: treatment. Eur.Heart J. N:24, 464-474

[23] Koeth O et al.(2008) Clinical, angiographic and cardiovascular magnetic resonance findings in consecutive patients with Takotsubo cardiomyopathy. Clin. Res. Cardiol. N:97, 623–627

[24] Gianni M et al.(2006) Apical ballooning syndrome or takotsubo cardiomyopathy: a systematic review. Eur. Heart J. N: 27, 1523–1529

[25] Hsich EM and Piña IL. (2009). Heart Failure in Women: A Need for Prospective Data. J Am Coll Cardiol N.54; 491-498

[26] Liu K et al. (1989) Ethnic differences in blood pressure, pulse rate, and related characteristics in young adults. The CARDIA study. Hypertension N:14:218-26

[27] Linde C.(2000) Women and arrhythmias. Pacing Clin Electrophysiol N: 23:1550-60

[28] Kadish AH. (1995) The effects of gender on cardiac electrophysiology and arrhythmias. In: Zipes DP, Jalife J, editors. Cardiac electrophysiology: from cell to bedside. 2nd ed. Philadelphia: WB Saunders; p. 1268-75

[29] Huikuri HV et al. (1996) Sex-related differences in autonomic modulation of heart rate in middle-aged subjects. Circulation N:94,122-5

[30] Burke JH et al.(1997) Gender-specific differences in the QT interval and the effect of autonomic tone and menstrual cycle in healthy adults. Am J Cardiol N:79,178-81

[31] Stramba-Badiale M et al.(1997) Gender and the relationship between ventricular repolarization and cardiac cycle length during 24-h Holter recordings. Eur Heart J N:18:1000-6

[32] Lehmann MH et al. (1997) Age-gender influence on the rate-corrected QT interval and the QT-heart rate relation in families with genotypically characterized long QT syndrome. J Am Coll Cardiol N:29, 93-9

[33] Locati EH et al.(1998) Age- and sex-related differences in clinical manifestations in patients with congenital long-QT syndrome: findings from the International LQTS Registry. Circulation N: 97, 2237-44

[34] Yarnoz MJ and Curtis AB.(2008) More reasons why men and women are not the same (gender differences in electrophysiology and arrhythmias). Am. J. Cardiol. N: 101 1291–1296

[35] Rollo P et al.(2001) Gender and Cardiac Arrhythmias Tex Heart Inst J 28, 265-75

[36] Lee RJ, Shinbane JS.(1997) Inappropriate sinus tachycardia. Diagnosis and treatment. Cardiol Clin N:15,599-605

[37] Morillo CA, Klein GJ, Thakur RK, Li H, Zardini M, Yee R.(1994) Mechanism of 'inappropriate' sinus tachycardia. Role of sympathovagal balance. Circulation N:90,873-7

[38] Rodriguez LM et al. (1992) Age at onset and gender of patients with different types of supraventricular tachycardias.Am J Cardiol N:70:1213-5

[39] Benjamin EJ et al.(1994) Independent risk factors for atrial fibrillation in a population-based cohort. The Framingham Heart Study. JAMA N:271,840-4

[40] Myerburg RJ et al. (1999) Cycling of inducibility of paroxysmal supraventricular tachycardia in women and its implications for timing of electrophysiologic procedures. Am J Cardiol N:83:1049-54

[41] Rosano GM et al.(1996) Cyclical variation in paroxysmal supraventricular tachycardia in women. Lancet N:347, 786–788

[42] Yarnoz MJ, Curtis AB.(2008) More reasons why men and women are not the same (gender differences in electrophysiology and arrhythmias. Am. J. Cardiol. N:101, 1291–1296

[43] Dagres N et al. (2007) Gender-related differences in presentation, treatment, and outcome of patients with atrial fibrillation in Europe: a report from the Euro Heart Survey on Atrial Fibrillation. J Am Coll Cardiol N: 49, 572–577

# 6

# Low-Level Exposure to Lead as a Cardiovascular Risk Factor

Anna Skoczynska and Marta Skoczynska
*Wroclaw Medical University,*
*Poland*

## 1. Introduction

Cardiovascular diseases are the main cause of death in many developed and developing countries around the world. Cardiovascular end points (myocardial infarction, stroke or sudden death) are strictly connected with prevalence of classic cardiovascular risk factors, such as smoking, sedimentary lifestyle, obesity, atherosclerotic lipid pattern and arterial hypertension. Also, many 'new' factors have been identified, e.g. hyperhomocysteinemia, increased fraction of small, dense LDL or lipoprotein (a), increased C-reactive protein, increased apo-B/apo-A ratio or some enzymes' increased activities (Skoczynska, 2006). However, traditional risk factors alone (nonmodifiable and modifiable alike) do not fully explain high incidence and mortality from these diseases. The effectiveness of different strategies concentrating on reducing known risk factors does not translate to a satisfactory reduction of incidence and mortality from myocardial infarction or stroke. It is essential to introduce strategies concerning 'new' risk-factors, as well as to identify those that remain unknown.

Heavy metals, such as lead, cadmium and mercury, are the most abundant xenobiotics in human environment. These metals are present in the air, house dust, soil, water, consumer products and some herbal remedies. Main toxicological problems result from these metals' accumulation in soil, water, plants and animals, which is responsible for human exposure to toxic metals many years after the cessation of the emission. The intrauterine exposure, which is especially dangerous, as metals pass the placental barrier (Bellinger et al., 1987), as well as lead exposure in early childhood (Roy et al., 2009), affects strongly immature tissues, mainly the central nervous system. Lead exposure during pregnancy has a clear impact on mental and behavioral development (Hu et al., 2006; Nie et al., 2011). It has been documented that there is no safe lead blood level and that its toxic action is present at levels much lower than previously suspected. Another problem is the existence of combined exposure to heavy metals, toxic and essential alike, in human natural environment. The disturbance in the homeostasis of trace metals (zinc, copper, calcium, iron, selenium) affects lead toxicity in the cardiovascular system (Faure et al., 1991; Kuliczkowski et al., 2004; Skoczynska et al., 1994).

Although the knowledge on low lead exposure effects on the heart and blood vessels is incomplete, it seems justified to put forward a thesis that environmental exposure to lead is a risk factor for developing a cardiovascular event. In case of this thesis' positive verification, conducted studies, aside from contributing new facts to the knowledge on lead toxicity, may become a set-point for solving practical issues, i.e. means for identification and reduction of lead exposure sources, diagnosis and monitoring of lead toxicity, prophylaxis and treatment of individuals with an increased body lead burden. This would allow to achieve long-term social benefits, such as a decrease in incidence and mortality from cardiovascular diseases.

## 2. The global decrease in exposure to lead

Together with industrialization and motorization, the world lead production had been rising till 1980s, when it reached over 3.8 million tons per year (Kelly & Matos, 2005). However, since the 1990s, in general, the exposure to lead around the world has declined. It has been caused by the elimination of leaded petrol, the decrease in sales of lead containing water pipes and canned foods, and the recall from production of lead containing paints.

In 1991, US Centers for Disease Control and Prevention (CDC) adopted the blood lead level of 10 µg/dL as a threshold for lead toxicity. In 1995, the same value was assumed by the World Health Organization. The United States National Health and Nutrition Examination Surveys (NHANES) have documented a dramatic decline in blood lead concentrations in US adults and children (Muntner et al., 2005). A decline in blood lead level has been found also in Australia (Rossi, 2008).

Despite legislative changes, in some developing countries the exposure to lead persists on an unchanged level. Only in 2000, in about 100 countries there was an exposure to leaded petrol. Lead is also used in the production of paints that are employed in maritime industry or to paint external building parts (Tong et al., 2000). In industrialized Asian, South and Latin American regions, also lead mining, smelting, battery factories, cottage industries, crystal glass foundries and glazed ceramics manufacturing are important antropogenic lead sources. In the nineties, in some industrial areas of China, the proportion of children with blood lead level exceeding 10 µg/dL reached 99% but in non-industrial regions was about 50% (Shen et al. 1996). Among children older than 18 months, living in the area of Mexico City, 44% had blood lead level higher than 10 µg/dL (Romieu et al., 1995). Similarly, in populations of children living in industrial regions of India, these proportions were disturbingly high and ranged from 40% to 62% (Conference on Lead Poisoning, Bangalore, 1999).

Still, the worst situation concerns Africa and is caused by lack of legislative regulations, low number of epidemiologic studies and little toxicological information (Mathee et al., 2006).

In many developed European countries, i.e. Belgium, Germany, Sweden and the United Kingdom, there was a decline in blood lead level between 1978 and 1988 (Tong et al., 2000). The research project entitled Public Health Impact of long-term, low-level Mixed Element exposure (PHIME) in a susceptible population revealed that the European population has been subjected to a dramatically lower exposure to lead since the abolition of lead from petrol. In spite of this fact, at PHIME Seminar 'Effects of exposure to metals; no margin of safety in Europe' at the European Environment Agency on 10th of February 2011, it was emphasized that 'lead pollution sources must continually be hunted down and stopped'. This recommendation is based on the observation that the level of exposure to lead associated with a reduced IQ in children seems to be much lower than previously known (Report of PHIME, 2011).

The exposure to lead in populations of Central-Eastern European countries is still dangerously high (Bogunia et al., 2007; Pawlas et al., 2008; Trzcinka-Ochocka et al., 2005). It is a consequence of political and economical neglect in the last decades. One of the main problems is lack of information on the factual level of environmental lead exposure.

## 3. The dependence of circulatory system changes on body lead burden

Lead does not fulfill any physiological function in the body and can be toxic even at a small blood concentration. At present, it is well documented that some neurological and cardiovascular effects of lead emerge at a blood lead level lower than adopted as a threshold, i.e. below 10 µg/dL. It has been estimated that blood lead level in a natural, non-contaminated environment amounts to 0.016 µg/dL, i.e. about 600 times lower than the standard adopted for children by the CDC (Flegal & Smith, 1992). In the 1980s-90s, it was shown that lead-induced hypertension develops as a result of the environmental exposure associated with the blood lead concentration of 10-40 µg/dL (Cheng et al., 2001; Harlan et al., 1985; Pirkle et al., 1985). Simultaneously, lead-induced changes in blood pressure were not large. Results of 31 meta-analyses showed only a slight increase in blood pressure at a doubled blood lead level; on average 1 mmHg for systolic and 0.6 mmHg for diastolic pressure (Nawrot & Staessen, 2002).

Also other studies performed in the 1980s-90s showed a toxic action of lead at a relatively low exposure, i.e. corresponding to the blood lead concentration of less than 25 µg/dL (Tong et al., 1998). In 2006, in *Circulation*, Menke et al. published data from NHANES analysis showing the association between blood lead level and mortality from both myocardial infarction and stroke. This association was significant at the lead level lower than 10 µg/dL (Menke et al., 2006).

The dependence of changes in the circulatory system on blood lead level is not clear. On the basis of literature, it seems likely that there is an inverse relationship, i.e. a lower exposure is associated with greater cardiovascular changes, similarly to the case of neurotoxic effects of lead in children (Lanphear et al., 2005).

In population studies of people exposed to lead, lead is determined in blood, urine and bone. The most frequently measured indicator of exposure is the blood concentration. Due to a relatively short half-life of lead in the blood (approximately 30 days), this biomarker does not reflect the body lead burden but rather a recent exposure to external or intrinsic sources (e.g. lead released into the blood from storage sites, in conditions such as acidosis, fever or infection). Therefore, a more reliable indicator of quantities of lead accumulated in the body is the bone concentration. Lead is measured in the skeletal system (in the tibia or in the patella) using the method of K-shell x-ray fluorescence (KXRF) (Arora et al., 2009).

The positive correlation between blood lead level and arterial pressure has been well documented. However, lead concentration in the patella better correlates with the occurrence of coronary heart disease than arterial hypertension. Also, it has been suggested that blood lead level is a better predictor of cardiovascular diseases in young people, and lead concentration in the skeleton in elderly (Weisskopf et al., 2009).

## 4. The lead effect on the cardiovascular system

### 4.1 Lead and arterial blood pressure

On the basis of numerous population studies in different settings, including prospective studies, it has been well documented that lead induces arterial hypertension. The majority of cross-sectional and prospective studies showed a significant association between blood lead level and systolic or diastolic blood pressure (Apostoli et al., 1992; Ding et al., 1998; Hu et al., 1996; Malvezzi et al., 2001; Micciolo et al., 1994; Schwartz, 1991; Takebayashi et al., 2011; Tsao et al., 2000; Weiss et al., 1988). These associations have been found in populations with different geographic, ethnic, and socioeconomic backgrounds (Martin et al., 2006). A positive correlation was also established between umbilical blood lead level and the occurence of arterial hypertension in pregnancy (Rabinowitz et al., 1987). The development of hypertension in workers chronically exposed to high lead levels has been interpreted as a consequence of lead-induced nephropathy (Agency for Toxic Substances and Disease Registry, 1999; U.S. Environmental Protection Agency, 2006). However, in workers occupationally exposed to lower than nephrotoxic lead levels, low blood lead concentration was found as a predictor of an increased systolic blood pressure (Sirivarasai et al., 2004; Telisman et al., 2001). Similarly, prospective studies showed a correlation between lead bone concentration and systolic blood pressure (Cheng et al. 2001; Glenn et al., 2003).

The impact of confounding factors on the relationship between body lead burden and arterial blood pressure can be reduced in experimental studies. Results of many studies performed on numerous experimental models, on various experimental animals (rats, rabbits, calf), have confirmed the hypertensive effect of small doses of lead and explained various mechanisms of this action. These mechanisms result from lead action on the central and peripheral nervous system (Hoffer et al., 1987; Nehru & Sidhu 2001; Silbergeld 1992; Reckziegel et al., 2011), the vessel wall (Ding et al., 1998; Dursun et al., 2005), the renin-angiotensin system (Rodriguez-Iturbe et al., 2005; Sharifi et al., 2004), the kallikrein system (Carmignani et al., 1999), metabolic processes (Skoczynska et al., 1993; Skoczynska et al., 2004), the generation of free radicals (Stohs & Bagchi 1995; Vaziri et al. 2001; Vaziri & Sica 2004), and intracellular signalling pathways (Carmignani et al., 2000), leading to an increase in the vascular tone, and the peripheral vascular resistance (Fig. 1).

It has been concluded that the evidence is sufficient to infer a causal relationship between lead exposure and arterial hypertension (Brown et al., 2011; Navas-Acien et al., 2007; Weisskopf et al., 2009). However, the most important mechanisms explaining the hypertensive effect of chronic low exposure to environmental lead still need an explanation. Hypertension induced by high doses of lead can be partially explained by the nephrotoxic action of this metal (Batuman, 1993; Navas-Acien et al., 2009). It is possible that also in low-lead exposed individuals an impaired renal function is responsible for a persistent increase in blood pressure, as an inverse association between the glomerular filtration rate and blood lead has been observed in people with blood lead levels as low as 10 µg/dL (Fadrowski et al., 2010), or even 5 µg/dL (Ekong et al., 2006). One of the problems to examine in the future is the exploration of dose – response relationship and the determination of the latency period for lead – induced hypertension.

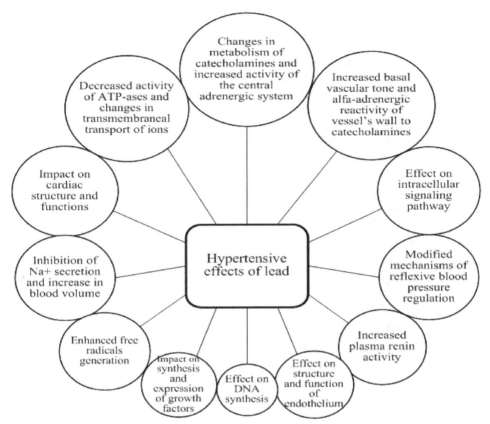

Fig. 1. Cardiovascular mechanisms of the hypertensive effect of low doses of lead (Skoczynska, 2006)

## 4.2 Lead and atherosclerosis

Aside from arterial hypertension, small amounts of lead cause also metabolic, functional and structural changes in the vessel wall. Some of these changes can accelerate the process of atherosclerosis. In the 1980s, in animal models, low-lead doses induced atherosclerosis was obtained (Revis et al., 1980,1981). Long-term lead exposure, measured by body lead store, was identified as a potential risk of intracranial carotid atherosclerosis in human (Lee et al., 2009). Some of the documented pro-atherosclerotic changes include: changes in lipid metabolism (Gatagonova, 1994; Kasperczyk et al., 2005a), endothelial dysfunctions (Ding et al., 1998; Vaziri et al., 2001), disturbances in essential metals' homeostasis (De Castro et al., 2010; Othman and Missiry, 1998; Wang et al., 2011), as well as an increase in free radicals' generation (Stohs and Bagchi 1995; Vaziri et al. 2001), a procoagulant state (Fujiwara et al., 2000; Kaji et al., 1991) and an inflammatory response (Heo et al., 1998) (Fig. 2).

In our previous studies performed on experimental animals exposed to small doses of lead, we have shown that an increased vessel wall reactivity to the catecholamines vasoconstricting action (Skoczynska et al., 1986; Skoczynska et al., 1987; Skoczynska et al.,

2001), an impaired vasodilatatory effect of acetylcholine (Skoczynska et al., 2005) and changes in vasoactive mediators blood levels (Skoczynska et al., 2003) are preceded by atherogenic dyslipidemia (Skoczynska et al., 1993), an increased lipid peroxidation, especially in the brain (Skoczynska et al.,1994), changes in the renin-angiotensin system (Wrobel & Skoczynska, 2002), and copper and zinc homeostasis (Skoczynska et al., 1994). In copper foundry workers exposed to lead, we have observed changes in vasoactive mediators blood levels (Skoczynska et al., 2002), hypertriglyceridemia (Skoczynska et al., 2007), an increased serum lipid peroxidation (Turczyn et al., 2010) and changes in copper and zinc homeostasis (Skoczynska et al., 2001).

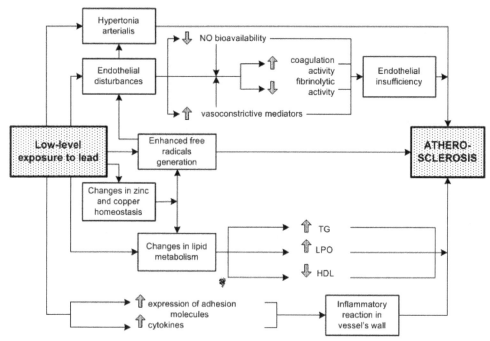

Fig. 2. Possible mechanisms of the pro-atherosclerotic action of lead (Skoczynska, 2006)

### 4.3 Lead and intermediate or immediate cardiovascular end points

Lead-induced changes in the circulatory system affect the occurrence of cardiovascular end points in lead exposed populations. Intermediate indicators of these events are functional and structural changes in the heart, such as changes in the left ventricular mass, heart rate, heart rate variability or electrocardiographic abnormalities. The 24-hour electrocardiographic evaluation performed in our centre in groups of men occupationally exposed to lead (copper foundry workers) showed that various heart rhythm disorders were more frequent as compared to the controls. A more frequent incidence of tachycardia (Gajek et al., 2004; Poręba et al., 2010a), a decreased heart rate variability (Poręba et al., 2011), and abnormal parameters of heart rate turbulence (Poręba et al., 2010a) were observed. In another group of men with arterial hypertension, occupationally exposed to lead, the study has demonstrated a significantly more frequent manifestation of left ventricular diastolic dysfunction and an increase in local arterial stiffness (Poręba et al., 2010b). However, lead exposed workers without hypertension also had an impaired diastolic function, compared with nonexposed controls (Beck & Steinmetz-Beck, 2005). In our earlier study, it was estimated that a ten-year risk of fatal cardiovascular disease (SCORE) in crystal glassworks' employees exposed to lead was higher in comparison to other workers (Doroszko et al., 2008). Also lipid disturbances were associated with the occupational exposure to lead (Skoczynska et al., 2007). All these changes were related to a relatively high blood lead level (above 40 μg/dL). Our newest experimental studies, using nuclear magnetic resonance, seem to confirm an increased incidence of left ventricular diastolic dysfunction in rats poisoned with small doses of lead (data in press).

In other studies, steel workers (Kasperczyk et al.,2005b) or battery workers (Tepper et al., 2001) exposed to lead displayed a higher left ventricular mass and/or a lower ejection fraction, compared to administrative workers from the same factories. On the other hand, in other studies, the interventricular septum and the left ventricular wall thickness determined in refinery workers with high blood lead level were similar to those determined in workers with lower blood lead concentration. Simultaneously, the decrease of diastolic cardiac function was more significant in the lead poisoned group (Zou et al., 1995). It may be concluded that results of studies performed on populations occupationally exposed to lead are inconsistent and the data on how lead affects the heart is insufficient. It remains unknown, for example, if lead, regardless of its hypertensive effect, leads to left ventricular diastolic dysfunction or changes heart rate variability.

There is no conclusion regarding the exact nature of lead influence on ECG. Since the 1970s, it has been known that lead increases heart sensitivity to noradrenaline arrhythmogenic action and causes bradycardia. Lead negative chronotropic action was associated with the blocking of heart beta adrenoreceptors activity (Bertel et al., 1978; Tsao et al. 2000). In various electrocardiographic studies, a significantly higher prevalence of heart ventricles repolarization disorders and heart rhythm disturbances was observed in groups of workers exposed to lead, in comparison to controls (Gatagonova 1995; Sroczynski et al., 1990). Among 775 men who participated in the Normative Aging Study, bone lead levels were found to be positively associated with heart rate, corrected QT and QRS intervals, especially in younger men. Additionally, a risk of intraventricular or atrioventricular block increased in men with elevated bone lead levels, whereas blood lead level was not associated with any of the electrocardiographic disturbances (Cheng et al., 1998; Eum et al., 2011). Authors of these studies suggest that the cumulative exposure to low lead levels causes electrocardiographic conduction disturbances. These disorders may be associated with the occurrence of different variants of genes involved in iron metabolism, such as hemochromatosis or heme oxygenase-1 genes. Park et al. found evidence that these genes' variants increase the impact of low-level lead exposure on the prolonged QT interval (Park et al., 2009). However, intermediate cardiovascular outcome varied across studies, and findings were incoherent.

Similarly, results of epidemiologic studies on the association between environmental low-lead exposure and immediate cardiovascular disease end points (coronary heart disease, stroke and cardiovascular disease other than arterial hypertension) are inconsistent. One of the first studies that analyzed a correlation between blood lead level and the incidence of coronary heart disease or stroke was The British Regional Heart Study. In this study, 7371 men aged 40 to 59 from 24 British towns were followed-up for 6 years. After allowing confounding effects of cigarette smoking and a town of residence, there was no evidence that blood lead level is a risk factor for major ischemic heart disease or stroke (Pocock et al., 1988). Also the study performed among 1052 inhabitants of Copenhagen County, who had the mean blood lead concentration of about 7 µg/dL in women and 18 µg/dL in men, and were observed for over 14 years, demonstrated a significant (p<0.03) risk for total mortality associated with blood lead but the risk for fatal and nonfatal cardiovascular disease or coronary complications was not significant (Møller & Kristensen, 1992).

On the contrary, studies published during 2002-2006 showed an increased cardiovascular mortality in the general population environmentally exposed to lead among individuals with blood lead levels from 20 µg/dL to 5 µg/dL.

The Second National Health and Nutrition Examination Survey (NHANES II), a national cross-sectional survey of the general US population conducted from 1976 to 1980, showed that individuals with blood lead levels of 20 to 29 µg/dL between 1976 and 1980 (15% of the US population at the time) experienced significantly increased all-cause, circulatory, and cardiovascular mortality from 1976 through 1992. After including the role of potential confounders, individuals with baseline blood lead levels of 20 to 29 µg/dL had a 46% increase in all-cause mortality (rate ratio (RR), 1.46; 95% confidence interval (CI), 1.14-1.86) and a 39% increase in circulatory mortality (RR, 1.39; 95% CI, 1.01-1.91), when compared to those with blood lead levels of less than 10 µg/dL (<0.5 µmol/L). All-cause mortality for those with blood lead levels of 10 to 19 µg/dL (0.5-0.9 µmol/L) was intermediately increased and statistically insignificant (Lustberg & Silbergeld, 2002).

The association between blood lead levels and increased all-cause and cardiovascular mortality was observed also at blood lead levels substantially lower than 20 µg/dL. In the Third National Health and Nutrition Examination Survey, which from 1988 to 1994 recruited 13,946 adult participants who were followed-up for up to 12 years for all-cause and cause-specific mortality, the geometric mean blood lead level in study participants was 2.58 µg/dL. After the multivariate adjustment, hazard ratios (95% CI) of participants in the highest tertile of blood lead (≥ 3.62 µg/dL) and those in the lowest tertile (< 1.94 µg/dL) were 1.25 (1.04 to 1.51; P(trend) across tertiles = 0.002) for all-cause mortality and 1.55 (1.08 to 2.24; P(trend) across tertiles = 0.003) for cardiovascular mortality. Blood lead level was significantly related to both myocardial infarction and stroke mortality, and the association was evident at levels ≥ 2 µg/dL) (Menke et al., 2006).

The second study based on the Third NHANES US community concerned 9,757 participants ≥ 40 years old put in three categories, depending on blood lead level: <5 µg/dL (the reference category), 5 to <10 and ≥10 µg/dL. The relative risk of mortality from all causes was 1.24 (95% confidence interval (CI), 1.05-1.48) for those with blood levels of 5 to <10 µg/dL and 1.59 (95% CI, 1.28-1.98) for those with blood levels ≥ 10 µg/dL (p for trend < 0.001) (Schober et al., 2006). To conclude, both studies based on the Third NHANES have documented an association between blood lead below 10 µg/dL and mortality among U.S. adults.

Also occupational exposure seems to be associated with an increased risk of cardiovascular diseases. In 1963, Dingwall-Fordyce and Lane published results of an analysis of the causes of death among workers who had been exposed to lead. There were 425 pensioners, 184 of whom had died; additionally, 153 deaths occurred among an unknown number of employees who had not yet reached the retirement age. This analysis provided evidence that heavy exposure to lead was associated with an increased incidence of deaths from cerebrovascular catastrophes (Dingwall-Fordyce & Lane, 1963). The study of 1261 typesetters exposed to low lead doses, started in 1961 and followed until the end of 1984, confirmed the increased cerebral mortality in workers subjected to prolonged exposure. The all-cause standardized mortality ratio was 0.74, the cardiac mortality ratio was 0.63, whereas the ratio for cerebrovascular disease was 1.35 (at the edge of statistical significance). For printers employed for 30 years or more, the cardiovascular mortality ratio was 1.68 (95% CI: 1.18-2.31; $p = 0.002$) (Michaels et al., 1991). In turn, in the prospective study described by Robinson in 1974, over 20 years (1947-67) the risk of mortality in a group of 592 tetraethyl lead workers and in a group of 660 non-exposed workers was similar. No difference between the two groups in either total mortality or mortality from specific diseases was found (Robinson, 1974). Other retrospective observation which covered 4.556 workers occupationally exposed to lead, diagnosed during 1970-1992, revealed increased total mortality (670 deaths; SMR = 108; 95% CI: 100-116) in comparison to the general population. However, the risk of cardiovascular mortality was significantly increased only in the subcohort with high exposure (153 deaths; SMR = 129; 95% CI: 109-151) (Wilczynska et al., 1998).

In analyses of results obtained from 13,043 South Korean lead workers with mean geometrical blood lead level of 6.01 µg/dL, the impact fractions for cardiac disease among lead workers would be estimated as about 5-13 times higher than those of the general population. Manufacture of accumulators, manufacture of other electronic valves, tubes, and components, and manufacture of accessories for motor vehicles were identified as a relatively important industry. Other industrial processes of relative importance included battery assembly, acid treatment and other soldering (Kim et al., 2008). Also in population of 420 male bus drivers in Thailand, with blood lead level ranging from 2.5 to 16.2 µg/dL (the mean of 6.3 ± 2.2 µg/dL), using the second derivative finger photoplethysmogram (SDPTG) as a marker of the cardiovascular risk, and allowing age, body mass index and lifestyle factors, a significant correlation between blood lead and SDPTG-AI was found (Kaewboonchoo et al., 2010).

## 4.4 Lead and peripheral artery disease

There have been no prospective studies on the association of blood lead with peripheral arterial disease (PAD). However, the relative risk for PAD, comparing blood lead levels ≥ 2.47 µg/dL versus < 1.03 µg/dL, in a cross-sectional analysis of NHANES 1999–2002, was 1.92. Data was obtained from 1999 to 2000, from 2125 participants who were ≥ 40 years of age. Peripheral arterial disease was defined as a condition with an ankle brachial index lower than 0.9 in at least one leg (Muntner et al., 2005). After adjustment for demographic and cardiovascular risk factors, the odds ratios of peripheral arterial disease, comparing the second, third and fourth quartile of blood lead level with the lowest quartile, were 1.63, 1.92 and 2.88, respectively. It was concluded that blood lead (as well as cadmium) is associated with an increased prevalence of peripheral arterial disease in the general U.S. population (Navas-Acien et al., 2004). Simultaneously, lead levels in urine (contrary to cadmium) were not associated with PAD at the levels found in this population (Navas-Acien et al., 2005). In turn, the observed association of homocysteine level and PAD can be completely explained by confounding due to smoking, increased blood lead and cadmium levels and impaired renal function (Guallar et al., 2006). The disturbances in homocysteine metabolism (Poręba et al., 2005) and the negative linear correlation between blood lead levels and the ankle-brachial index (Doroszko et al., 2008) were found also in workers occupationally exposed to lead; however, the latter relationship was discovered only in a subgroup of workers with a normal lipid pattern. Results obtained by Schafer et al. showed that hyperhomocysteinemia could be a mechanism that underlies lead effects on the cardiovascular and central nervous systems, possibly offering new targets for prevention of long-term consequences of lead exposure (Schafer et al., 2005).

In 2009, Weisskopf et al. published results of the analysis of all observational studies from database searches and citations regarding lead, intermediate and immediate cardiovascular end points. Studies in general populations have identified a positive association between lead exposure and coronary heart disease, cardiac mortality, cerebral mortality and peripheral arterial disease. Estimates of the relative risk of cardiovascular mortality in workers exposed to lead varied widely across occupational studies; with positive, inverse or null correlations. The positive association between lead levels and cardiovascular mortality occurred in workers with the heaviest exposure. Authors concluded that the evidence is suggestive but not sufficient to infer a causal relationship of lead exposure and clinical cardiovascular outcomes. There is also a suggestive but insufficient evidence to infer a causal relationship of lead exposure and heart rate variability (Weisskopf et al., 2009).

## 5. Genetic polymorphisms and lead toxicity

Human sensitivity to toxic effect of heavy metals differs depending on age, sex, general health status, quantitative and qualitative alimental deficiency, diet, smoking, lifestyle, place of inhabitancy and socioeconomical status, hygienic habituation, total occupational and environmental exposure to xenobiotics. Some of the critical effects of lead result from lead interference with enzymatic processes responsible for the synthesis of heme. These include the inhibition of delta-aminolevulinic acid dehydratase (ALAD), changes in the concentration of delta-aminolevulinic acid in urine (ALA-U), blood (ALA-B) or plasma (ALA-P), changes in the concentration of coproporhyrin in urine and zinc protoporphyrin (ZP) in blood. As a result of exposure to lead, there is a decrease in activity of blood pyrimidine nucleotidase (P5'N) and nicotinamide adenine dinucleotide synthetase (NADS), as well as changes in nucleotides' blood content. All these effects have been used as biomarkers of lead toxicity (Skoczynska, 2006). Genetic polymorphisms that affect lead toxicokinetics and toxicodynamics may be important factors modifying the risk of harmful effects of lead in vulnerable populations.

Differences in lead effect on the heme synthesis pathway, observed between different representatives of the same population exposed to lead, may be determined by different types of the ALAD gene. In turn, the differences between heme precursors levels in different ALAD genotypes can be related to a varied lead affinity to different ALAD isozymes. Thus, ALAD1 homozygotes (a genotype more frequent than ALAD 1-2) might be more susceptible to disturbances in heme metabolism caused by lead exposure than ALAD2 carriers (Sakai et al., 2000; Suzen et al., 2003). ALAD 1-1 subjects might be also more susceptible to the cytogenetic effect of lead than ALAD 1-2 subjects (Alexander et al., 1998; Dyudu & Suzen 2003). ALAD polymorphisms may be also involved in the emergence of lead-induced arterial hypertension. In terms of exposure to large doses of lead, ALAD polymorphisms are associated with lead-induced renal hyperfiltration (Weaver et al., 2003). It has been shown, that ALAD 1-2 variants affect the presence of the association between renal function and bone (the tibia or the patella) lead level. Similarly, variant B of the vitamin D receptor gene modifies renal sufficency, although only in young population exposed to high doses of lead (Weaver et al., 2006). Also the impact of endothelial nitric oxide synthase (eNOS) gene polymorphisms on kidney function has been demonstrated in employees exposed chronically to lead: the presence of the Asp allele was associated with higher serum creatinine than the genotype Glu/Glu (Weaver et al., 2003). Lead and selected genes, i.e. vitamin D receptor (VDR) and ALAD genes, may influence blood pressure and risk of hypertension. In a group of workers, 798 exposed to lead and 135 non-exposed, VDR genotypes (BB and Bb vs. Bb), lead concentration in the blood and in the tibia, and the amount of lead bound by dimercapto-succinic acid were all positive predictors of systolic blood pressure. Lead exposed individuals with the VDR B allele, mainly heterozygotes, had systolic blood pressures that were 2.7-3.7 mm Hg higher than in workers with the bb genotype. VDR genotype was also associated with diastolic blood pressure; lead workers with the VDR B allele had diastolic blood pressures that were 1.9-2.5 mm Hg higher than in lead workers with the VDR bb genotype (p = 0.04). In addition, compared to lead workers with the VDR bb genotype, workers with the VDR B allele had a higher prevalence of hypertension (adjusted odds ratio (95% confidence interval) = 2.1 (1.0, 4.4), p = 0.05) and a larger increase in blood pressure with age (Lee et al., 2001).

In the analysis described by Scinicariello et al., on the basis of data obtained from adults who participated in the Third NHANES, whose DNA was available (n=6,016), multivariable logistic and linear regressions stratified by race/ethnicity were used to examine whether blood pressure was associated with the ALAD gene and blood lead levels. Blood lead level was associated with systolic pressure in non-Hispanic whites and with hypertension, systolic and diastolic pressures in non-Hispanic blacks, but not in Mexican Americans. Non-Hispanic white ALAD2 carriers of the highest blood lead level quartile had a significantly higher adjusted prevalence odds ratio for hypertension compared with ALAD1 homozygous individuals. In addition, a significant interaction between lead concentration and the ALAD2 allele, in relation to systolic blood pressure, was shown in non-Hispanic whites and non-Hispanic blacks (Scinicariello et al., 2010).

Also a mutation of the hemochromatosis gene (HFE H63D) has been associated with changes in blood pressure, examined as the pulse pressure (the difference between systolic and diastolic blood pressure) within the Normative Aging Study between 1991-2001. Baseline bone lead levels, markers of the cumulative lead exposure, are associated with steeper increases in pulse pressure in men with at least one H63D allele (p-interaction = 0.03 for tibia and 0.02 for patella), compared with men with only wild types or C282Y variant (Zhang et al., 2010). HFE variants are associated also with increased blood lead levels in young children (Hopkins et al., 2008).

Lead induces arterial hypertension in the consequence of low exposure, which may be not manifested by a toxic effect on the marrow, kidneys or other organs. The existence of lead hypertensive effect, in the range of blood concentration lower than 40 µg/dL, has been supported by numerous experimental and population studies. However, the presence of a significant correlation between blood lead level and systolic and/or diastolic blood pressure has not been confirmed by all of performed epidemiologic tests. These discrepancies can be explained by the fact that lead-induced hypertension results rather from the past than from the current exposure, and hence arterial pressure values should be rather related to bone than to blood lead level. The occurrence of polymorphisms of genes involved in lead toxic effect may stand for another explanation. Interactions between lead toxicity and ALAD or HFE genes polymorphisms were observed in occupational and epidemiologic studies. These polymorphisms, occurring singularly or in an association with other polymorphisms (e.g. the vitamin D receptor gene), seem to be involved in lead-induced hypertension. Results of experimental studies indicate that the correlation between lead exposure, arterial blood pressure and the presence of polymorphisms of angiotensin converting enzyme and beta(2)adrenergic receptor genes should be analyzed in the general population. It is likely that studies of these polymorphisms, gene-to-gene interactions and interactions between genes and environmental factors may provide the identification of causes of so called spontaneous hypertension (Skoczynska, 2008).

## 6. Problems related to lead toxicity

It has been established that low level exposure to lead induces arterial hypertension. However, the data of many studies is suggestive but insufficient to infer that low level exposure to lead increases the occurrence of cardiovascular end points. The causal interference between lead exposure and immediate as well as some of intermediate end points needs a further explanation. The dose-effect relationship in the cardiovascular action of lead also remains unclear. It is possible that only low and recent exposure to lead is associated with arterial hypertension. Perhaps, there is an inverse relationship between blood lead levels and blood pressure values, similarly as in neurotoxic effects of lead in young organisms. It is also possible that cardiac end points are associated with long-term exposure to lead, which would be implied by the existent relationship between the patella lead and the occurrence of coronary heart disease.

Subsequently, blood lead level, most often determined spectrophotometrically, is variable and depends not only on external but also internal exposure. Factors such as fever, alcohol and acidosis cause a mobilization of lead from organs and from the skeleton. A single measurement of blood lead should be therefore verified, which is frequently practiced in occupationally exposed but would be difficult to apply to the general population. In turn, bone (the tibia or the patella) lead concentration, an established marker of accumulated lead, is determined using the method of K-shell x-ray fluorescence. This marker is more stable in comparison to blood lead but more difficult and expensive to measure.

In the population analysis of data on lead cardiovascular effects, it is indispensable to determine the role of confounding factors. The presence of a greater number of these factors cause incoherence in studies' results. Factors such as race, education, income, urban versus rural location and socioeconomic status should be considered. There are especially great difficulties in establishing how hypertension impacts relations between low exposure to lead and other than hypertension lead effects. Hypertension may result from lead action or occur independently but in each case constitutes a factor that confounds relations between lead and e.g. coronary heart disease or stroke. Similarly, disturbances in lipid and homocysteine metabolism or trace metals homeostasis may be simultaneously confounding factors and results of lead action.

## 7. Chelation treatment for lead poisoning

The chelation treatment has historically been used to reduce body lead burden in patients with severe symptoms of poisoning with lead. Chelating agents are organic compounds capable of linking together metal ions to form complex ring-like structures, which are subsequently excreted with urine. Effectiveness of chelation depends on whether the chelating agent is able to reach the intracellular site where the heavy metal is firmly bound. This intracellular availability is conditioned by many factors, e.g. ionic diameter, intra/extracellular compartmentalization and excretion pathway. Hydrophilic chelators are most effective in metals' excretion with urine, but they weaken complex intracellular metal deposits, whereas lipophilic chelators can redistribute toxic metals to lipid-rich organs, e.g. the brain (Andersen & Aaseth, 2002).

The chelation is usually performed using calcium disodium ethylenediamine tetra acetic acid (CaNa$_2$EDTA) and a preceeded administration of calcium. A contraindication to chelation is hypocalcemia or renal insufficiency. Also D-penicillamine and British anti-lewisite (BAL) have been used as antidotes for acute and chronic poisoning. 2, 3-dimercaprol (BAL) has long been the mainstay of chelation therapy for lead or arsenic poisoning. A thiol chelating agent, meso-2,3,-dimercaptosuccinic acid (DMSA), an analogue of BAL, has been tried successfully in animals as well as in a few cases of human lead and arsenic intoxication. DMSA could be a safe and effective method of treatment, but one of the major disadvantages of chelation with DMSA is its inability to remove lead from the intracellular sites because of its lipophobic nature (Kalia & Flora, 2005).

Even after many years of chelation, an effective treatment of patient poisoned with lead is difficult to obtain. New trends in chelation therapy including combined treatment are promising. This includes the use of structurally different chelators or a combination of an adjuvant and a chelator to provide better clinical and biochemical recovery, in addition to lead mobilization. Kalia et al. compared the therapeutic efficacy of captopril and DMSA, either individually, or in combination, against arsenite induced oxidative stress and metal mobilization in rats. Interestingly, combined administration of captopril and DMSA had a remarkable effect in depleting total arsenic concentration from blood and soft tissues. In addition, captopril administration during chelation treatment had beneficial effects particularly on the protection of inhibited blood ALAD activity (Kalia et al., 2007).

The therapeutic efficacy of melatonin or N-acetylcysteine (NAC) in reducing lead concentration in blood and other soft tissues was studied individually and in combination with DMSA. Administration of melatonin and NAC individually provided protection to the antioxidant defense, which disturbed by lead may significantly compromise a normal cellular function. Administration of melatonin and NAC (a thiol containing antioxidant) provided an increase in tiobarbituric acid levels, reduced glutathione and oxidized glutathione contents in tissues, which suggests these drugs' ability to act as free radical scavengers and to protect cells against toxic insult. In turn, a combined treatment of DMSA and NAC provided more pronounced efficacy in restoring altered biochemical variables and in reducing body lead burden than monotherapy with DMSA. The results suggest the involvement of ROS in lead toxicity and a pronounced beneficial role of NAC in therapeutic implications of lead poisoning, when co-administered with a thiol chelator (DMSA). They also support the hypothesis that cellular redox status may be significantly reversed by utilizing a thiol containing an antioxidant compound. Authors concluded that combined therapy with an antioxidant moiety and a thiol-chelating agent may be a better choice for treating plumbism (Flora et al., 2004a).

It has been suggested that a concomitant administration of an antioxidant could play a significant and important role in abating a number of toxic effects of lead, when administered with thiol chelators. Flora et al. also investigated the effect of taurine, an amino acid and a known antioxidant, either alone or in combination with DMSA, in the treatment of subchronic lead intoxication in male rats. DMSA was able to increase the activity of ALAD, while both taurine and DMSA were able to significantly increase GSH level and bring them towards normal. In animals treated with taurine, there has been a reduction of changes of biochemical parameters indicative of oxidative stress, especially in the brain. The data also implied a promising role of taurine during chelation of lead, as a possible potentiator of the depletion of blood, liver and brain lead, compared to DMSA alone (Flora et al., 2004b).

Chelation is a beneficial therapy in case of chronic intoxication with heavy metals. This therapy is of smaller significance in case of acute poisoning, which is a result of a complex clinical situation. Acute metal intoxication usually proceeds with multiorgan distress syndrome, determining contraindications to treatment with chelators. Symptoms of kidney or liver dysfunction limit credibility of indicators monitoring chelator's effectiveness. As a rule, patients need the intensive care and symptomatic treatment. However, the moment chelators are allowed to include, the chelation therapy can determine the prognosis. In workers occupationally exposed to heavy metals, chelation can serve as a prognostic procedure, useful in occupational risk estimation. It also enables to undertake appropriate actions. Temporary or lasting discontinuation of work in exposition to lead, before clinical symptoms appear, results in a significant decrease in the occupational lead poisoning.

However, due to metal accumulation in tissues, chelation is not a fully effective therapy and needs repeated doses of drugs, usually administered through the parenteral way. A combined therapy, an antioxidant plus chelator, does not seem to be the best choice for all of the patients poisoned with metals. This therapy can be beneficial only if an antioxidant is simultaneously a chelator, as it is in case of N-acetylcysteine. Then, the additive impact of both chelators is expected. The effectiveness of the therapy with an antioxidant is significantly dependent on patient's oxidative status at the beginning of the treatment. This effect, due to the antioxidant potential, can be beneficial as well as aggravating. It concerns especially metals which do not undergo Fenton's reaction: cadmium, lead, mercury. Additionally, the use of antioxidants without chelators, i.e. in the prevention of cardiovascular diseases, showed only equivocal benefits resulting from the antioxidant supplementation. Moreover, some of patients showed an increased number of cardiovascular end points and incidence of neoplasms. New long-term chelators, consisting of structurally different components (including N-acetylcysteine), are needed.

To summarize, chelation is a common therapy in case of poisoning with toxic metals but it is only partially satisfactory because of metal accumulation in tissues. A combined therapy with long term, structurally different chelators could become a viable alternative in the future.

In developed countries, workers occupationally exposed to lead at high concentrations (i.e. copper founders) are subjected to biological monitoring. Chelation, which is practised as a part of the monitoring, decreases body burden with toxic metals. In the nearest future, it is essential to began a study on the effect of chelation on arterial blood pressure and cardiovascular end points in workers exposed to lead.

## 8. Plan for the future

Current investigations, which will continue after previous clinical, epidemiologic and experimental studies, are to explain whether environmental exposure to lead is a risk factor for development of vascular changes in the heart, brain and legs. They are also designed to explain the role of homocysteine and lead-iron interactions in cardiac and vascular effects of lead. The final purpose of project is the assessment of environmental exposure to lead as a lowering average life expectation factor.

Further cross-sectional and prospective studies, combined epidemiological and toxicological, on the presence of the relationship between blood lead concentrations and prevalence of coronary heart disease, stroke and peripheral artery disease are needed. Confounding factors' (male sex, age over 65, smoking, hypertension, diabetes and abnormal lipid pattern) influence on studied relations should be considered. DNA isolation should be conducted in order to determine the frequency of genetic polymorphisms that may influence the presence of a relationship between blood lead levels and ischemic heart disease or stroke. It should also be researched whether polymorphisms of determined genes (e.g. beta receptor and vitamin D receptor genes, or PPAR alpha and lipoprotein lipase genes) affect lead-induced hypertension or lead-induced changes in the lipid pattern. Moreover, the determination of iron and homocysteine role in lead toxic effects is needed.

Obtained results may confirm the thesis that environmental exposure to lead is a risk factor for developing a cardiovascular event. In case of a positive verification, conducted studies may become a set-point for solving practical issues, i.e. providing means of reducing sources of lead exposure and/or lead toxicity (chelators, antioxidants). Probably, current environmental safety standards for blood lead level ought to be lowered. A criterion for elevated lead exposure screening needs to be verified not only in children but also in adults. The risk assessment of lead exposure impact should include lead cardiovascular effects. The risk assessment of cardiovascular end points should include the information on lead exposure.

## 9. References

Alexander B.H., Checkoway H., Costa-Mallen P., Faustman E.M., Woodes J.S., Kelsey K.T., VanNetten C., Costa L.G. Interaction of blood lead and delta-aminolevulinic acid dehydratase genotype on markers of heme synthesis and sperm production in lead smelter workers. Environ Health Perspect. 1998; 106(4):213-6.

Andersen O., Aaseth J. Molecular mechanisms of in vivo metal chelation: implications for clinical treatment of metal intoxications. Environ Health Perspect. 2002; 5:887-90.

Apostoli P., Maranelli G., Micciolo R. Is hypertension a confounding factor in the assessment of blood lead reference values? Sci Total Environ. 1992; 120: 127-134.

Arora M., Weuve J., Weisskopf M.G., Sparrow D., Nie H., Garcia R.I., Hu H. Cumulative lead exposure and tooth loss in men: the normative aging study. Environ Health Perspect. 2009 Oct;117(10):1531-4. Epub 2009 Jun 15.

Batuman V. Lead nephropathy, gout and hypertension. Am J Med Sci. 1993; 305: 241-247.

Beck B., Steinmetz-Beck A. Echocardiographic evaluation of left ventricular function in persons with chronic professional exposure to lead. Adv Clin Exp Med. 2005; 14(5):905-916

Bellinger D., Leviton A., Waternaux C., Needleman H., Rabinowitz M. Longitudinal analyses of prenatal and postnatal lead exposure and early cognitive development. N Engl J Med. 1987 Apr 23;316(17):1037-43.

Bertel O., Bühler F.R., Ott J. Lead-induced hypertension: blunted beta-adrenoceptor-mediated functions. Br Med J. 1978 Mar 4;1(6112):551

Bogunia M., Kwapuliński J., Bogunia E., Brodziak B., Ahnert B., Nogaj E., Kowol J., Rzepka J., Winiarska H., Wojtanowska M. Lead content in blood of children living near zinc smelter plant exposure on environmental tobacco smoking (ETS). Przegl. Lek. 2007;64(10):723-8.

Brown M.J., Raymond J., Homa D., Kennedy C., Sinks T. Association between children's blood lead levels, lead service lines, and water disinfection, Washington, DC, 1998-2006. Environ Res. 2011 Jan;111(1):67-74. Epub 2010 Nov 26.

Carmignani M., Boscolo P., Poma A., Volpe A.R. Kininergic system and arterial hypertension following chronic exposure to inorganic lead. Immunopharmacology, 1999, 44(1-2), 105-10.

Carmignani M., Volpe A.R., Boscolo P., Qiao N., Di Gioacchino M., Grilli A. Catcholamine and nitric oxide systems as targets of chronic lead exposure in inducing selective functional impairment.Life Sci. 2000; 68(4): 401-15.

Cheng Y., Schwartz J., Sparrow D., Aro A., Weiss S.T., Hu H. Bone lead and blood lead levels in relation to baseline blood pressure and the prospective development of hypertension: the Normative Aging Study. Am J Epidemiol. 2001 15;153(2):164-71.

Cheng Y., Schwartz J., Vokonas P.S., Weiss S.T., Aro A., Hu H. Electrocardiographic conduction disturbances in association with low-level lead exposure (the Normative Aging Study). Am J Cardiol. 1998 Sep 1;82(5):594-9.

De Castro C.S., Arruda A.F., Da Cunha L.R., SouzaDe J.R., Braga J.W., Dórea J.G. Toxic metals (Pb and Cd) and their respective antagonists (Ca and Zn) in infant formulas and milk marketed in Brasilia, Brazil. Int J Environ Res Public Health. 2010 Nov;7(11):4062-77.

Ding Y., Vaziri N.D., Gonick H.C.: Lead - induced hypertension. II. Response to sequential infusions of L-arginine, superoxide dismutase, and nitroprusside. Environ Res. 1998; 76:107-113.

Dingwall-Fordyce I., Lane R.E. A follow-up study of lead workers. Br J Ind Med. 1963 Oct;20:313-5.

Doroszko A., Skoczynska A., Drożdż K., Kreczyńska B. Cardiovascular risk in workers ocupationally exposed to lead. Part II. The impact of lead on the cardiovascular function on the basis of ECG, ABI and intima media thickness evaluation. Med.Pracy 2008; 59(5): 355-363. 29.

Dursun N., Arifoglu C., Süer C., Keskinol L. Blood pressure relationship to nitric oxide, lipid peroxidation, renal function, and renal blood flow in rats exposed to low lead levels. Biol Trace Elem Res. 2005 May; 104(2):141-9.

Duydu Y., Suzen H.S. Influence of delta-aminolevulinic acid dehydratase (ALAD) polymorphism on the frequency of sister chromatid exchange (SCE) and the number of high-frequency cells (HFCs) in lymphocytes from lead-exposed workers. Mutat Res. 2003; 540(1):79-88.

Eum K.D., Nie L.H., Schwartz J., Vokonas P.S., Sparrow D., Hu H., Weisskopf M.G. Prospective cohort study of lead exposure and electrocardiographic conduction disturbances in the Department of Veterans Affairs Normative Aging Study. Environ Health Perspect. 2011 Jul; 119(7):940-4. Epub 2011 Mar 16.

Fadrowski J., Navas-Acien A., Tellez-Plaza M., Guallar E., Weaver V.M., Furth S.L. Blood lead level and kidney function in US adolescents: The Third National Health and Nutrition Examination Survey. Arch Intern Med. 2010; 170(1):75-82.

Faure P., Roussel A.M., Richard M.J., Foulon T., Groslambert P., Hadjian A., Favier A. Effect of an acute zinc depletion on rat lipoprotein distribution and peroxidation. Biol Trace Elem Res. 1991 Feb; 28(2):135-46.

Flegal A.R., Smith D.R. Current needs for increased accuracy and precision in measurements of low levels of lead in blood. Environ Res. 1992 Aug; 58(2):125-33.

Flora S.J., Pande M., Bhadauria S., Kannan G.M. Combined administration of taurine and meso 2,3-dimercaptosuccinic acid in the treatment of chronic lead intoxication in rats. Hum Exp Toxicol. 2004; 23:157-66 (a).

Flora S.J., Pande M., Kannan G.M., Mehta A. Lead induced oxidative stress and its recovery following co-administration of melatonin or N-acetylcysteine during chelation with succimer in male rats. Cell Mol Biol (Noisy-le-grand). 2004; 50 Online Pub:OL543-51 (b).

Fujiwara Y., Yamamoto C., Kaji T. Proteoglycans synthesized by cultured bovine aortic smooth muscle cells after exposure to lead: lead selectively inhibits the synthesis of versican, a large chondroitin sulfate proteoglycan. Toxicology, 2000; 154: 9-19.

Gajek J., Zyśko D., Chlebda E. Heart rate variability in workers chronically exposed to lead. Kardiol Pol. 2004; 61(7):21-30.

Gatagonova T.M. Bioelectrical activity of the myocardium and cardiac pump function in workers engaged in lead production. Gig Sanit. 1995 May-Jun; (3):16-9.

Gatagonova T.M. Characteristics of the serum lipids in workers of lead industry. Med Tr Prom Ekol. 1994; (12):17-21.

George Foundation. Project lead-free: a study of lead poisoning in major Indian cities. In: Proceedings of the International Conference on Lead Poisoning, Bangalore, India, 8-10 February 1999. Bangalore, The George Foundation, 1999: 79-86.

Glenn B.S., Stewart W.F., Links J.M., Todd A.C., Schwartz B.S. The longitudinal association of lead with blood pressure. Epidemiology 2003; 14(1):30-6.

Guallar E., Silbergeld E.K., Navas-Acien A., Malhotra S., Astor B.C., Sharrett A.R., Schwartz B.S. Confounding of the relation between homocysteine and peripheral arterial disease by lead, cadmium, and renal function. Am J Epidemiol. 2006 Apr 15; 163(8):700-8. Epub 2006 Feb 16.

Harlan W.R., Landis J.R., Schmouder R.L., Goldstien N.G., Harlan L.C. Blood lead and blood pressure. JAMA. 1985; 253: 530–534.

Heo Y., Lee W.T.: Lawrence D.A.: Differential effects of lead and cAMP on development and activities of Th1- and Th2-lymphocytes. Toxicol. Sci., 1998, 43, 172-178.

Hoffer B.J., Olson L., Palmer M.R. Toxic effects of lead in the developing nervous system: in oculo experimental models. Environ Health Perspect. 1987; 74:169-75.

Hopkins M.R., Ettinger A.S., Hernández-Avila M., Schwartz J., Téllez-Rojo M.M., Lamadrid-Figueroa H., Bellinger D., Hu H., Wright R.O. Variants in iron metabolism genes predict higher blood lead levels in young children. Environ Health Perspect. 2008 Sep; 116(9):1261-6.

Hu H., Hashimoto D., Besser M. Levels of lead in blood and bone of women giving birth in a Boston hospital.Arch Environ Health. 1996; 51(1): 52-8.

Hu H., Téllez-Rojo M.M., Bellinger D., Smith D., Ettinger A.S., Lamadrid-Figueroa H., Schwartz J., Schnaas L., Mercado-García A., Hernández-Avila M. Fetal lead exposure at each stage of pregnancy as a predictor of infant mental development. Environ Health Perspect. 2006 Nov; 114(11):1730-5.

Kaewboonchoo O., Morioka I., Saleekul S., Miyai N., Chaikittiporn C., Kawai T. Blood lead level and cardiovascular risk factors among bus drivers in Bangkok, Thailand. Ind Health. 2010; 48(1):61-5.

Kaji T., Sakamoto M. Stimulation of heparan sulphate release from cultured endothelial cells by plasmin. Blood Coagul Fibrinolysis. 1991; 2(3): 419-23.

Kalia K., Flora S.J. Strategies for safe and effective therapeutic measures for chronic arsenic and lead poisoning. J Occup Health. 2005; 47:1-21.

Kalia K., Narula G.D., Kannan G.M., Flora S.J. Effects of combined administration of captopril and DMSA on arsenite induced oxidative stress and blood and tissue arsenic concentration in rats. Comp Biochem Physiol C Toxicol Pharmacol. 2007; 144:372-9.

Kasperczyk J. Lipids, lipid peroxidation and 7-ketocholesterol in workers exposed to lead. Hum Exp Toxicol. 2005 Jun; 24(6):287-95.

Kasperczyk S., Przywara-Chowaniec B., Kasperczyk A., Rykaczewska-Czerwińska M., Wodniecki J., Birkner E., Dziwisz M., Krauze-Wielicka M. Function of heart muscle in people chronically exposed to lead. Ann Agric Environ Med. 2005; 12(2):207-10.(b)

Kelly T.D. & Matos G.R. Historical statistics for mineral and material commodities in the United States. In: U.S. Geological Survey, 140, 2005, Lead: 20.08.2011, at http://pubs.usgs.gov/ds/2005/140/.

Kim K.R., Lee S.W., Paik N.W., Choi K. Low-level lead exposure among South Korean lead workers, and estimates of associated risk of cardiovascular diseases. J Occup Environ Hyg. 2008 Jun; 5(6):399-416.

Kuliczkowski W., Jołda-Mydłowska B., Kobusiak-Prokopowicz M., Antonowicz-Juchniewicz J., Kosmala W. Effect of heavy metal ions on function of vascular endothelium in patients with ischemic heart disease. Pol Arch Med Wewn. 2004 Jun; 111(6):679-85.

Lanphear B.P., Hornung R., Khoury J., Yolton K., Baghurst P., Bellinger D.C., Canfield R.L., Dietrich K.N., Bornschein R., Greene T., Rothenberg S.J., Needleman H.L., Schnaas L., Wasserman G., Graziano J., Roberts R. Low-level environmental lead exposure and children's intellectual function: an international pooled analysis. Environ Health Perspect. 2005 Jul; 113(7):894-9.

Lead-related nephrotoxicity: a review of the epidemiologic evidence. Ekong E.B., Jaar B.G., Weaver V.M. Lead-related nephrotoxicity: a review of the epidemiologic evidence. Kidney Int. 2006 Dec; 70(12):2074-84.

Lee B.K., Lee G.S., Stewart W.F., Ahn K.D., Simon D., Kelsey K.T., Todd A.C., Schwartz B.S. Associations of blood pressure and hypertension with lead dose measures and polymorphisms in the vitamin D receptor and delta-aminolevulinic acid dehydratase genes. Environ Health Perspect. 2001: 109(4):383-9.

Lee T.H., Tseng M.C., Chen C.J., Lin J.L. Association of high body lead store with severe intracranial carotid atherosclerosis. Neurotoxicology. 2009 Nov; 30(6):876-80. Epub 2009 Jul 16.

Lustberg M. & Silbergeld E. Blood lead levels and mortality. Arch Intern Med. 2002; 162:2443-2449.

Malvezzi C.K., Moreira E.G., Vassilieff I, Vassilieff V.S., Cordellini S.: Effect of L-arginine, DMSA and the association of L-arginine and DMSA on tissue lead mobilization and blood pressure level in plumbism. Brazilian J of Medical and Biological Research. 2001; 34: 1341-1346.

Martin D., Glass T.A., Bandeen-Roche K., Todd A.C., Shi W., Schwartz B.S. Association of blood lead and tibia lead with blood pressure and hypertension in a community sample of older adults. Am J Epidemiol. 2006 Mar 1; 163(5):467-78. Epub 2006 Jan 18.

Mathee A., Röllin H., von Schirnding Y., Levin J., Naik I. Reductions in blood lead levels among school children following the introduction of unleaded petrol in South Africa. Reductions in blood lead levels among school children following the introduction of unleaded petrol in South Africa

Menke A., Muntner P., Batuman V., Silbergeld E.K., Guallar E. Blood lead below 0.48 µmol/L (10 µg/dL) and mortality among US adults. Circulation. 2006; 114: 1388–1394.

Micciolo R., Canal L., Maranelli G., Apostoli P. Non-occupational lead exposure and hypertension in northern Italy. Int J Epidemiol. 1994; 23: 312-320.

Michaels D., Zoloth S.R., Stern F.B. Does low-level lead exposure increase risk of death? A mortality study of newspaper printers. Int J Epidemiol. 1991 Dec;20(4):978-83.

Møller L. & Kristensen T.S. Blood lead as a cardiovascular risk factor. Am J Epidemiol. 1992; 136: 1091–1100.

Muntner P., Menke A., DeSalvo K.B., Rabito F.A., Batuman V. Continued decline in blood lead levels among adults in the United States: the National Health and Nutrition Examination Surveys. Arch Intern Med. 2005 Oct; 10;165(18):2155-61.

Navas-Acien A., Guallar E., Silbergeld E.K., Rothenberg S.J. Lead exposure and cardiovascular disease--a systematic review. Environ Health Perspect. 2007 Mar; 115(3):472-82.

Navas-Acien A., Selvin E., Sharrett A.R., Calderon-Aranda E., Silbergeld E., Guallar E. Lead, cadmium, smoking, and increased risk of peripheral arterial disease. Circulation. 2004; 109: 3196–3201.

Navas-Acien A., Silbergeld E.K., Sharrett R., Calderon-Aranda E., Selvin E., Guallar E. Metals in urine and peripheral arterial disease. Environ Health Perspect. 2005 Feb; 113(2):164-9.

Navas-Acien A., Tellez-Plaza M., Guallar E., Muntner P., Silbergeld E., Jaar B., Weaver V. Blood cadmium and lead and chronic kidney disease in US adults: a joint analysis. Am J Epidemiol. 2009 Nov 1; 170(9):1156-64. Epub 2009 Aug 21.

Nawrot T.S., Thijs L., Den Hond E.M., Roels H.A., Staessen J.A. An epidemiological re-appraisal of the association between blood pressure and blood lead: a meta-analysis. J Hum Hypertens. 2002 Feb;16(2):123-31.

Nehru B., Sidhu P. Behavior and neurotoxic consequences of lead on rat brain followed by recovery. Biol Trace Elem Res. 2001; 84(1-3):113-21.

Nie L.H., Wright R.O., Bellinger D.C., Hussain J., Amarasiriwardena C., Chettle D.R., Pejović-Milić A., Woolf A., Shannon M. Blood lead levels and cumulative blood lead index (CBLI) as predictors of late neurodevelopment in lead poisoned children. Biomarkers. 2011 Sep; 16(6):517-24. Epub 2011 Aug 9.

Othman A.I., El Missiry M.A. Role of selenium against lead toxicity in male rats. j Biochem Mol Toxicol. 1998; 12(6):345-9.

Park S.K., Hu H., Wright R.O., Schwartz J., Cheng Y., Sparrow D., Vokonas P.S., Weisskopf M.G. Iron metabolism genes, low-level lead exposure, and QT interval. Environ Health Perspect. 2009 Jan; 117(1):80-5. Epub 2008 Aug 22.

Pawlas K., Pawlas N., Kmiecik-Malecka E., Malecki A. The relationship between children's blood lead level and postural stability. J Human Kinetics; 2008, 20:71-80.

Pirkle J.L., Schwartz J., Landis J.R., Harlan W.R. The relationship between blood lead levels and blood pressure and its cardiovascular risk implications. Am J Epidemiol. 1985; 121: 246–258.

Pocock S.J., Shaper A.G., Ashby D., Delves H.T., Clayton B.E. The relationship between blood lead, blood pressure, stroke, and heart attacks in middle-aged British men. Environ Health Perspect. 1988 Jun; 78:23-30.

Poręba R., Gać P., Poręba M., Andrzejak R. The relationship between occupational exposure to lead and manifestation of cardiovascular complications in persons with arterial hypertension. Toxicol Appl Pharmacol. 2010 Nov 15; 249(1):41-6. (b)

Poręba R., Gać P., Poręba M., Derkacz A., Andrzejak R. Tachycardia as an independent risk factor in chronic lead poisoning. In: Sobieszczańska M, Jagielski J, Macfarlane PW (Eds.). Electrocardiology 2009. JAKS Publishing Company, Wroclaw 2010, pp. 251-261. (a)

Poręba R., Poręba M., Gać P., Steinmetz-Beck A., Beck B., Pilecki W., Andrzejak R., Sobieszczańska M. Electrocardiographic changes in workers occupationally exposed to lead. Ann Noninvasive Electrocardiol. 2011; 16(1):33-40.

Poręba R., Skoczyńska A., Derkacz A., Szymańska-Chabowska A., Andrzejak R. Serum homocysteine level in person occupationaly exposed to lead. Adv.Clin.Exp.Med. 2005 Vol.14 no.3; s.537-543.

Rabinowitz M., Bellinger D., Leviton A., Needleman H., Schoenbaum S. Pregnancy hypertension, blood pressure during labor, and blood lead levels. Hypertension. 1987; 10(4):447-51.

Reckziegel P., Dias V.T., Benvegnú D., Boufleur N., Silva Barcelos R.C., Segat H.J., Pase C.S., Dos Santos C.M., Flores E.M., Bürger M.E. Locomotor damage and brain oxidative stress induced by lead exposure are attenuated by gallic acid treatment. Toxicol Lett. 2011; 203(1):74-81. Epub 2011 Mar 22.

Report of the PHIME Seminar at European Environment Agency *"Effects of exposure to metals; no margin of safety in Europe"* on 10th of February 2011.

Revis N.W., Major T.C., Horton C.Y. The effects of calcium, magnesium, lead, or cadmium on lipoprotein metabolism and atherosclerosis in the pigeon. J Environ Pathol Toxicol. 1980 Sep; 4(2-3):293-303.

Revis N.W., Zinsmeister A.R., Bull R. Atherosclerosis and hypertension induction by lead and cadmium ions: an effect prevented by calcium ion. Proc Natl Acad Sci U S A. 1981 Oct; 78(10):6494-8.

Robinson T.R. 20-year mortality of tetraethyl lead workers. J Occup Med. 1974 Sep;16(9):601-5.

Rodríguez-Iturbe B., Sindhu R.K., Quiroz Y., Vaziri N.D. Chronic exposure to low doses of lead results in renal infiltration of immune cells, NF-kappaB activation, and overexpression of tubulointerstitial angiotensin II. Antioxid Redox Signal. 2005 Sep-Oct; 7(9-10):1269-74.

Romieu I., Carreon T., Lopez L., Palazuelos E., Rios C., Manuel Y., Hernandez-Avila M. Environmental urban lead exposure and blood lead levels in children of Mexico City. Environ Health Perspect. 1995 Nov; 103(11):1036-40.

Rossi E. Low level environmental lead exposure--a continuing challenge. Clin Biochem Rev. 2008 May; 29(2):63-70.

Roy A., Bellinger D., Hu H., Schwartz J., Ettinger A.S., Wright R.O., Bouchard M., Palaniappan K., Balakrishnan K. Lead exposure and behavior among young children in Chennai, India Environ Health Perspect. 2009 Oct; 117(10):1607-11. Epub 2009 Jun 26.

Sakai T., Morita Y., Araki T., Kano M., Yoshida T. Relationship between delta-aminolevulinic acid dehydratase genotypes and heme precursors in lead workers. Am J Ind Med. 2000; 38(3):355-60.

Schafer J.H., Glass T.A., Bressler J., Todd A.C., Schwartz B.S. Blood lead is a predictor of homocysteine levels in a population-based study of older adults. Environ Health Perspect. 2005 Jan; 113(1):31-5. 25.

Schober S.E., Mirel L.B., Graubard B.I., Brody D.J., Flegal K.M. Blood lead levels and death from all causes, cardiovascular disease, and cancer: results from the NHANES III mortality study. Environ Health Perspect. 2006; 114(10):1538-41

Schwartz J. Lead, blood pressure, and cardiovascular disease in men and women. Environ Health Perspect. 1991, 91:71-5.

Scinicariello F., Yesupriya A., Chang M.H., Fowler B.A. Modification by ALAD of the association between blood lead and blood pressure in the U.S. population: results from the Third National Health and Nutrition Examination Survey. Environ Health Perspect. 2010 Feb; 118(2):259-64.

Sharifi A.M., Darabi R., Akbarloo N., Larijani B., Khoshbaten A. Investigation of circulatory and tissue ACE activity during development of lead-induced hypertension. Toxicol Lett. 2004 Nov 2; 153(2):233-8.

Shen X., Rosen J.F., Guo D., Wu S. Childhood lead poisoning in China. Sci Total Environ. 1996 Mar 15; 181(2):101-9.

Silbergeld EK. Mechanisms of lead neurotoxicity, or looking beyond the lamppost. FASEB J. 1992 Oct; 6(13):3201-6.

Sirivarasai J., Kaojarern S., Wananukul W., Deechakwan W., Srisomerarn P.. Non-occupational lead and cadmium exposure and blood pressure in Thai men. Asia Pac J Public Health. 2004; 16:133-137.

Skoczynska A. Genetic aspects of hypertensive effects of lead. Med Pr. 2008; 59(4):325-32.

Skoczynska A. In: Lead as cardiovascular risk factor. Ed: W.Górnicki Wyd. Med. 2006

Skoczynska A., Gruber K., Belowska-Bień K., Mlynek V. Risk of cardiovascular diseases in lead-exposed workers of crystal glassworks. Part I. Effect of lead on blood pressure and lipid metabolism. Med Pr. 2007;58(6):475-83.

Skoczynska A., Juzwa W., Smolik R., Szechiński J., Behal F.J. Response of the cardiovascular system to catecholamines in rats given small doses of lead.Toxicology. 1986; 39(3):275-89.

Skoczynska A., Martynowicz H., Poręba R., Antonowicz-Juchniewicz J., Sieradzki A., Andrzejak R. Trehalase concentration in urine as a marker of renal dysfuncton in workers occupationally exposed to lead. Med Pr. 2001; 52: 247-252.

Skoczynska A., Martynowicz H., Rupnik A., Turczyn B., Wojakowska A., Górecka H. Glycosaminoglycans content in the organs of rats chronically treated with lead. Metal Ions Biol Med. 2004, 8, 364-367.

Skoczynska A., Poręba R., Derkacz A. Endothelial dysfunction in workers exposed to lead. In: Atherosclerosis: risk factors, diagnosis and treatment. Monduzzi Editore, International Proceedings Division, Salzburg. 2002; July 7-10: 77-81.

Skoczynska A., Smolik R. The effect of combined exposure to lead and cadmium on serum lipids and lipid peroxides level in rats. Int J Occup Med Environ Health, 1994, 7, 263-271

Skoczynska A., Smolik R., Jeleń M. Lipid abnormalities in rats given small doses of lead. Arch Toxicol 1993, 67, 200-4.

Skoczynska A., Smolik R., Milian A. The effect of combined exposure to lead and cadmium on the concentration of zinc and copper in rat tissues. Int J Occup Med Environ Health. 1994; 7(1):41-9.

Skoczynska A., Stojek E. The impact of subchronic lead poisoning on the vascular effect of nitric oxide in rats. Environ Toxicol Pharmacol. 2005; 19: 99-106.

Skoczynska A., Stojek E., Górecka H., Wojakowska A. The serum vasoactive agents in lead-treated rats. Int J Occup Med Environ Health. 2003; 16: 169-177.

Skoczynska A., Szechiński J., Juzwa W., Smolik R., Běhal F. Carotid sinus reflexes in rats given small doses of lead. Toxicology 1987, 43, 161-171.

Skoczynska A., Wróbel J., Andrzejak R. Lead-cadmium interaction effect on the responsiveness of rat mesenteric vessels to norepinephrine and angiotensin II. Toxicology, 2001; 162: 157-170.

Sroczyński J., Biskupek K., Piotrowski J., Rudzki H. Effect of occupational exposure to lead, zinc and cadmium on various indicators of the circulatory system of metallurgical workers. Med Pr. 1990; 41(3):152-8.

Stohs S.J., Bagchi D. Oxidative mechanisms in the toxicity of metal ions. Free Rad Biol Med. 1995; 18: 321-336.

Suzen H.S., Duydu Y., Avdin A., Isimer A., Vural N. Influence of the delta-aminolewulinic acid dehydratase (ALAD) polymorphism on biomarkers of lead exposure in Turkish storage battery manufacturing workers. Am J Ind Med. 2003; 43(2):165-71.

Takebayashi T. Epidemiologic review of long-term, low-level exposure to environmental chemicals and cardiovascular disease: an exposure-response relationship. Nippon Eiseigaku Zasshi. 2011; 66(1):13-21.

Telisman S., Jurasović J., Pizent A., Cvitković P. Blood pressure in relation to biomarkers of lead, cadmium, copper, zinc, and selenium in men without occupational exposure to metals. Environ Res. 2001; 87(2):57-68.

Tepper A., Mueller C., Singal M., Sagar K. Blood pressure, left ventricular mass, and lead exposure in battery manufacturing workers. Am J Ind Med. 2001 Jul; 40(1):63-72.

Tong S., Baghurst P.A., Sawyer M.G., Burns J., McMichael A.J. Declining blood lead levels and changes in cognitive function during childhood: the Port Pirie Cohort Study. JAMA. 1998 Dec 9; 280(22):1915-9.

Tong S., von Schirnding Y.E., Prapamontol T. Environmental lead exposure: a public health problem of global dimensions. Bull World Health Organ. 2000; 78(9):1068-77.

Trzcinka-Ochocka M., Jakubowski M., Raźniewska G. Asessment of occupational exposure to lead in Poland. Med Pr. 2005; 56(5):395-404.

Tsao D.A., Yu H.S., Cheng J.T., Ho C.K., Chang H.R. The change of beta-adrenergic system in lead-induced hypertension. Toxicol Appl Pharmacol. 2000; 164(2):127-33.

Turczyn B., Skoczynska A., Wojakowska A. Serum and urinary glycosaminoglycans in workers chronically exposed to lead. Med. Pr. 2010; 61(5):553-60.

Vaziri N.D., Ding Y., Ni Z.: Compensatory up-regulation of nitric oxide synthase isoforms in lead-induced hypertension; reversal by a superoxide dismutase-mimetic drug. J Pharm Exp Ther. 2001; 298(2): 679-685.

Vaziri N.D., Sica D.A. Lead-induced hypertension: role of oxidative stress. Curr Hypertens Rep. 2004 Aug; 6(4):314-20.

Wang L., Zhou X., Yang D., Wang Z. Effects of lead and/or cadmium on the distribution patterns of some essential trace elements in immature female rats. Hum Exp Toxicol. 2011 Apr 18. (Epub ahead of print).

Weaver V.M., Lee B.K., Todd A.C., Ahn K.D., Shi W., Jaar B.G., Kelsey K.T., Lustberg M.E., Silbergeld E.K., Parsons P.J., Wen J., Schwartz B.S. Effect modification by dela-aminolevulinic acid dehydratase, vitamin D receptor, and nitric oxide synthase gene polymorphisms on associations between patella lead and renal function in lead workers. Environ. Res. 2006, 102(1):61-9.

Weaver V.M., Schwartz B.S., Ahn K.D., Stewart W.F., Kelsey K.T., Todd A.C., Wen J., Simon D.J., Lustberg M.E., Parsons P.J., Silbergeld E.K., Lee B.K. Associations of renal function with polymorphisms in the delta-aminolevulinic acid dehydratase, vitamin D receptor, and nitric oxide synthase genes in Korean lead workers. Environ Health Perspect. 2003; 111(13):1613-9.

Weiss S.T., Munoz A., Stein A., Sparrow D., Speizer F.E. The relationship of blood lead to systolic blood pressure in a longitudinal study of policemen. Environ Health Perspect. 1988; 78: 53-6.

Weisskopf M.G., Jain N., Nie H., Sparrow D., Vokonas P., Schwartz J., Hu H. A prospective study of bone lead concentration and death from all causes, cardiovascular diseases, and cancer in the Department of Veterans Affairs Normative Aging Study. Circulation. 2009 Sep; 22;120(12):1056-64. Epub 2009 Sep 8.

Wilczyńska U., Szeszenia-Dabrowska N., Sobala W. Mortality of men with occupational lead poisoning in Poland. Med Pr. 1998; 49(2):113-28.

Wrobel J., Skoczynska A. The activity of angiotensin converting enzyme in vascular mesenteric bed of rats poisoned with lead and cadmium. Med Pr. 2002; 53(2):131-6.

Zhang A., Park S.K., Wright R.O., Weisskopf M.G., Mukherjee B., Nie H., Sparrow D., Hu H. HFE H63D polymorphism as a modifier of the effect of cumulative lead exposure on pulse pressure: the Normative Aging Study. Environ Health Perspect. 2010 Sep; 118(9):1261-6. Epub 2010 May 14.

Zou H.J., Ding Y., Huang K.L., Xu M.L., Tang G.F., Wu M.H., Wang S.Y. Effects of lead on systolic and diastolic cardiac functions. Biomed Environ Sci. 1995 Dec;8(4):281-8.

# 7

# New Cardiovascular Risk Factors and Physical Activity

Nicolás Terrados[1,2] and Eduardo Iglesias-Gutiérrez[2]
*[1]Regional Sports Medicine Unit of the Principality of Asturias, Avilés,*
*[2]Department of Functional Biology,*
*The University of Oviedo, Asturias,*
*Spain*

## 1. Introduction

A cardiovascular risk factor (CRF) is a biological characteristic or behaviour that increases the possibility of cardiovascular disease (CVD) (1). The concept of risk factors first appeared some fifty years ago with the publication of the Framingham Study (2). Since that time, advances in the field of epidemiology have made large scale clinical studies possible and have led to the identification of a series of cardiovascular disease risk factors that induce the formation of atheromatous plaques. The establishment of a specific biological characteristic, environmental factor or habit as a CRF requires: a standardised methodology; concordant prospective studies; an added effect when various risk factors concur in an individual; and, that the modification of the factor (in the case that the factor is modifiable) results in a diminution of the risk (3).

Historically, there has been clear evidence of a series of 'traditional' CRFs (Table 1), such as hypercholesterolemia, hypertension, hyperglycaemia, nicotine poisoning, sedentarism, etc. which have been used in the stratification of individual risk (4). In the recent past, a number of important studies have proposed the inclusion of new or 'emergent' CRFs in the evaluation and stratification of cardiovascular risk and this has implications for preventive and therapeutic strategies.

Numerous documents and reports that include recommendations for the prevention of CVD and control of the main cardiovascular risk factors have been published by national and international scientific institutions and organisations (from the USA, Europe (5) etc.). Following the latest recommendations of the world renowned National Cholesterol Education Program (NCEP) (4), Table 1 lists the most significant 'traditional' CRFs whilst Table 2 shows the 'emergent' factors. Some of the 'new' factors have been recognised for decades though they have been subject to debate and controversy, and consensus has not been reached on their inclusion in cardiovascular risk evaluation.

The NCEP Panel III identifies three classes of CRFs that influence the possibilities of suffering CVD, although only the first two are relevant to the modification of treatment objectives: major CRFs, factors linked to lifestyles and emergent risk factors.

Age and sex (men ≥ 45 years old, women ≥ 55 years old)

Nicotine poisoning

Arterial hypertension (BP ≥ 140/90 mmHg or undergoing antihypertensive treatment)

Increase LDL cholesterol

Fall in HDL cholesterol (< 40 mg/dl)*

Family history of premature coronary heart disease
    Male first degree relatives < 55 years
    Female first degree relatives < 65 years
Diabetes mellitus**

Lifestyle (overweight/obesity, sedentarism, atherogenic diet)***

---

* Adapted from Panel III of the National Cholesterol Education Program (4).
*If HDL cholesterol is ≥ 60 mg/dl, it is considered as a 'negative' risk factor".
**Diabetes mellitus carries a risk equivalent to a secondary prevention situation.
***These factors are not computed in the algorithms for stratification of risk.
AP: arterial pressure; LDL: low density lipoproteins; HDL: high density lipoproteins.

Table 1. Major ('traditional') cardiovascular risk factors, (4).

Panel III recognises that, in addition to the main CRFs, CVD is influenced by the presence of other factors which modification can have a positive effect on some of the major CRFs and reduce risk; these therefore represent direct treatment objectives. These factors act through other intermediate elements or worsen independent risk factors such as, obesity, sedentarism, a family history of premature CVD, psychosocial conditions or being male. Although they do not figure in algorithm calculations on the stratification of risk (6), two of them, obesity and sedentarism, are considered as causal CRFs by the American Heart Association.

## 2. Traditional cardiovascular risk factors

### 2.1 Lipid risk factors

Hypercholesterolemia is one of the main cardiovascular risk factors that are modifiable. The *Multiple Risk Factor Intervention Trial* demonstrated the existence of a continuous and graded relationship between cholesterolemia and total mortality and mortality due to ischemic heart disease (7).

The three main classes of lipoproteins are: Low-density lipoproteins (LDL); High-density lipoproteins (HDL); and Very low-density lipoproteins (VLDL). There is another class of lipoproteins known as Intermediate-density lipoproteins (IDL) that is between VLDL and LDL, though in clinical practice, it is included in the LDL category.

With the exception of HDLs, that play a role in reverse cholesterol transport and therefore exercise a vasoprotector action, lipid particles are more atherogenic the more cholesterol that they transport. Chylomicrons carry such a small quantity of cholesterol that their increase in hyperchylomicronemia (Type I dyslipidemia) is not associated with atherosclerosis lesions. In contrast, with the accumulation of VLDLs, a fifth of which are made up of cholesterol, an increase in atherogenesis is observed. Given that LDLs are particles with a higher level of cholesterol, they are the main cause of atherogenesis when they are in excess.

Although LDLs receive most attention in clinical management, there is a growing body of evidence that indicates that VLDLs play an important role in atherogenesis.

Levels of HDL cholesterol are inversely related with the risk of CVD; they seem to play a protective role against the onset of atherosclerosis as they capture free cholesterol from the peripheric tissues such as the cells of the vascular wall. This cholesterol is transformed into cholesterol esters, a part of which is transferred to the VLDLs by the cholesterol esters transfer proteins (CETP) and returned to the liver by IDLs and LDLs and another part is transferred directly to the liver by the HDL particles. The liver reuses the cholesterol for the synthesis of VLDLs, for the synthesis of bile salts or excretes it directly into the bile. Therefore, HDLs tend to reduce cholesterol levels.

## 2.2 Non-lipid risk factors

### Hypertension

Hypertension is a principal and independent CRF, but its damaging effect is increased when associated with other coronary risk factors such as smoking, diabetes and dyslipidemia. The Sixth Report of the Joint National Committee on Prevention, Detection, Evaluation, and Treatment of High Blood Pressure defines hypertension as a systolic arterial pressure of $\geq140$mmHg or diastolic $\geq90$mmHg or the need for antihypertensive treatment (8). A number of studies, for example the Framingham study, have demonstrated an increase in total mortality and cardiovascular risk in cases of increased levels of arterial pressure (diastolic and systolic), with a continuous and gradual relationship (9,10,11). The association applies to men and women, young and old alike.

### Smoking

Smoking contributes clearly to CVD. The relationship between smoking and the risk of CVD is dose dependent and affects men and women equally. Observational studies suggest that stopping smoking leads to a substantial reduction of the risk of a cardiovascular event.

### Diabetes

Diabetes is defined as the presence of a level of glucose, on an empty stomach, more than, or equal to, 126 mg/dL (12). The risk of cardiovascular disease is significantly increased for sufferers of diabetes mellitus type 1 and type 2 (13). The increase of risk attributed to hyperglycaemia is independent of other risk factors such as obesity, overweight or dyslipidemia that are often observed in diabetics.

80% of diabetes mellitus patient mortality is caused by complications associated with atherosclerosis with ischemic heart disease being responsible in 75% of cases (14). In addition, the risk of acute myocardial infarction in diabetes mellitus type 2 patients with no previous history of myocardial infarction is similar to non-diabetics who have previously suffered a heart attack (15).

Although it is probable that strict control of diabetes reduces micro-vascular disorders and other complications such as renal disease and retinopathies, statistics relative to the effects of glycemic control on coronary episodes are uncertain. Diabetics often present dyslipidemia, characterised by moderate hypercholesterolemia and hypertriglyceridemia with low concentrations of HDL cholesterol that involve increased cardiovascular risk. This is frequently associated with central obesity, hyperinsulinism and AHT. Therefore, the association of numerous CRFs explains why many individuals already exhibit disorders when they are diagnosed with diabetes mellitus.

## 3. Emergent cardiovascular risk factors

Traditional factors can strongly predict the risk of cardiovascular disease but not completely (16). Thus, recently new biomarkers have emerged, although their predictive value still needs to be validated in multiple cohorts and different populations.

**Lipid Risk Factors**

    Total cholesterol quotient/HDL cholesterol

    Apolipoproteins

    HDL subclasses

    Triglycerides

    "Small and dense" LDL particles

    Residual or remnant lipoproteins

**Non-lipid Risk Factors**

    Markers of inflammation

    Homocysteinaemia

    Impaired fasting glycaemia

    Thrombogenic / hemostatic factors

LDL: Low-density lipoproteins; HDL: High-density lipoproteins

Table 2. Emergent cardiovascular risk factors

### 3.1 Apolipoproteins

### Apolipoprotein A

A apolipoproteins are a group of proteins that are variably distributed among different lipoproteins. Apo A-I is the most abundant apolipoprotein in plasma and is nearly 90% of the HDL and 60-70% of the protein fraction of the sub-fractions HDL2 and HDL3, respectively. Apo A-I is initially synthesised in the liver and intestine as a protein precursor which is degraded to its mature form in plasma; it is a simple polypeptide chain that contains 243 amino acids. This protein participates in the reverse transport of cholesterol.

The apolipoprotein apo A-II is the second highest concentration protein component of HDL, although it is absent in the HDL2 sub-fraction and plasma levels do not correlate with HDL-cholesterol levels.

The measurement of the concentration of apo A-I in serum perfectly reproduces the predictive value of coronary disease of the concentration of HDL in serum. Nevertheless, this correlation is not valid in subjects with hypertriglyceridemia, in which the fraction of HDL is enriched with triglycerides and cholesterol is almost absent.

### Apolipoprotein B

B apolipoprotein is a protein of great molecular weight, present in chylomicrons, VLDL, and LDL lipoproteins. There are two molecular forms in plasma, apo B-100 (apo B) and apo B-48. Apo B is a unique polypeptide chain of 4536 amino acids (one of the biggest plasma proteins), synthesised in the liver and secreted in VLDLs. It is quantitatively maintained during the conversion of VLDL to IDL until LDL, of which it is the only protein component, and for this reason, levels of apo B are correlated with levels of these lipoproteins. Studies have established the relationship between B concentrations in serum and cardiovascular risk (17,18,19).

Given that each particle of VLDL, IDL and LDL only contains one apo B molecule, its concentration in serum reflects the risk associated with all these atherogenic particles. Although considered as a risk factor by the NCEP, its determination is not recommended in clinical practice, due to the unavailability of clinical guides or risk stratification algorithms based on its concentration, although it can be useful in some situations.

Nevertheless, from an experimental point of view, it can offer important additional information. The concentration of apo B in serum provides data on the number of particles, especially LDL particles, as they contain approximately 90% of total circulating apo B. It has been suggested that a LDL/ decreased apo B relationship is an indicator of the predominance of small and dense LDL particles (20).

The estimation of LDL cholesterol using the Friedewald formula is inexact when levels of triglycerides are higher than 300mg/dL and, if no validated direct method or ultracentrifugation is available, the concentration of apo B can be used as an alternative for the stratification of risk and the setting of therapeutic objectives (21). A modification of the Friedewald formula has been described for the calculation of LDL cholesterol that includes apo B. The LDL cholesterol obtained in this way has been shown to be more independent of hypertriglyceridemia than calculations made with the Friedewald formula (22).

The results of some studies have shown that the relationship between apo B/apo A-I is better for evaluating cardiovascular risk than the total cholesterol/HDL cholesterol relationship or LDL cholesterol/HDL (23,24). The number of particles and, in particular, the balance between them, that is to say, the apo B/apo A-I relationship, may be more important than the lipid quantity carried by each particle.

### 3.2 Triglycerides

In spite of the evidence put forward by some epidemiological studies on the relationship between hypertriglyceridemia and the incidence of CVD (25,26), the results of other, more recent, multivariate works do not allow the definitive classification of triglycerides as an independent CRF (4). This is due to the close relationship between increased levels of triglycerides and other lipid CRFs (the presence of residual lipoproteins or remnants of VLDLs and chylomicrons in plasma, the predominance of 'small and dense' particles of LDL in plasma or decreased plasma concentration of HDL cholesterol), non-lipid CRFs (hypertension) and emergent CRFs (glucose intolerance, prothrombotic state). The NCEP Panel III states that increases in levels of triglycerides (>200mg/dL) are associated with a higher risk of CVD. It is also commonly associated with other lipid and non-lipid risk factors and indicates that therapeutic objectives should be based on lifestyle changes (loss of weight, physical exercise, stopping smoking).

### 3.3 Lipoprotein(a)

In recent years, lipoprotein (a) (Lp(a)) has attracted enormous interest as a cardiovascular risk factor (27,28). Lp(a) is a spherical lipoprotein, rich in cholesterol esters and phospholipids, it has a composition that is similar to LDL and contains a specific glycoprotein, apolipoprotein (a), linked by a disulphide bridge to the apolipoprotein B-100. In addition, it has great structural homology to the plasminogen fibrinolytic proenzyme (Figure 1) (29).

A variety of mechanisms that may explain the relationship between lp(a) and cardiovascular disease have been described in published works. Firstly, it is argued that as lp(a) is an LDL particle it plays a role in the initiation, progression and possible rupture of the atheromatous plaque. Secondly, it is suggested that this particle competes with the plasminogen particle and inhibits thrombolytic activity (30). Finally, cell line studies with rats have shown that lipoprotein (a) inhibits NO synthesis (31).

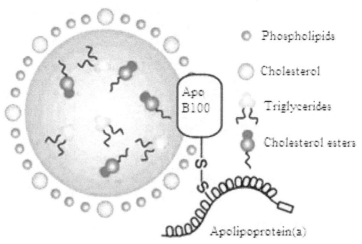

Fig. 1. Structure of lipoprotein (a).

Although an increase in the plasma concentration of lp(a) implies a higher risk of CVD, mainly in individuals at greater global risk (32), the principal consensus documents, such as the NCEP Panel III and the latest European STORE project proposal, do not include it among cardiovascular risk factors that are computable for the evaluation of overall risk. This is due to the fact that some studies do not corroborate independent prediction, based on lp(a) levels, of suffering CVD (33,34) and there is no evidence that elimination benefits the patient (35).

### 3.4 Ultra-sensitive CRP

The inflammatory process characterises all phases of atherothrombotic development. There are many studies that relate a variety of elements that intervene in the inflammatory process with the risk of CVD. These elements include: the intercellular-1 adhesion molecule (ICAM-1); the vascular-1 adhesion molecule (VCAM-1); E-selectin; P-selectin; proinflammatory cytokines, such as interleucine-6 (IL-6), and the tumor necrosis factor-alpha (TNF-α). All of the aforementioned have been shown to be predictors of CRFs (36). In clinical practice, difficulties in determining these markers and the short half-life of these molecules in circulatory blood mean that it is not possible to include them in the daily clinical routine. Of the other markers of inflammation that have been suggested, such as, serum amyloid A, the leukocyte count, fibrinogen, nitrotyrosine, myeloperoxidase and c-reactive protein (CRP), only the latter has been consolidated as a candidate due to its stability, analysis precision and accessibility (37). The AHA (American Heart Association) and CDC (Centers for Disease Control) say that of all the markers of inflammation, only ultra-sensitive CRP (US-CRP) has the characteristics necessary for use in clinical practice (38).

Ultra-sensitive CRP (US-CRP) is currently the best characterised inflammation biomarker and has been established as a potential marker of cardiovascular risk. US-CRP in plasma is a firm candidate for use in clinical practice as it is considered as an independent predictor of coronary illness for the general population, for both sexes and for patients that have already presented clinical manifestations of CVD (36,37). However, sufficient evidence that reducing CRP levels prevents CHD events is lacking (16, 39).

CRP is a member of the pentraxin family of proteins which are characterised by having a pentameric structure and radial symmetry, formed by five protomers of 24 kD and 206 amino acids that are linked among themselves by non covalent bonds and have the capacity to bond to a great variety of substances, such as, phosphocholine, fibronectin, chromatin, histones and ribonucleoproteins (40).

The differentiation of monocytes and macrophages, that takes place during atherosclerotic process, frees proinflammatory molecules that include interleukin-6 (IL-6) which activates, in the liver, the liberation of inflammation markers like CRP. High levels (>10 mg/dl) are registered in bacterial infections though ultra-sensitive analysis can detect very low levels (0-3 mg/dl) that are associated with the atherosclerotic process. Their half-life is more than 24 hours and their blood levels are not altered by diet.

### 3.5 Homocysteine

In the last decade, numerous studies have been published that relate increases homocysteinaemia (Hcy) to CVD (41-45). Nevertheless, the mechanism that controls this relationship is not completely understood. Homocysteine has a direct cytotoxic effect on endothelial cells in cultivation. An alteration in endothelial function has been observed, evaluated by echo-Doppler, in individuals with moderate hyperhomocysteinaemia and improvements have been noted on reducing the concentration of homocysteine by means of folic acid treatment. It should be remembered that levels of plasma homocysteine are related to levels of vitamin $B_{12}$ and folic acid (46).

Homocysteine can promote LDL oxidation through the production of reactive oxygen species such as hydrogen peroxide and studies have described the promotion of the multiplication of smooth muscle cells and a reduction in DNA synthesis in endothelial cells. A large number of prospective and retrospective studies support the hypothesis that an excess of plasma homocysteine is associated with a higher risk of coronary illness, peripheral and cerebrovascular disease (44,47-49).

### 3.6 Asymmetric dimethylarginine

The relationship established between a high concentration of asymmetric dimethylarginine (ADMA) and endothelial dysfunction and the possible relationship between high ADMA values and the incidence of cardiovascular accidents, has led a number of research groups to study the association between high ADMA and death by any cause.

Some studies indicate that ADMA plasma levels may predict the risk of cardiovascular events. In 2001, Valkonen et al. (50) showed that subjects with ADMA levels of more than 0.62 μmol/L (percentile 75) had almost four times more risk of suffering an acute cardiovascular event. Similar results have been described by other authors in cases of patients with unstable angina; it was noted that those patients with higher ADMA levels (>0,62 μmol/L, percentile 75) had five times more risk of suffering a cardiovascular event (51).

Zoccali et al. (52) showed that in haemodialysis patients, ADMA plasma levels are an independent predictor of mortality and cardiovascular risk. In their multivariate study, only ADMA and age were significantly predictive, independent of the incidence of cardiovascular episodes (such as chest angina and heart attack) and death by any cause. Patients whose concentration of plasma ADMA was above the percentile 75, had three times more risk of suffering a cardiovascular episode than patients whose initial ADMA levels were lower than the average.

There are currently a number of case studies, controls and prospective clinical trials taking place with a variety of patient populations that are aimed at gaining greater understanding of the role of ADMA as an independent risk factor for CVD and mortality. The data generated by these studies will help in determining the significance of ADMA as a risk factor and explore its diagnostic importance in different illnesses and diseases.

### 4. Cardiovascular risk factors and physical activity

There is much research on the effect of physical activity on the alteration of risk factors associated with heart disease. The most beneficial effect of exercise is on the level of oxidative metabolism which influences levels of lipids in the blood. Aerobic exercise reduces levels of triglycerides and total cholesterol and may increase levels of HDLs, especially if accompanied by weight loss. Although reductions in total cholesterol and LDL cholesterol generated by physical exercise seem to be relatively small (in general, they are less than 10%), there are important increases in HDL cholesterol and significant reductions in triglycerides. Transversal studies with trained athletes and non-trained subjects unequivocally demonstrate that individuals with higher levels of aerobic activity have higher HDL levels and lower levels of triglycerides (53), even after a single session of exercise (54). Nevertheless, results from longitudinal studies, over relatively long periods of time, are much less clear. Many studies on physical exercise have described an increase in HDL and a reduction in triglycerides (53,55), but others have described very small changes or no changes at all. However, almost all studies have shown that proportions of LDL/HDL and total cholesterol/HDL fall after endurance training and this means less cardiovascular risk

There are reliable data that demonstrate the effectiveness of physical exercise on the reduction in blood pressure in patients with mild or moderate hypertension. Endurance training can reduce systolic and diastolic arterial pressure (DAP) by approximately 10 mmHg in individuals with moderate essential hypertension.

With regards to the other traditional cardiovascular risk factors, physical exercise can play a role in the reduction and control of weight and in the control of diabetes. Exercise has also been shown to be effective in the control and reduction of stress and anxiety (56).

Whilst the effect of exercise on 'traditional' CRFs is well documented, the effect of exercise on 'emergent' CRFs has not been studied in depth and results are not well known. It must not be forgotten that is very important the change in the volume of blood that affects plasma concentrations, independently of changes in total lipids, both in terms of lipids and the other biochemical parameters expressed as a concentration, for the evaluation of changes engendered by physical exercise. The failure to correctly take this factor into account could explain some of the controversies concerning studies on CRFs and physical exercise.

The beneficial effects of exercise, leading to the reduction of levels of apolipoprotein B, have been widely reported, but this has not been the case with the relationship between exercise and levels of apolipoprotein A-I (57,58). Some authors have found that long-term, regular physical exercise does not seem to modify levels of apolipoproteins in comparison with sedentary groups (59). There is relatively little information available on levels of lipoprotein (a) in young people although some studies have confirmed a favourable relationship between regular physical exercise and levels of lipoprotein (a) (57,59), whilst others found no difference in lipoprotein (a) concentration between healthy sedentary individuals and professional endurance athletes (60).

The previously mentioned studies have been undertaken by different authors with different population groups and there are no published works that, at the same time, analyse the influence of intense physical exercise and the influence of continuous physical exercise (training) on levels of apolipoproteins A-I, B and lipoproteins (a), in the same population group.

The beneficial effects of physical exercise also seem to be related to the effect on the inflammatory process. In the short term, intense physical exercise produces a transitory inflammatory response which is reflected in an increase in acute phase reactants and cytokines that is proportional to the amount of exercise and muscle damage. Nevertheless, regular physical activity (training) is associated with a chronic anti-inflammatory response that influences levels of acute phase reactants such as ultra-sensitive CRP and also affects lipids and lipoproteins (61-64). However, Sadepghipour *et al.* in 2010 found no relationship between CRP and physical activity in schoolchildren (65).

Some factors (BMI, the sex of the subject, the moment when the post-exercise sample is taken, diet, etc.), can have an influence on the values measured of ultra-sensitive CRP in response to physical exercise (62). Another issue that must be taken into account is that many studies that have examined the effects of intense physical exercise on levels of ultra-sensitive CRP have not made a concentration correction in accordance with the changes in plasma volume after exercise (62). Results should be individually corrected according to the post-exercise levels of hemoconcentration or hemodilution (66).

### Effect of exercise on Traditional and Emergent cardiovascular risk factors

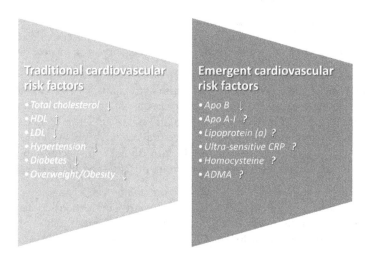

With regards to homocysteine, studies with large population groups have shown that regular physical exercise can reduce homocysteine plasma levels (47,67,68). However, other studies have concluded that intense physical exercise increases levels of Hcy (69,70). More recent studies, undertaken by our work group (71), demonstrate increased plasma homocysteine levels, both in total and reduced, after intense exercise. This increase is independent of the type of exercise and the vitamin levels but could be related to changes in renal function (71). The mechanism of this effect is not clearly understood though a study on alterations in the redox state of the homocysteine might lead to the comprehension of the underlying process. Furthermore, a study on its relationship with plasma concentrations of NO, ADMA and their proximate metabolites might lead to an understanding of how intense physical exercise produces an increase in levels of homocysteine, as long as regular, moderate physical exercise (training) seems to be a beneficial modulator of homocysteine. Also related to homocysteine, is the proven fact that regular physical exercise produces a series of beneficial effects on oxidative metabolism which result in less oxidative stress and a greater defensive capacity against oxidative damage; this is caused by the increase in activity of endogenous antioxidant systems and the greater resistance of the LDL particles to oxidation (71,72). All this signifies a reduction in oxidised LDL levels and systematic markers of inflammation, as explained by Arquer *et al.*, in 2010 (72).

In spite of the fact that the role of ADMA as a cardiovascular risk marker is reflected in an increasing number of clinical studies and scientific publications, very few studies have looked at the effect of intense or sustained (training) physical exercise on ADMA plasma levels, with contradictory results. While Schlager *et al.*, in 2011, found that supervised exercise training, twice a week during six months, in peripheral arterial disease patients decreases ADMA (73), Seljeflot *et al.*, in 2011, observed no effect of 4 weeks of exercise training in ADMA concentration in patients with chronic heart failure, speculating that the duration of the exercise protocol could be insufficient to find any effects of exercise into significant changes in ADMA (74).

It is therefore recommended that studies should be undertaken on the effect of intense and sustained (training) physical exercise on emergent cardiovascular risk factors, especially on homocysteine and ADMA.

## 5. Conflict of interests

The authors have no conflicts of interest

## 6. Acknowledgements

This work has been made possible by the support of the Ministry of Science and Innovation, Carlos III Institute of Health, F.I.S. (PI020665)

## 7. References

[1] Kannel W, Dawber TR, Kagan A, Revotskie N, and Stokes J III. Factors of risk in the development of coronary heart disease-six year follow-up experience. Ann Intern Med. 1961; 55:33-50.

[2] Dawber TR, Meadors GF, Moore FE Jr. Epidemiological approaches to heart disease: the Framingham Study. Am J Public Health Nations Health. 1951; 41(3):279-81.

[3] Wilson PW, D'Agostino RB, Levy D, Belanger AM, Silbershatz H, Kannel WB. Prediction of coronary heart disease using risk factors categories. Circulation. 1998; 97(18):1837-47.

[4] Expert Panel on Detection, Evaluation, and Treatment of High Blood Cholesterol in Adults. Executive Summary of the Third Report of the National Cholesterol Education Program (NCEP) Expert Panel on Detection, Evaluation, and Treatment of High Blood Cholesterol in Adults (Adult Treatment Panel III). JAMA. 2001; 285(19):2486-97.

[5] De Backer G, Ambrosioni E, Borch-Johnsen K, Brotons C, Cifkova R, Dallongeville J, Ebrahim S, Faergeman O, Graham I, Mancia G, Manger Cats V, Orth-Gomér K, Perk J, Pyörälä K, Rodicio JL, Sans S, Sansoy V, Sechtem U, Silber S, Thomsen T, Wood D; Third Joint Task Force of European and Other Societies on Cardiovascular Disease Prevention in Clinical Practice. European guidelines on cardiovascular disease prevention in clinical practice. Third Joint Task Force of European and

Other Societies on Cardiovascular Disease Prevention in Clinical Practice. Eur Heart J. 2003; 24(17):1601-10.

[6] Grundy SM. Primary prevention of coronary heart disease: integrating risk assessment with intervention. Circulation. 1999; 100(9):988-98.

[7] Stamler J, Wentworth DN, Neaton JD. Is relationship between serum cholesterol and risk of premature death from coronary heart disease continuous and graded? Findings in 356.222 primary screenees of the Multiple Risk Factor Intervention Trial (MRFIT) JAMA. 1986; 256(20):2823-8.

[8] The sixth report of the Joint National Committee on Prevention, Detection, Evaluation, and Treatment of High Blood Pressure. Arch Intern Med. 1997; 157(21):2413-46.

[9] MacMahon S, Peto R, Cutler J, Collins R, Sorlie P, Neaton J, Abbott R, Godwin J, Dyer A, Stamler J. Blood pressure, stroke, and coronary heart disease. Part 1, prolonged differences in blood pressure: prospective observational studies corrected for the regression dilution bias. Lancet. 1990; 335(8692):765-74.

[10] Staessen JA, Fagard R, Thijs L, Celis H, Arabidze GG, Birkenhäger WH, Bulpitt CJ, de Leeuw PW, Dollery CT, Fletcher AE, Forette F, Leonetti G, Nachev C, O'Brien ET, Rosenfeld J, Rodicio JL, Tuomilehto J, Zanchetti A. Randomised double-blind comparison of placebo and active treatment for older patients with isolated systolic hypertension. The Systolic Hypertension in Europe (Syst-Eur) Trial Investigators. Lancet 1997; 350(9080):757-64.

[11] Franklin SS, Khan SA, Wong ND, Larson MG, Levy D. Is pulse pressure useful in predicting risk for coronary heart disease? The Framingham Heart Study. Circulation. 1999; 100(4):354-60.

[12] Expert Committee on the Diagnosis and Classification of Diabetes Mellitus. Report of the expert committee on the diagnosis and classification of diabetes mellitus. Diabetes Care. 2003;26(Suppl 1):S5-20.

[13] Kannel WB, McGee DL. Diabetes and cardiovascular disease: the Framingham Study. JAMA. 1979; 241(19):2035-8.

[14] Laakso M, Lehto S. Epidemiology of risk factors for cardiovascular disease in diabetes and impaired glucose tolerance. Atherosclerosis. 1998; 137(Suppl 1):S65-73.

[15] Haffner SM, Letho S, Ronnemaa T, Pyorala K, Laakso M. Mortality from coronary heart disease in subjects with type II diabetes and non diabetic subjects with and without prior myocardial infarction. N Engl J Med. 1998; 339(4):229-33.

[16] Garg A. What is the role of alternative biomarkers for coronary heart disease? Clin Endocrinol (Oxf). 2011;75(3):289-93.

[17] Tornvall P, Bavenholm P, Landou C, de Faire U, Hamsten A. Relation of plasma levels and composition of apolipoprotein B-containing lipoproteins to angiographically defined coronary artery disease in young patients with myocardial infarction. Circulation. 1993; 88(5 Pt 1):2180-9.

[18] Sniderman AD. Apolipoprotein B and apolipoprotein AI as predictors of coronary artery disease. Can J Cardiol. 1988; 4(Suppl A):24A-30A.

[19] Sedlis SP, Schechtman KB, Ludbrook PA, Sobel BE, Schonfeld G. Plasma apoproteins and the severity of coronary artery disease. Circulation. 1986; 73(5):978-86.

[20] Wägner AM, Jorba O, Rigla M, Alonso E, Ordóñez-Llanos J, Pérez A. LDL-cholesterol/apolipoprotein B ratio is a good predictor of LDL phenotype B in type 2 diabetes. Acta Diabetol. 2002; 39(4):215-20.

[21] Sniderman AD, Furberg CD, Keech A, Roeters van Lennep JE, Frohlich J, Jungner I, Walldius G. Apolipoproteins versus lipids as indices of coronary risk and as targets for statin treatment. Lancet. 2003; 361(9359):777-80.

[22] Planella T, Cortes M, Martinez-Bru C, Gonzalez-Sastre F, Ordonez- Llanos J. Calculation of LDL-Cholesterol by using apolipoprotein B for classification of nonchylomicronemic dyslipemia. Clin Chem. 1997; 43(5):808-15.

[23] Walldius G, Jungner I, Aastveit AH, Holme I, Furberg CD, Sniderman AD. The apo B/apo A-I ratio is better than cholesterol ratios to estimate the balance between plasma proatherogenic and antiatherogenic lipoproteins and to predict coronary risk. Clin Chem Lab Med. 2004;42(12): 1355-63.

[24] Walldius G, Jungner I . The apoB/apoA-I ratio: a strong, new risk factor for cardiovascular disease and a target for lipid-lowering therapy--a review of the evidence. J Intern Med. 2006; 259(5):493-519.

[25] Austin MA, Hokanson JE, Edwards KL. Hypertriglyceridemia as a cardiovascular risk factor. Am J Cardiol. 1998; 81(4A):7B-12B.

[26] Assmann G, Schulte H, Funke H, von Eckardstein A. The emergence of triglycerides as a significant independent risk factor in coronary artery disease. Eur Heart J. 1998; 19(Suppl M):M8-M14.

[27] Moliterno DJ, Lange RA, Meidell RS, Willard JE, Leffert CC, Gerard RD, Boerwinkle E, Hobbs HH, Hillis LD. Relation of plasma lipoprotein(a) to infarct artery patency in survivors of myocardial infarction. Circulation. 1993;88(3):935-40.

[28] Seman LJ, DeLuca C, Jenner JL, Cupples LA, McNamara JR, Wilson PWF, Castelli WP, Ordovas JM, Schaefer EJ. Lipoprotein(a)-cholesterol and coronary heart disease in the Framingham Heart Study. Clin Chem. 1999; 45(7):1039-46.

[29] Utermann G. The mysteries of lipoprotein (a). Science. 1989;246(4932):904-10.

[30] Rubiés-Prat J. Lipoproteína(a): del genotipo al riesgo cardiovascular, pasando por el fenotipo. Clin Invest Arterioscler. 2004; 16:151-3.

[31] Moeslinger T, Fiedl R, Volf I, Brunner M, Koller E, Spieckermann PG. Inhibition of nitric oxide synthesis by oxidized lipoprotein (a) in a murine cell line. FEBS Lett. 2000; 478(1-2):95-9.

[32] Von Eckardstein A, Schulte H, Cullen P, Assmann G. Lipoprotein(a) further increases the risk of coronary events in men with high global cardiovascular risk. J Am Coll Cardiol. 2001; 37(2):434-9.

[33] Nishino M, Malloy MJ, Naya-Vigne J, Russell J, Kane JP, Redberg RF. Lack of association of lipoprotein(a) levels with coronary calcium deposits in asymptomatic postmenopausal women. J Am Coll Cardiol. 2000; 35(2):314-20.

[34] Moliterno DJ, Jokinen EV, Miserez AR, Lange RA, Willard JE, Boerwinkle E, Hillis LD, Hobbs HH. No association between plasma lipoprotein(a) concentrations and the presence or absence of coronary atherosclerosis in African Americans. Arterioscler Thromb Vasc Biol. 1995; 15(7):850-5.

[35] Marcovina SM, Koschinsky ML, Albers JJ, Skarlatos S. Report of the National Heart, Lung, and Blood Institute Workshop on lipoprotein(a) and cardiovascular disease: recent advances and future directions. Clin Chem. 2003; 49(11):1785-96.

[36] Ridker PM, Hennekens CH, Buring JE, Rifai N. C-reactive protein and other markers of inflammation in the prediction of cardiovascular disease in women. N Engl J Med. 2000; 342(12):836-43.

[37] Shishehbor MH, Bhatt DL. Inflammation and atherosclerosis. Curr Atheroscler Rep. 2004; 6(2):131-9.

[38] Pearson TA, Mensah GA, Alexander RW, Anderson JL, Cannon RO 3rd, Criqui M, Fadl YY, Fortmann SP, Hong Y, Myers GL, Rifai N, Smith SC Jr, Taubert K, Tracy RP, Vinicor F; Centers for Disease Control and Prevention; American Heart Association. Markers of inflammation and cardiovascular disease: application to clinical and public health practice: A statement for healthcare professionals from the Centers for Disease Control and Prevention and the American Heart Association. Circulation. 2003; 107(3):499-511.

[39] Buckley DI, Fu R, Freeman M, Rogers K, Helfand M. C-reactive protein as a risk factor for coronary heart disease: a systematic review and meta-analyses for the U.S. Preventive Services Task Force. Ann Intern Med. 2009, 151(7):483-95.

[40] Healy H, Westhuyzen J. Biology and relevance of C-reactive protein in cardiovascular and renal disease. Ann Clin Lab Sci. 2000; 30(2):133-43.

[41] Refsum H, Ueland PM, Nygard O, Vollset SE. Homocysteine and cardiovascular disease. Annu Rev Med. 1998; 49:31-62.

[42] Kang SS, Wong PWK, Malinow MR. Hyperhomocyst(e)inemia as a risk factor for occlusive vascular disease. Annu Rev Nutr. 1992; 12:279-98.

[43] Malinow MR, Bostom AG, Krauss RM. Homocyst(e)ine, diet, and cardiovascular diseases: a statement for healthcare professionals from the Nutrition Committee, American Heart Association. Circulation. 1999; 99(1):178-82.

[44] Bostom AG, Rosenberg IH, Silbershatz H, Jacques PF, Selhub J, D'Agostino RB, Wilson PWF, Wolf PA. Nonfasting plasma total homocysteine levels and stroke incidence in elderly persons: the Framingham Study. Ann Intern Med. 1999; 131(5):352-5.

[45] Stehouwer CDA, Weijenberg MP, van den Berg M, Jakobs C, Feskens EJM, Kromhout D. Serum homocysteine and risk of coronary heart disease and cerebrovascular disease in elderly men: a 10-year follow-up. Arterioscler Thromb Vasc Biol. 1998; 18(12):1895-901.

[46] Woo KS, Chook P, Lolin YI, Sanderson JE, Metreweli C, Celermajer DS Folic acid improves arterial endothelial function in adults with hyperhomocysteinemia. J Am Coll Cardiol. 1999; 34(7):2002-6.

[47] Nygard O, Vollset SE, Refsum H, Stensvol I, Tverdal A, Nordrehaug E, Ueland M, Kvale G. Total plasma homocysteine and cardiovascular risk profile. The Hordaland Homocysteine Study. JAMA. 1995; 274(19):1526-33.

[48] Genest JJ, McNamara JR, Salem DN, Wilson PW, Schaefer EJ, Malinow MR Plasma homocyst(e)ine levels in men with premature coronary artery disease. J Am Coll Cardiol. 1990; 16(5):1114-9.

[49] Stampfer MJ, Malinow MR, Willett WC, Newcomer LM, Upson B, Ullmann D et al. A prospective study of plasma homocyst(e)ine and risk of myocardial infarction in US physicians. JAMA. 1992;268(7):877-81.

[50] Valkonen VP, Päivä H, Salonen JT, Lakka TA, Lehtimäki T, Laakso J, Laaksonen R. Risk of acute coronary events and serum concentration of asymmetrical dimethylarginine. Lancet. 2001; 358(9299): 2127-28

[51] Lu TM, Ding YA, Lin SJ et al: Plasma levels of asymmetrical dimethylarginine and adverse cardiovascular events after percutaneous coronary intervention. Eur Heart J. 2003; 24(21):1912-9.

[52] Zoccali C, Bode-Böger S, Mallamaci F, Benedetto F, Tripepi G, Malatino L, Cataliotti A, Bellanuova I, Fermo I, Frölich J, Böger R. Plasma concentration of asymmetrical dimethylarginine and mortality in patients with end-stage renal disease: a prospective study. Lancet. 2001; 358(9299): 2113-17.

[53] Pitsavos C, Panagiotakos DB, Tambalis KD, Chrysohoou C, Sidossis LS, Skoumas J, Stefanadis C. Resistance exercise plus to aerobic activities is associated with better lipids' profile among healthy individuals: the ATTICA study. QJM. 2009, 102(9):609-16.

[54] Henderson GC, Krauss RM, Fattor JA, Faghihnia N, Luke-Zeitoun M, Brooks GA. Plasma triglyceride concentrations are rapidly reduced following individual bouts of endurance exercise in women. Eur J Appl Physiol. 2010, 109(4):721-30.

[55] Chomistek AK, Chiuve SE, Jensen MK, Cook NR, Rimm EB. Vigorous physical activity, mediating biomarkers, and risk of myocardial infarction. Med Sci Sports Exerc. 2011, Mar 25. [Epub ahead of print]

[56] Petruzzello SJ, Landers DM, Hatfield BD, Kubitz KA, Salazar W. A meta-analysis on the anxiety-reducing effects of acute and chronic exercise. Outcomes and mechanisms. Sports Med. 1991; 11(3):143-82.

[57] Taimela S, Viikari JS, Porkka KV, Dahlen GH. Lipoprotein (a) levels in children and young adults: the influence of physical activity. The Cardiovascular Risk in Young Finns Study. Acta Paediatr. 1994;83(12):1258-63.

[58] Mackinnon LT, Hubinger LM. Effects of exercise on lipoprotein(a). Sports Med. 1999; 28(1):11-24.

[59] Thomas NE, Baker JS, Davies B. Established and recently identified coronary heart disease risk factors in young people: the influence of physical activity and physical fitness. Sports Med. 2003; 33(9):633-50.

[60] Lippi G, Schena F, Salvagno GL, Montagnana M, Ballestrieri F, Guidi GC. Comparison of the lipid profile and lipoprotein(a) between sedentary and highly trained subjects. Clin Chem Lab Med. 2006;44(3):322-6.

[61] Kasapis C, Thompson PD. The effects of physical activity on serum C-reactive protein and inflammatory markers: a systematic review. J Am Coll Cardiol. 2005; 45(10):1563-9.

[62] Plaisance EP, Grandjean PW. Physical activity and high-sensitivity C-reactive protein. Sports Med. 2006; 36(5):443-58.

[63] Gonzales-Ordóñez AJ, Venta R, Terrados N, Arias A, Macias-Robles MD. Association between Sensitivity for Activated Protein C (APC) and Lipid or Lipoprotein Levels. Thrombosis and Haemostasis. 2002; 88: 1069-1070.

[64] Metsios GS, Stavropoulos-Kalinoglou A, Sandoo A, van Zanten JJ, Toms TE, John H, Kitas GD. Vascular function and inflammation in rheumatoid arthritis: the role of physical activity. Open Cardiovasc Med J. 2010; 4:89-96.

[65] Sadeghipour HR, Rahnama A, Salesi M, Rahnama N, Mojtahedi H. Relationship between C-reactive protein and physical fitness, physical activity, obesity and selected cardiovascular risk factors in schoolchildren. Int J Prev Med. 2010, 1(4):242-6.

[66] Dill DB, Costill DL. Calculation of percentage changes in volumen of blood, plasma, and red cells in dehydration. Journal of applied Physiology. 1974; 37(2):247-8.

[67] Bailey D, Davies B, Baker J. Training in hipoxia: modulation or metabolic and cardiovascular risk factors in men. Med Sci Sports Exerc. 2000; 32(6):1058-66.

[68] König D, Bissé E, Deibert P, Müller H-M, Wieland H, Berg A. Influence of training volume and acute physical exercise on the homocysteine levels in endurance-trained men: interactions with plasma folate and vitamin B12. Ann Nutr Metab. 2003; 47(3-4):114-8.

[69] Wright M, Francis K, Cornwell P. Effect of acute exercise on plasma homocysteine. J Sports Med Phys Fitness. 1998; 38(3):262-5.

[70] De Crée C, Malinow MR, van Kranenburg GP, Geurten PG, Longford NT, Keizer HA. Influence of exercise and menstrual cycle phase on plasma homocyst(e)ine levels in young women-a prospective study. Scand J Med Sci Sports. 1999; 9(5):272-8.

[71] Venta R, Cruz E, Valcárcel G, Terrados N. Plasma vitamins, amino acids, and renal function in postexercise hyperhomocysteinemia. Medicine and Science in Sports and Exercise. 2009; 41(8):1645-1651.

[72] Arquer A, Elosua R, y J Marrugat. Actividad física y estrés oxidativo. Apunts Med Esport. 2010. doi: 10.1016/j. apunts.2009.12.002

[73] Schlager O, Giurgea A, Schuhfried O, Seidinger D, Hammer A, Gröger M, Fialka-Moser V, Gschwandtner M, Koppensteiner R, Steiner S. Exercise training increases endothelial progenitor cells and decreases asymmetric dimethylarginine in peripheral arterial disease: A randomized controlled trial. Atherosclerosis. 2011, 217(1):240-8.

[74] Seljeflot I, Nilsson BB, Westheim AS, Bratseth V, Arnesen H. The L-arginine-asymmetric dimethylarginine ratio is strongly related to the severity of chronic heart failure. No effects of exercise training. J Card Fail. 2011, 17(2):135-42.

# 8

# Obstructive Sleep Apnoea Syndrome as a Systemic Low-Grade Inflammatory Disorder

Carlos Zamarrón[1], Emilio Morete[1] and Felix del Campo Matias[2]
*[1]Servicio de Neumología, Hospital Clínico Universitario, Santiago,*
*[2]Hospital Universitario Rio Hortega, Valladolid,*
*Spain*

## 1. Introduction

Obstructive sleep apnea syndrome (OSAS) is a common disorder characterized by recurrent upper airway collapse during sleep. A reduction or complete cessation of airflow occurs despite ongoing inspiratory efforts and leads to arousals, sleep fragmentation, and oxyhemoglobin desaturation (Remmers et al., 1978; Young et al., 1993).

Though clinically recognized for more than four decades (Gastaut et al., 1965), general awareness of OSAS has been slow to develop. OSAS has been associated with cardiovascular disease (Marin et al., 2005; Duran-Cantolla et al., 2010; Barbe et al., 2010), automobile accidents (Teran-Santos et al., 1999), chronic obstructive pulmonary disease (Chaouat et al., 1995), heart failure (Oldenburg et al., 2007) and health related quality of life deterioration (Pichel et al., 2004). OSAS often coexists with obesity and has been related to insulin resistance and metabolic syndrome (Choi et al., 2008).

Patients with OSAS experience repetitive episodes of hypoxia and reoxygenation during transient cessation of breathing that may have systemic effects. These patients also present increased levels of biomarkers linked to endocrine-metabolic and cardiovascular alterations (Zamarron et al., 2008). Moreover, OSAS may involve sleep fragmentation, tonic elevation of sympathetic neural activity, oxidative stress, inflammation, hypercoagulability and endothelial dysfunction (Bradley & Floras, 2009; Fava et al., 2011). All of this indicates that OSAS should be considered a systemic disease rather than a local abnormality.

The present review analyses the pathophysiology related to the systemic consequences of OSAS and the mechanisms involved in the association between OSAS and systemic diseases (Figure 1).

## 2. Sleep fragmentation

Extreme sleep habits can affect health and have been associated with increased inflammation. Significant changes in habitual sleep duration can lead to chronic low-grade systemic inflammation (Meisinger et al., 2005; Patel et al., 2009). Activation of pro-inflammatory pathways may represent a mechanism. In a recent study in pediatric OSAS patients, increased TNF-α levels were primarily driven by sleep fragmentation and body mass index. These levels were closely associated with the degree of sleepiness, as measured by the Multiple Sleep Latency Test. Surgical treatment of OSAS resulted in significant reductions in TNF-α levels with reciprocal prolongations in sleep latency (Gozal et al., 2010).

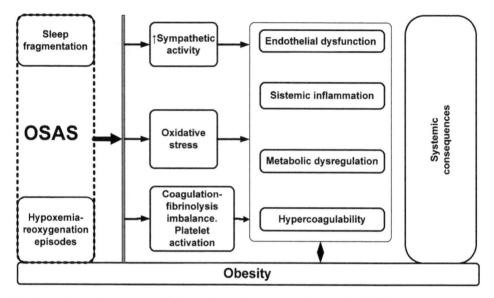

Fig. 1. A schematic summary of the proponed sequence of events in OSAS starting from episodic hypoxia and ending with systemic consequences.

Sleep fragmentation increases sympathetic nervous activity, which, in turn, results in a higher metabolic rate and elevated catecholamine secretion. Furthermore, severe sleep fragmentation can disturb nocturnal renin and aldosterone secretion profiles, and increase nighttime urine excretion. Moller et al. found that long-term CPAP reduced blood pressure, which was correlated with reductions in plasma renin and angiotensin II levels (Moller et al., 2003).

Although the mechanism of this altered inflammatory status in humans undergoing experimental sleep loss is unknown, it is likely that autonomic activation and metabolic changes play key roles (Mullington et al., 2010).

## 3. Enhanced sympathetic traffic

In OSAS patients, tonic activation of chemoreflex activity produces enhanced sympathetic traffic (Somers et al., 1988). Cyclic intermittent hypoxia (IH) and hypercapnia provides the causal link between upper airway obstruction during sleep and sympathetic activation during awakening. In a recent study in healthy humans, IH significantly increased sympathetic activity and daytime blood pressure after a single night of exposure. The baroreflex control of sympathetic outflow declined (Tamisier et al., 2011). Surges in sympathetic nervous system activity associated with apneic events have also been related to antifibrinolytic activity reflected by elevations in PAI-1 (von & Dimsdale, 2003). During apneic events, there is an up-regulation of the renin-angiotensin system and down-regulation of nitric oxide synthases (Fletcher et al., 1999; Prabhakar et al., 2001).

The increased sympathetic activity and IH associated with apneic episodes has been proposed as a possible mechanism behind the association between OSAS, systemic inflammation and cardiovascular disease. CPAP reduces sympathetic nerve activity (Maser et al., 2008), increases arterial baroreflex sensitivity (Marrone et al., 2011) and decreases vascular risk (Kohler et al., 2008).

## 4. Oxidative stress

There is an emerging consensus that OSAS is an oxidative stress disorder. In a recent study involving children with OSAS, Malakasioti found an increase of hydrogen peroxide levels in exhaled breath condensate, which is an indirect index of altered redox status in the respiratory tract (Malakasioti et al., 2011).

Apnea produces a decline in oxygen levels followed by reoxygenation when breathing resumes. The cyclical episodes of hypoxia-reoxygenation, analogous to cardiac ischemia/reoxygenation injury causing ATP depletion and xanthine oxidase activation, and increases the generation of oxygen-derived free radicals. CPAP therapy decreases the levels of oxidative stress in OSAS patients (Chin et al., 2000; Alonso-Fernandez et al., 2009).

Oxidative stress can profoundly regulate the cellular transcriptome through activation of transcription factors, including specificity protein-1, hypoxia-inducible factor-1, c-jun, and possibly nuclear factor-kappaB. Activation of redox-sensitive gene expression is suggested by the increase in some protein products of these genes, including VEGF (Teramoto et al., 2003), EPO (Marrone et al., 2008), endothelin-1 (Belaidi et al., 2009), inflammatory cytokines and adhesion molecules (Ohga et al., 1999; Dyugovskaya et al., 2002; Ohga et al., 2003).

Increased oxidative stress has been associated with development of cardiovascular diseases and can be promoted by the chronic intermittent hypoxia characteristic of OSAS (Park et al., 2007). A variety of studies suggest that oxidative stress is present in OSAS at levels relevant to tissues such as the arterial wall (Grebe et al., 2006; Barcelo et al., 2006). This process enhances lipid uptake into human macrophages and may contribute to atherosclerosis in OSAS patients (Lattimore et al., 2005). Furthermore, OSAS decreases blood antioxidant status in high BMI subjects and may change the relationship between oxidative stress markers (Wysocka et al., 2008). After CPAP, expression of eNOS and phosphorylated eNOS was found to be significantly increased whereas expression of nitrotyrosine and nuclear factor-kappaB significantly decreased (Jelic et al., 2010) but some studies shown that CPAP may not affect antioxidant defense (Alzoghaibi & Bahammam, 2011).

Recently, Nair reported that oxidative stress is mediated, at least in part, by excessive NADPH oxidase activity. This author suggests that pharmacological agents targeting NADPH oxidase may provide a therapeutic strategy in OSAS (Nair et al., 2011).

## 5. Systemic inflammation

Local and systemic inflammation is present in OSAS. Insofar as local inflammation, bronchial and nasal changes are especially relevant (Devouassoux et al., 2007). In a recent study, patients showed a significant increase in IL-8 and ICAM concentrations in both plasma and exhaled condensate. In addition, they showed a higher neutrophil percentage in induced sputum. These findings were significantly and positively correlated to AHI (Carpagnano et al., 2010), however, CPAP-therapy did have a significant effect (Lacedonia et al., 2011).

Several studies have reported changes in circulating levels of adhesion molecules in OSAS patients (El-Solh et al., 2002; Zamarron-Sanz et al., 2006). Dyugovskaya analysed polymorphonuclear apoptosis and expression of adhesion molecules in vitro in patients with moderate to severe OSAS. Decreased apoptosis and increased expression of adhesion molecules were observed. Although adhesion molecules may facilitate increased polymorphonuclear-endothelium interactions, decreased apoptosis may further augment these interactions and facilitate free radical and proteolytic enzymes (Dyugovskaya et al., 2008).

OSAS patients present increased levels of inflammatory mediators such as TNFα and IL-6 (Imagawa et al., 2004; Bravo et al., 2007) that decrease with CPAP treatment (Arias et al., 2008; Steiropoulos et al., 2009).

Systemic inflammation is increasingly being recognized as a risk factor for a number of complications including atherosclerosis (Ross, 1999) and is a well-established factor in the pathogenesis of cardiovascular disease (Hansson, 2005). Certain acute-phase proteins that have been associated in humans with cardiovascular disease, such as serum amyloid (Svatikova et al., 2003), C-reactive protein (Taheri et al., 2007; Punjabi & Beamer, 2007) which have been associated in humans with cardiovascular disease are elevated in OSAS patients and improve with CPAP treatment (Yokoe et al., 2003; Kuramoto et al., 2009).

The mechanisms by which inflammation contributes to OSAS-induced vascular dysfunction are not known. Reoxygenation after a brief period of hypoxia as experienced repetitively and systematically by OSAS patients may predispose to cell stress. It has been suggested that such events favor the activation of a proinflammatory response as mediated through the nuclear transcription factor nuclear factor-kappaB, a master regulator of inflammatory gene expression.

Inflammation may be an important link between increased sympathetic nervous system activity and vascular dysfunction in OSAS. Chronically elevated sympathetic activity produced an inflammatory response in several organs and vascular beds (Yu et al., 2005).

Some authors point to the role of the T-lymphocyte. This cell is known to play an important role in ANG II-induced hypertension and endothelial dysfunction via NADPH oxidase-induced superoxide production (Guzik et al., 2007).

Increased expression of inflammatory cytokines may contribute to endothelial dysfunction and subsequent cardiovascular complications (Ryan et al., 2005; Foster et al., 2007). Currently, some studies suggest that pentraxin 3, an acute phase response protein, is rapidly produced and released by several cell types, in particular by mononuclear phagocytes, and endothelial cells in response to primary inflammatory signals, may play a significant role in OSAS-associated vascular damage (Kasai et al., 2011). Arnaud report that some inhibition of molecules such as RANTES/CCL5, a cytokine that is a a selective attractant for memory T lymphocytes and monocytes may play a significant role in athesroscletoric remodeling OSAS-associated vascular damage (Arnaud et al., 2011)

However, mesenchymal stem cells triggered an early anti-inflammatory response in rats subjected to recurrent obstructive apneas, suggesting that these stem cells could play a role in the physiological response to counterbalance inflammation in OSAS (Carreras et al., 2010).

In a recent study on healthy human males, Querido et al. analysed the effect over 10 days of nightly IH in the following systemic inflammatory markers: serum granulocyte macrophage colony-stimulating factor, interferon-gamma, interleukin-1 β, interleukin-6, interleukin-8, leptin, monocyte chemotactic protein-1, vascular endothelial growth factor, intracellular adhesion molecule-1, and vascular cell adhesion molecule-1. There was no significant change in any of the markers. These findings suggest that a more substantial or a different pattern of hypoxemia might be necessary to activate systemic inflammation, that the system may need to be primed before hypoxic exposure, or that increases in inflammatory markers OSAS patients may be more related to other factors such as obesity or nocturnal arousal (Querido et al., 2011).

## 6. Hypercoagulability

Hypercoagulability resulting from increased coagulation or inhibited fibrinolysis is associated with an increased risk for cardiovascular disease (Zouaoui et al., 2006). This is another factor implicated in the association between this disease and OSAS (Peled et al., 2008).

A variety of findings support the existence of a relation between hypercoagulability, OSAS and cardiovascular disease. Firstly, patients with OSAS present higher plasma levels of several procoagulant factors such as fibrinogen (Reinhart et al., 2002; Tkacova et al., 2008), activated clotting factor FVII, FXIIa and thrombin/antithrombin III complexes (von et al., 2005) and the fibrinolysis-inhibiting enzyme plasminogen activator inihibitor (PAI-1) (von et al., 2006; Zamarron et al., 2008). Secondly, increased D-dimer levels in untreated OSAS have been correlated with severity of nocturnal hypoxemia, characteristic of OSAS (Shitrit et al., 2005). Thirdly, sleep fragmentation and sleep efficiency data have been associated with increased levels of von Willebrand factor and soluble tissue factor, two markers of a prothrombotic state (von et al., 2007).

OSAS is associated with platelet activation (Akinnusi et al., 2009). Platelet activation is a link in the pathophysiology of diseases prone to thrombosis and inflammation (Gasparyan et al., 2011). In these patients, platelet activation is associated with greater levels of oxygen desaturation (Oga et al., 2009;Rahangdale et al., 2011) that decreases after CPAP treatment (Varol et al., 2011).

In a current article, thromboelastography, a simple test of hemostasis, has been proposed for evaluating the risk of future cardiovascular disease in patients with OSAS (Othman et al., 2010).

## 7. Endothelial dysfunction

Endothelial dysfunction is an early marker of vascular abnormality preceding clinically overt cardiovascular disease (Giannotti & Landmesser, 2007; Halcox et al., 2009).

The intact endothelium regulates vascular tone and repair capacity, maintaining proinflammatory, anti-inflammatory, and coagulation homeostasis. Alteration of these homeostatic pathways results in endothelial dysfunction before structural changes in the vasculature. The hypoxia, hypercapnia, and pressor surges accompanying obstructive apneic events may serve as potent stimuli for the release of vasoactive substances and for impairment of endothelial function.

In OSAS, endothelial dysfunction could be caused by both hypoxia-reoxygenation cycles and chronic sleep fragmentation produced by repetitive arousals. A causal relationship between OSAS and endothelial dysfunction was demonstrated by a study in which flow-mediated dilation in the forearm was improved by CPAP treatment (Ip et al., 2004; Trzepizur et al., 2009). Levels of nitric oxide, a major vasodilator substance released by the endothelium, have been found to be decreased in OSAS patients, and these levels normalize with CPAP therapy (Haight & Djupesland, 2003).

A number of studies with OSAS patients indicate an associated endothelial dysfunction (Nieto et al., 2004). In patients with OSAS, increased production of superoxide by neutrophils (Schulz et al., 2000), increased biomarkers of lipid peroxidation (Lavie et al., 2004), and increased levels of 8-isoprostanes (Alonso Fernandez 2009; Carpagnano et al., 2003) have been observed.

Among the most important vasoconstrictive substances is endothelin-1, a peptide hormone secreted under the influence of hypoxia (Kanagy et al., 2001). Several studies have reported higher endothelin-1 levels in OSAS patients (Phillips et al 1999; Saarelainen & Hasan, 2000) however, Grimpen reports conflicting findings (Grimpen et al., 2000). This divergence might be explained by differences in study design. The groups studied by Phillips (Phillips et al., 1999) and Saarelainen (Saarelainen & Hasan, 2000) had more severe disease and, thus, underwent more severe oxygen desaturations that acted as a trigger for endothelin-1 secretion. Gjorup showed that hypertensive OSAS patients had greater nocturnal and diurnal endothelin-1 plasma levels than healthy controls, suggesting that OSAS does not affect plasma endothelin-1 levels in the absence of coexistent cardiovascular diseases (Gjorup et al., 2007).

The inconsistency of the above endothelin-1 levels likely reflects the predominantly abluminal release of endothelin. Using rat models of arterial hypertension, several authors have reported elevated vascular production of endothelin-1, while circulating levels remained similar to controls (Pohl & Busse, 1989; Rossi & Pitter, 2006). This demonstrates that circulating levels of endothelin-1 do not exclude elevated vascular production in OSAS.

In recent years, endothelial progenitor cells have gained a central role in vascular regeneration and endothelial repair capacity through angiogenesis and restoring endothelial function of injured blood vessels. Endothelial progenitor cells are decreased in patients with endothelial dysfunction and underlie an increased risk for cardiovascular morbidity in OSAS. Endothelial progenitor cells may have a potential role in the pathogenesis of vascular diseases that is pertinent to OSAS (Berger & Lavie, 2011).

It has recently been reported that OSAS patients presented increased oxidant production in the microcirculation and endothelial dysfunction, both of which improved with treatment (Patt et al., 2010)

## 8. OSAS and endocrine-metabolic consequences

Even though OSAS is generally less prevalent in women than men, differences diminish after the onset of menopause. This may be the result of declining estrogen and progesterone

(Resta et al., 2004; Anttalainen et al., 2006). Accordingly, estrogen replacement therapy in menopausal women lessens the prevalence of OSAS (Shahar et al., 2003; Wesstrom et al., 2005).

On the other hand, men diagnosed with OSAS may manifest decreased libido and a decline in morning serum testosterone levels (Teloken et al., 2006; Hoekema et al., 2006). At first, this was thought to reflect an associated dysfunction of the pituitary-gonadal axis related to sleep fragmentation and hypoxia (Meston et al., 2003). However, the correction of hypoxia and sleep fragmentation in OSAS patients treated with CPAP does not lead to complete recovery, suggesting that existence of other underlying causes. In a recent study, with the exception of prolactine, CPAP therapy produced no significant changes the serum level of sexual hormones including FSH and LH (Macrea et al., 2010). Some authors claim that obesity is the major contributing factor to the reduced pituitary gonadal function in OSAS (Luboshitzky et al., 2005).

## 9. Obesity

Central, or visceral, obesity is associated with the greatest risk for OSAS (Shinohara et al., 1997). The mechanism by which obesity can favor the onset of OSAS is not well-known, but it could be that central obesity precipitates or exacerbates OSAS because fat deposits in the upper airway affect distensibility (Isono, 2009). The increased volume of abdominal fat could predispose to hypoventilation during sleep and/or reduce the oxygen reserve, favoring oxygen desaturation during sleep (Schwartz et al., 2008). In addition, the disrupted sleep patterns characteristic of OSAS predispose to metabolic effects and weight gain. Patel investigated the association between self-reported usual sleep duration and subsequent weight gain in the Nurses' Health Study. They showed that a habitual sleep time of less than 7 hours is associated with a modest increase in future weight gain and incident obesity (Patel et al., 2006).

In recent years, much attention has been focused on the interaction between OSAS and products released by adipose tissue such as leptin, adiponectin, resistin and grelin (Ronti et al., 2006).

Leptin is an adipocyte-derived hormone that regulates body weight through control of appetite and energy expenditure (Proulx et al., 2002). Furthermore, leptin is a cytokine and is therefore also involved in the inflammatory process. Several studies have shown increased levels of leptin in OSAS (Phillips et al., 2000; Tokuda et al., 2008), suggesting its role in the disease (Ip et al., 2000). The mechanisms underlying the relation between leptin and OSAS are very diverse, and may involve overnight changes in apnea levels (Patel et al., 2004; Sanner et al., 2004), sleep hypoxemia (Tatsumi et al., 2005), and hypercapnia (Shimura et al., 2005).

A direct relationship between OSAS and leptin is supported by the fact that effective OSAS treatment with CPAP also influences leptin levels (Shimizu et al., 2002; Cuhadaroglu et al., 2009). Although the precise mechanism explaining the effect of CPAP has not yet been elucidated, it can be inferred that reduction in sympathetic activity (Snitker et al., 1997), and improvement in insulin sensitivity play a role (Brooks et al., 1994).

Leptin levels have been proposed as a prognostic marker for OSAS (Ozturk et al., 2003) and have been implicated in the pathogenesis of OSAS-related cardiovascular disease (Kapsimalis et al., 2008; Tokuda et al., 2008; Al et al., 2009).

Leptin can also act as a respiratory stimulant, and impairment of the leptin signaling pathway causes respiratory depression in mice (O'Donnell et al., 2000). This hormone has been associated with obesity hypoventilation syndrome in humans (Phipps et al., 2002) and may reflect a compensatory response to hypoventilation (Makinodan et al., 2008).

OSAS has independently been associated with reduced levels of adiponectin (Masserini et al., 2006; Zhang et al., 2006; Carneiro et al., 2009) which may favour cardiovascular disease development. The recurrent hypoxia-reoxygenation attacks in OSAS patients may activate oxidative stress and lead to low levels of adiponectin (Vatansever et al., 2010).

Some authors have observed that serum adiponectin levels may be independent of the degree of OSAS (Tokuda et al., 2008). Decreased adiponectin may result from increased sympathetic activity (Delporte et al., 2002), and higher levels of cytokines such as IL-6 and TNFα (Fasshauer et al., 2003). In fact, there are conflicting reports as to whether CPAP treatment of OSAS effectively normalizes adiponectin levels (de Lima et al., 2010).

Obesity has been implicated in the relation between OSAS and adiponectin (Makino et al., 2006), In a recent study involving media under hypoxic conditions in an ex-vivo mouse model, adiponectin secretion was measured. In obese mice, hypoxic stress reduced adiponectin in the supernatant of mesenteric fat tissue, but not subcutaneous fat tissue. These findings suggest that abdominal obesity, representing abundant mesenteric fat tissue susceptible to hypoxic stress, partly explains adiponectin levels in OSAS patients, and that reduction of visceral fat accumulation may combat OSAS-related atherosclerotic cardiovascular diseases in abdominal obesity (Nakagawa et al., 2011).

Resistin is a white adipose tissue hormone whose function has yet to be established. In a study of 20 obese OSAS patients, Harsch found that CPAP treatment of OSAS had no significant influence on resistin levels (Harsch et al., 2004). In OSAS patients, hypoxic stress during sleep may enhance resistin production, possibly mediating systemic inflammatory processes. Through its effect on OSAS, CPAP therapy may help control resistin production (Yamamoto et al., 2008).

OSAS may decrease serum resistin levels in subjects with excess body mass and also may contribute to glucose metabolism, but has no influence on leptin levels (Wysocka et al., 2009)

Ghrelin is a hormone that influences appetite and fat accumulation and its physiological effects are opposite to those of leptin. No clear relation has been found between ghrelin and OSAS. In a study of 30 obese OSAS patients, Harsch found that plasma ghrelin levels were significantly higher in OSAS patients than in controls. These elevated ghrelin levels could not be explained by obesity alone, since they rapidly decreased with CPAP therapy (Harsch et al., 2003). In another study of 30 untreated obese patients with moderate-severe OSAS, significantly higher levels of serum leptin were found in OSAS patients than in controls, but ghrelin levels were no different (Ulukavak et al., 2005).

In a recent study of 55 consecutive OSAS patients, the study group presented significantly higher serum ghrelin levels than controls. There was a significant positive correlation between ghrelin and AHI. No significant difference was noted in the levels of leptin, adiponectin, and resistin (Li et al., 2010).

Increased ghrelin levels have been found to support the presence of increased appetite and caloric intake in obese patients with OSAS, which in turn may further promote the severity of the underlying conditions (Spruyt et al., 2010). In obese children, OSAS is associated with daytime sleepiness, elevation of proinflammatory cytokines, increased leptin, and decreased adiponectin (Tsaoussoglou et al., 2010).

## 10. OSAS and insulin resistance

A variety of studies based on animal models indicate that hypoxia can alter glucose homeostasis (Cheng et al., 1997; Li et al., 2006). Polotsky described that long-term exposure to intermittent hypoxia increased levels of insulin and glucose intolerance in obese, leptin-deficient mice (Polotsky et al., 2003). Humans exposed to hypoxia present worsened glucose tolerance (Braun et al., 2001).

Insulin resistance is a central part of the metabolic syndrome, a condition that is reaching epidemic proportions in Western Society and now emerging in developing countries (Prentice, 2006). Most studies involving OSAS and insulin resistance demonstrate an association between these two diseases, independently of obesity (Tassone et al., 2003; McArdle et al., 2007). In a large population-based study involving normoglycemic hypertensive men, Resnick found that the severity of OSAS was associated with increased insulin resistance (Resnick et al., 2003). The magnitude of these beneficial effects is modulated by the hours of CPAP adherence and the degree of obesity (Tasali et al., 2011).

Insulin resistance is associated to states of inflammation (Reaven, 2005). Monocyte chemoattractant protein-1 levels are elevated in OSAS and may be involved in the pathogenesis of insulin resistance in these patients (Piemonti et al., 2003; Hayashi et al., 2006).

## 11. Metabolic syndrome and OSAS

Metabolic syndrome is an emerging public health problem that represents a constellation of cardiovascular risk factors (Batsis et al., 2007). The clinical identification of metabolic syndrome is based on measures of abdominal obesity, atherogenic dyslipidemia, elevated blood pressure, and glucose intolerance (Executive Summary of the NCEP., 2001).

Although the etiology of this syndrome is largely unknown, it is likely to be comprised of a complex interaction between genetic, metabolic, and environmental factors (Nestel, 2003). Several recent studies suggest that a proinflammatory state may also be an important component (Aso et al., 2005; Gude et al., 2009). The close association between OSAS and metabolic syndrome is called "Syndrome Z"(Wilcox et al., 1998)

The prevalence of metabolic syndrome is markedly higher among OSAS patients. Ambrosetti et al. studied 89 consecutive OSAS patients and found metabolic syndrome in 53% of them (Ambrosetti et al., 2006). Another recent study found a prevalence of 68% (Drager et al., 2009). Obese OSAS patients may have an increased rate of metabolic syndrome and higher levels of serum lipids, fasting glucose, leptin and fibrinogen than obese subjects without OSAS. Thus, clinicians should be encouraged to systematically evaluate the presence of metabolic abnormalities in OSAS and vice versa (Basoglu et al., 2011).

Both clinical and animal studies suggest that an independent relationship may exist between OSAS and hyperlipidemia. Hypoxic stress produced by OSAS potentially increases the risk of hyperlipidemia. In rodent models, hyperlipidemia can result from exposure to intermittent hypoxia (Li et al., 2005). In a sample of nearly 5,000 subjects from the Sleep Heart Health study, there was a positive association between OSAS severity and increased serum total cholesterol and triglycerides, as well as decreased serum HDL, in people under the age of 65 (Newman et al., 2001).

In a population-based sample of four hundred women aged 20-70 years the frequency of metabolic syndrome increased from 10.5% in women with AHI <5 to 57.1% in women with AHI ≥ 30. AHI and minimal saturation level remained significantly associated with metabolic syndrome also when adjusting for the waist-to-hip-ratio (Theorell-Haglow et al., 2011).

Both OSAS and metabolic syndrome may exert negative synergistic effects on the cardiovascular system through multiple mechanisms (Bonsignore & Zito, 2008; Levy et al., 2009).

Intermittent hypoxia, the hallmark feature of OSAS, leads to a preferential activation of inflammatory pathways. Oxidative stress, cardiovascular inflammation, endothelial dysfunction, and metabolic abnormalities in OSAS could accelerate atherogenesis (Quercioli et al., 2010). Further studies are required to determine the precise role of inflammation in the cardiovascular pathogenesis of OSAS, particularly its interaction with oxidative stress, obesity and metabolic dysfunction (Kent et al., 2011)

## 12. Conclusions

OSAS patients experience hypoxia–reoxygenation episodes, hypercapnia and arousal from sleep with modifications in the autonomic nervous system, oxidative stress and inflammation. OSAS is frequently associated to endocrine metabolic alterations and obesity.

Inflammatory processes play an important role in the pathogenesis of atherosclerosis and circulating levels of several inflammation markers have been associated with future cardiovascular risk. OSAS plays a mediating role between obesity and cardiovascular disease. Clinical and experimental data suggest a relationship between OSAS and adipose tissue pathophysiology which appears biologically plausible, however, further research is still needed. Multiple factors have been proposed to activate proinflammatory pathways in obesity, including generation of reactive oxygen species, and release of inflammatory cytokines potentially activated by OSAS-related hypoxic stress. All of this indicates that, more than a local abnormality, OSAS should be considered a systemic disease.

## 13. References

Executive Summary of The Third Report of The National Cholesterol Education Program (NCEP) Expert Panel on Detection, Evaluation, And Treatment of High Blood Cholesterol In Adults (Adult Treatment Panel III) (2001). *JAMA, 285,* 2486-2497.

Akinnusi, M. E., Paasch, L. L., Szarpa, K. R., Wallace, P. K., & El Solh, A. A. (2009). Impact of nasal continuous positive airway pressure therapy on markers of platelet activation in patients with obstructive sleep apnea. *Respiration, 77,* 25-31.

Al, L. N., Mulgrew, A., Cheema, R., Vaneeden, S., Butt, A., Fleetham, J. et al. (2009). Pro-atherogenic cytokine profile of patients with suspected obstructive sleep apnea. *Sleep Breath.,* 13:391-5

Alonso-Fernandez, A., Garcia-Rio, F., Arias, M. A., Hernanz, A., de la, P. M., Pierola, J. et al. (2009). Effects of CPAP on oxidative stress and nitrate efficiency in sleep apnoea: a randomised trial. *Thorax, 64,* 581-586.

Alzoghaibi, M. A. & Bahammam, A. S. (2011). The effect of one night of continuous positive airway pressure therapy on oxidative stress and antioxidant defense in hypertensive patients with severe obstructive sleep apnea. *Sleep Breath, 13,391-5* May 13. [Epub ahead of print]

Ambrosetti, M., Lucioni, A. M., Conti, S., Pedretti, R. F., & Neri, M. (2006). Metabolic syndrome in obstructive sleep apnea and related cardiovascular risk. *J.Cardiovasc.Med.(Hagerstown.), 7,* 826-829.

Anttalainen, U., Saaresranta, T., Aittokallio, J., Kalleinen, N., Vahlberg, T., Virtanen, I. et al. (2006). Impact of menopause on the manifestation and severity of sleep-disordered breathing. *Acta Obstet.Gynecol.Scand., 85,* 1381-1388.

Arias, M. A., Garcia-Rio, F., Alonso-Fernandez, A., Hernanz, A., Hidalgo, R., Martinez-Mateo, V. et al. (2008). CPAP decreases plasma levels of soluble tumour necrosis factor-alpha receptor 1 in obstructive sleep apnoea. *Eur.Respir.J., 32,* 1009-1015.

Arnaud, C., Beguin, P. C., Lantuejoul, S., Pepin, J. L., Guillermet, C., Pelli, G. et al. (2011). The Inflammatory Pre-Atherosclerotic Remodeling Induced by Intermittent Hypoxia is Attenuated by RANTES/CCL5 Inhibition. *Am.J.Respir.Crit. Care. Med.,* Jun 16. [Epub ahead of print]

Aso, Y., Wakabayashi, S., Yamamoto, R., Matsutomo, R., Takebayashi, K., & Inukai, T. (2005). Metabolic syndrome accompanied by hypercholesterolemia is strongly associated with proinflammatory state and impairment of fibrinolysis in patients with type 2 diabetes: synergistic effects of plasminogen activator inhibitor-1 and thrombin-activatable fibrinolysis inhibitor. *Diabetes Care, 28,* 2211-2216.

Barbe, F., Duran-Cantolla, J., Capote, F., de la, P. M., Chiner, E., Masa, J. F. et al. (2010). Long-term effect of continuous positive airway pressure in hypertensive patients with sleep apnea. *Am.J.Respir.Crit Care Med., 181,* 718-726.

Barcelo, A., Barbe, F., de la, P. M., Vila, M., Perez, G., Pierola, J. et al. (2006). Antioxidant status in patients with sleep apnoea and impact of continuous positive airway pressure treatment. *Eur.Respir.J., 27,* 756-760.

Basoglu, O. K., Sarac, F., Sarac, S., Uluer, H., & Yilmaz, C. (2011). Metabolic syndrome, insulin resistance, fibrinogen, homocysteine, leptin, and C-reactive protein in obese patients with obstructive sleep apnea syndrome. *Ann.Thorac.Med., 6,* 120-125.

Batsis, J. A., Nieto-Martinez, R. E., & Lopez-Jimenez, F. (2007). Metabolic syndrome: from global epidemiology to individualized medicine. *Clin.Pharmacol.Ther., 82,* 509-524.

Belaidi, E., Joyeux-Faure, M., Ribuot, C., Launois, S. H., Levy, P., & Godin-Ribuot, D. (2009). Major role for hypoxia inducible factor-1 and the endothelin system in promoting myocardial infarction and hypertension in an animal model of obstructive sleep apnea. *J.Am.Coll.Cardiol., 53,* 1309-1317.

Berger, S. & Lavie, L. (2011). Endothelial progenitor cells in cardiovascular disease and hypoxia-potential implications to obstructive sleep apnea. *Transl.Res., 158,* 1-13.

Bonsignore, M. R. & Zito, A. (2008). Metabolic effects of the obstructive sleep apnea syndrome and cardiovascular risk. *Arch.Physiol. Biochem., 114,* 255-260.

Bradley, T. D. & Floras, J. S. (2009). Obstructive sleep apnoea and its cardiovascular consequences. *Lancet, 373,* 82-93.

Braun, B., Rock, P. B., Zamudio, S., Wolfel, G. E., Mazzeo, R. S., Muza, S. R. et al. (2001). Women at altitude: short-term exposure to hypoxia and/or alpha(1)-adrenergic blockade reduces insulin sensitivity. *J.Appl.Physiol, 91,* 623-631.

Bravo, M. D., Serpero, L. D., Barcelo, A., Barbe, F., Agusti, A., & Gozal, D. (2007). Inflammatory proteins in patients with obstructive sleep apnea with and without daytime sleepiness. Sleep Breath, 11,177-85.

Brooks, B., Cistulli, P. A., Borkman, M., Ross, G., McGhee, S., Grunstein, R. R. et al. (1994). Obstructive sleep apnea in obese noninsulin-dependent diabetic patients: effect of continuous positive airway pressure treatment on insulin responsiveness. *J.Clin.Endocrinol.Metab, 79,* 1681-1685.

Carneiro, G., Togeiro, S. M., Ribeiro-Filho, F. F., Truksinas, E., Ribeiro, A. B., Zanella, M. T. et al. (2009). Continuous Positive Airway Pressure Therapy Improves Hypoadiponectinemia in Severe Obese Men with Obstructive Sleep Apnea without Changes in Insulin Resistance. *Metab Syndr.Relat. Disord.,* 7:537-42

Carpagnano, G. E., Kharitonov, S. A., Resta, O., Foschino-Barbaro, M. P., Gramiccioni, E., & Barnes, P. J. (2003). 8-Isoprostane, a marker of oxidative stress, is increased in exhaled breath condensate of patients with obstructive sleep apnea after night and is reduced by continuous positive airway pressure therapy. *Chest, 124,* 1386-1392.

Carpagnano, G. E., Spanevello, A., Sabato, R., Depalo, A., Palladino, G. P., Bergantino, L. et al. (2010). Systemic and airway inflammation in sleep apnea and obesity: the role of ICAM-1 and IL-8. *Transl.Res., 155,* 35-43.

Carreras, A., Almendros, I., Montserrat, J. M., Navajas, D., & Farre, R. (2010). Mesenchymal stem cells reduce inflammation in a rat model of obstructive sleep apnea. *Respir.Physiol. Neurobiol., 172,* 210-212.

Chaouat, A., Weitzenblum, E., Krieger, J., Ifoundza, T., Oswald, M., & Kessler, R. (1995). Association of chronic obstructive pulmonary disease and sleep apnea syndrome. *Am.J.Respir.Crit Care Med., 151,* 82-86.

Cheng, N., Cai, W., Jiang, M., & Wu, S. (1997). Effect of hypoxia on blood glucose, hormones, and insulin receptor functions in newborn calves. *Pediatr.Res., 41,* 852-856.

Chin, K., Nakamura, T., Shimizu, K., Mishima, M., Nakamura, T., Miyasaka, M. et al. (2000). Effects of nasal continuous positive airway pressure on soluble cell adhesion molecules in patients with obstructive sleep apnea syndrome. *Am.J.Med., 109,* 562-567.

Choi, K. M., Lee, J. S., Park, H. S., Baik, S. H., Choi, D. S., & Kim, S. M. (2008). Relationship between sleep duration and the metabolic syndrome: Korean National Health and Nutrition Survey 2001. *Int.J.Obes.(Lond), 32,* 1091-1097.

Cuhadaroglu, C., Utkusavas, A., Ozturk, L., Salman, S., & Ece, T. (2009). Effects of nasal CPAP treatment on insulin resistance, lipid profile, and plasma leptin in sleep apnea. *Lung, 187,* 75-81.

De Lima, A. M., Franco, C. M., de Castro, C. M., Bezerra, A. A., Ataide, L., Jr., & Halpern, A. (2010). Effects of nasal continuous positive airway pressure treatment on oxidative stress and adiponectin levels in obese patients with obstructive sleep apnea. *Respiration, 79*, 370-376.

Delporte, M. L., Funahashi, T., Takahashi, M., Matsuzawa, Y., & Brichard, S. M. (2002). Pre- and post-translational negative effect of beta-adrenoceptor agonists on adiponectin secretion: in vitro and in vivo studies. *Biochem.J., 367*, 677-685.

Devouassoux, G., Levy, P., Rossini, E., Pin, I., Fior-Gozlan, M., Henry, M. et al. (2007). Sleep apnea is associated with bronchial inflammation and continuous positive airway pressure-induced airway hyperresponsiveness. *J.Allergy. Clin.Immunol., 119*, 597-603.

Drager, L. F., Queiroz, E. L., Lopes, H. F., Genta, P. R., Krieger, E. M., & Lorenzi-Filho, G. (2009). Obstructive sleep apnea is highly prevalent and correlates with impaired glycemic control in consecutive patients with the metabolic syndrome. *J.Cardiometab.Syndr., 4*, 89-95.

Duran-Cantolla, J., Aizpuru, F., Montserrat, J. M., Ballester, E., Teran-Santos, J., Aguirregomoscorta, J. I. et al. (2010). Continuous positive airway pressure as treatment for systemic hypertension in people with obstructive sleep apnoea: randomised controlled trial. *BMJ, 341*, c5991.

Dyugovskaya, L., Lavie, P., & Lavie, L. (2002). Increased adhesion molecules expression and production of reactive oxygen species in leukocytes of sleep apnea patients. *Am.J.Respir.Crit Care Med., 165*, 934-939.

Dyugovskaya, L., Polyakov, A., Lavie, P., & Lavie, L. (2008). Delayed neutrophil apoptosis in patients with sleep apnea. *Am.J.Respir.Crit Care Med., 177*, 544-554.

El-Solh, A. A., Mador, M. J., Sikka, P., Dhillon, R. S., Amsterdam, D., & Grant, B. J. (2002). Adhesion molecules in patients with coronary artery disease and moderate-to-severe obstructive sleep apnea. *Chest, 121*, 1541-1547.

Fasshauer, M., Kralisch, S., Klier, M., Lossner, U., Bluher, M., Klein, J. et al. (2003). Adiponectin gene expression and secretion is inhibited by interleukin-6 in 3T3-L1 adipocytes. *Biochem.Biophys.Res.Commun., 301*, 1045-1050.

Fava, C., Montagnana, M., Favaloro, E. J., Guidi, G. C., & Lippi, G. (2011). Obstructive sleep apnea syndrome and cardiovascular diseases. *Semin.Thromb.Hemost., 37*, 280-297.

Fletcher, E. C., Bao, G., & Li, R. (1999). Renin activity and blood pressure in response to chronic episodic hypoxia. *Hypertension, 34*, 309-314.

Foster, G. E., Poulin, M. J., & Hanly, P. J. (2007). Intermittent hypoxia and vascular function: implications for obstructive sleep apnoea. *Exp.Physiol, 92*, 51-65.

Gasparyan, A. Y., Ayvazyan, L., Mikhailidis, D. P., & Kitas, G. D. (2011). Mean platelet volume: a link between thrombosis and inflammation? *Curr.Pharm.Des, 17*, 47-58.

Gastaut, H., Tassinari, C. A., & Duron, B. (1965). [Polygraphic study of diurnal and nocturnal (hypnic and respiratory) episodal manifestations of Pickwick syndrome]. *Rev.Neurol.(Paris), 112*, 568-579.

Giannotti, G. & Landmesser, U. (2007). Endothelial dysfunction as an early sign of atherosclerosis. *Herz, 32*, 568-572.

Gjorup, P. H., Sadauskiene, L., Wessels, J., Nyvad, O., Strunge, B., & Pedersen, E. B. (2007). Abnormally increased endothelin-1 in plasma during the night in obstructive sleep apnea: relation to blood pressure and severity of disease. *Am.J.Hypertens., 20*, 44-52.

Gozal, D., Serpero, L. D., Kheirandish-Gozal, L., Capdevila, O. S., Khalyfa, A., & Tauman, R. (2010). Sleep measures and morning plasma TNF-alpha levels in children with sleep-disordered breathing. *Sleep, 33*, 319-325.

Grebe, M., Eisele, H. J., Weissmann, N., Schaefer, C., Tillmanns, H., Seeger, W. et al. (2006). Antioxidant vitamin C improves endothelial function in obstructive sleep apnea. *Am.J.Respir.Crit Care Med., 173*, 897-901.

Grimpen, F., Kanne, P., Schulz, E., Hagenah, G., Hasenfuss, G., & Andreas, S. (2000). Endothelin-1 plasma levels are not elevated in patients with obstructive sleep apnoea. *Eur.Respir.J., 15*, 320-325.

Gude, F., Rey-Garcia, J., Fernandez-Merino, C., Meijide, L., Garcia-Ortiz, L., Zamarron, C. et al. (2009). Serum levels of gamma-glutamyl transferase are associated with markers of nocturnal hypoxemia in a general adult population. *Clin.Chim.Acta.* 407,67-71

Guzik, T. J., Hoch, N. E., Brown, K. A., McCann, L. A., Rahman, A., Dikalov, S. et al. (2007). Role of the T cell in the genesis of angiotensin II induced hypertension and vascular dysfunction. *J.Exp.Med., 204*, 2449-2460.

Haight, J. S. & Djupesland, P. G. (2003). Nitric oxide (NO) and obstructive sleep apnea (OSA). *Sleep Breath., 7*, 53-62.

Halcox, J. P., Donald, A. E., Ellins, E., Witte, D. R., Shipley, M. J., Brunner, E. J. et al. (2009). Endothelial function predicts progression of carotid intima-media thickness. *Circulation, 119*, 1005-1012.

Hansson, G. K. (2005). Inflammation, atherosclerosis, and coronary artery disease. *N.Engl.J.Med., 352*, 1685-1695.

Harsch, I. A., Koebnick, C., Wallaschofski, H., Schahin, S. P., Hahn, E. G., Ficker, J. H. et al. (2004). Resistin levels in patients with obstructive sleep apnoea syndrome--the link to subclinical inflammation? *Med.Sci.Monit., 10*, CR510-CR515.

Harsch, I. A., Konturek, P. C., Koebnick, C., Kuehnlein, P. P., Fuchs, F. S., Pour, S. S. et al. (2003). Leptin and ghrelin levels in patients with obstructive sleep apnoea: effect of CPAP treatment. *Eur.Respir.J., 22*, 251-257.

Hayashi, M., Fujimoto, K., Urushibata, K., Takamizawa, A., Kinoshita, O., & Kubo, K. (2006). Hypoxia-sensitive molecules may modulate the development of atherosclerosis in sleep apnoea syndrome. *Respirology., 11*, 24-31.

Hoekema, A., Stel, A. L., Stegenga, B., van der Hoeven, J. H., Wijkstra, P. J., van Driel, M. F. et al. (2006). Sexual Function and Obstructive Sleep Apnea-Hypopnea: A Randomized Clinical Trial Evaluating the Effects of Oral-Appliance and Continuous Positive Airway Pressure Therapy. *J.Sex Med.,* 4 Pt 2):1153-62

Imagawa, S., Yamaguchi, Y., Ogawa, K., Obara, N., Suzuki, N., Yamamoto, M. et al. (2004). Interleukin-6 and tumor necrosis factor-alpha in patients with obstructive sleep apnea-hypopnea syndrome. *Respiration, 71*, 24-29.

Ip, M. S., Lam, K. S., Ho, C., Tsang, K. W., & Lam, W. (2000). Serum leptin and vascular risk factors in obstructive sleep apnea. *Chest, 118*, 580-586.

Ip, M. S., Tse, H. F., Lam, B., Tsang, K. W., & Lam, W. K. (2004). Endothelial function in obstructive sleep apnea and response to treatment. *Am.J.Respir.Crit. Care. Med., 169*, 348-353.

Isono, S. (2009). Obstructive sleep apnea of obese adults: pathophysiology and perioperative airway management. *Anesthesiology, 110*, 908-921.

Jelic, S., Lederer, D. J., Adams, T., Padeletti, M., Colombo, P. C., Factor, P. H. et al. (2010). Vascular inflammation in obesity and sleep apnea. *Circulation, 121,* 1014-1021.

Kanagy, N. L., Walker, B. R., & Nelin, L. D. (2001). Role of endothelin in intermittent hypoxia-induced hypertension. *Hypertension, 37,* 511-515.

Kapsimalis, F., Varouchakis, G., Manousaki, A., Daskas, S., Nikita, D., Kryger, M. et al. (2008). Association of sleep apnea severity and obesity with insulin resistance, C-reactive protein, and leptin levels in male patients with obstructive sleep apnea. *Lung, 186,* 209-217.

Kasai, T., Inoue, K., Kumagai, T., Kato, M., Kawana, F., Sagara, M. et al. (2011). Plasma pentraxin3 and arterial stiffness in men with obstructive sleep apnea. *Am.J.Hypertens., 24,* 401-407.

Kent, B. D., Ryan, S., & McNicholas, W. T. (2011). Obstructive sleep apnea and inflammation: Relationship to cardiovascular co-morbidity. *Respir.Physiol Neurobiol., 178,*475-81.

Kohler, M., Pepperell, J. C., Casadei, B., Craig, S., Crosthwaite, N., Stradling, J. R. et al. (2008). CPAP and measures of cardiovascular risk in males with OSAS. *Eur.Respir.J., 32,* 1488-1496.

Kuramoto, E., Kinami, S., Ishida, Y., Shiotani, H., & Nishimura, Y. (2009). Continuous positive nasal airway pressure decreases levels of serum amyloid A and improves autonomic function in obstructive sleep apnea syndrome. *Int.J.Cardiol., 135,* 338-345.

Lacedonia, D., Salerno, F. G., Carpagnano, G. E., Sabato, R., Depalo, A., & Foschino-Barbaro, M. P. (2011). Effect of CPAP-therapy on bronchial and nasal inflammation in patients affected by obstructive sleep apnea syndrome. *Rhinology, 49,* 232-237.

Lattimore, J. D., Wilcox, I., Nakhla, S., Langenfeld, M., Jessup, W., & Celermajer, D. S. (2005). Repetitive hypoxia increases lipid loading in human macrophages-a potentially atherogenic effect. *Atherosclerosis, 179,* 255-259.

Lavie, L., Vishnevsky, A., & Lavie, P. (2004). Evidence for lipid peroxidation in obstructive sleep apnea. *Sleep, 27,* 123-128.

Levy, P., Pepin, J. L., Arnaud, C., Baguet, J. P., Dematteis, M., & Mach, F. (2009). Obstructive sleep apnea and atherosclerosis. *Prog.Cardiovasc.Dis., 51,* 400-410.

Li, A. M., Ng, C., Ng, S. K., Chan, M. M., So, H. K., Chan, I. et al. (2010). Adipokines in children with obstructive sleep apnea and the effects of treatment. *Chest, 137,* 529-535.

Li, J., Bosch-Marce, M., Nanayakkara, A., Savransky, V., Fried, S. K., Semenza, G. L. et al. (2006). Altered metabolic responses to intermittent hypoxia in mice with partial deficiency of hypoxia-inducible factor-1alpha. *Physiol. Genomics, 25,* 450-457.

Li, J., Thorne, L. N., Punjabi, N. M., Sun, C. K., Schwartz, A. R., Smith, P. L. et al. (2005). Intermittent hypoxia induces hyperlipidemia in lean mice. *Circ.Res., 97,* 698-706.

Luboshitzky, R., Lavie, L., Shen-Orr, Z., & Herer, P. (2005). Altered luteinizing hormone and testosterone secretion in middle-aged obese men with obstructive sleep apnea. *Obes.Res., 13,* 780-786.

Macrea, M. M., Martin, T. J., & Zagrean, L. (2010). Infertility and obstructive sleep apnea: the effect of continuous positive airway pressure therapy on serum prolactin levels. *Sleep Breath., 14,* 253-257.

Makino, S., Handa, H., Suzukawa, K., Fujiwara, M., Nakamura, M., Muraoka, S. et al. (2006). Obstructive sleep apnoea syndrome, plasma adiponectin levels, and insulin resistance. *Clin.Endocrinol.(Oxf)*, 64, 12-19.

Makinodan, K., Yoshikawa, M., Fukuoka, A., Tamaki, S., Koyama, N., Yamauchi, M. et al. (2008). Effect of serum leptin levels on hypercapnic ventilatory response in obstructive sleep apnea. *Respiration*, 75, 257-264.

Malakasioti, G., Alexopoulos, E., Befani, C., Tanou, K., Varlami, V., Ziogas, D. et al. (2011). Oxidative stress and inflammatory markers in the exhaled breath condensate of children with OSA. *Sleep Breath.*.

Marin, J. M., Carrizo, S. J., Vicente, E., & Agusti, A. G. (2005). Long-term cardiovascular outcomes in men with obstructive sleep apnoea-hypopnoea with or without treatment with continuous positive airway pressure: an observational study. *Lancet*, 365, 1046-1053.

Marrone, O., Salvaggio, A., Bue, A. L., Bonanno, A., Riccobono, L., Insalaco, G. et al. (2011). Blood Pressure Changes After Automatic and Fixed CPAP in Obstructive Sleep Apnea: Relationship with Nocturnal Sympathetic Activity. *Clin.Exp.Hypertens.*, 33,373-80.

Marrone, O., Salvaggio, A., Gioia, M., Bonanno, A., Profita, M., Riccobono, L. et al. (2008). Reticulocytes in untreated obstructive sleep apnoea. *Monaldi Arch.Chest, Dis.*, 69, 107-113.

Maser, R. E., Lenhard, M. J., Rizzo, A. A., & Vasile, A. A. (2008). Continuous positive airway pressure therapy improves cardiovascular autonomic function for persons with sleep-disordered breathing. *Chest*, 133, 86-91.

Masserini, B., Morpurgo, P. S., Donadio, F., Baldessari, C., Bossi, R., Beck-Peccoz, P. et al. (2006). Reduced levels of adiponectin in sleep apnea syndrome. *J.Endocrinol.Invest*, 29, 700-705.

McArdle, N., Hillman, D., Beilin, L., & Watts, G. (2007). Metabolic risk factors for vascular disease in obstructive sleep apnea: a matched controlled study. *Am.J.Respir.Crit. Care. Med.*, 175, 190-195.

Meisinger, C., Heier, M., & Loewel, H. (2005). Sleep disturbance as a predictor of type 2 diabetes mellitus in men and women from the general population. *Diabetologia*, 48, 235-241.

Meston, N., Davies, R. J., Mullins, R., Jenkinson, C., Wass, J. A., & Stradling, J. R. (2003). Endocrine effects of nasal continuous positive airway pressure in male patients with obstructive sleep apnoea. *J.Intern.Med.*, 254, 447-454.

Moller, D. S., Lind, P., Strunge, B., & Pedersen, E. B. (2003). Abnormal vasoactive hormones and 24-hour blood pressure in obstructive sleep apnea. *Am.J.Hypertens.*, 16, 274-280.

Mullington, J. M., Simpson, N. S., Meier-Ewert, H. K., & Haack, M. (2010). Sleep loss and inflammation. *Best.Pract.Res.Clin.Endocrinol.Metab*, 24, 775-784.

Nair, D., Dayyat, E. A., Zhang, S. X., Wang, Y., & Gozal, D. (2011). Intermittent hypoxia-induced cognitive deficits are mediated by NADPH oxidase activity in a murine model of sleep apnea. *PLoS.One.*, 6, e19847.

Nakagawa, Y., Kishida, K., Kihara, S., Yoshida, R., Funahashi, T., & Shimomura, I. (2011). Nocturnal falls of adiponectin levels in sleep apnea with abdominal obesity and impact of hypoxia-induced dysregulated adiponectin production in obese murine mesenteric adipose tissue. *J.Atheroscler.Thromb.*, 18, 240-247.

Nestel, P. (2003). Metabolic syndrome: multiple candidate genes, multiple environmental factors--multiple syndromes? *Int.J.Clin.Pract.Suppl*, 3-9.

Newman, A. B., Nieto, F. J., Guidry, U., Lind, B. K., Redline, S., Pickering, T. G. et al. (2001). Relation of sleep-disordered breathing to cardiovascular disease risk factors: the Sleep Heart Health Study. *Am.J.Epidemiol.*, 154, 50-59.

Nieto, F. J., Herrington, D. M., Redline, S., Benjamin, E. J., & Robbins, J. A. (2004). Sleep apnea and markers of vascular endothelial function in a large community sample of older adults. *Am.J.Respir.Crit Care Med.*, 169, 354-360.

O'Donnell, C. P., Tankersley, C. G., Polotsky, V. P., Schwartz, A. R., & Smith, P. L. (2000). Leptin, obesity, and respiratory function. *Respir.Physiol*, 119, 163-170.

Oga, T., Chin, K., Tabuchi, A., Kawato, M., Morimoto, T., Takahashi, K. et al. (2009). Effects of obstructive sleep apnea with intermittent hypoxia on platelet aggregability. *J.Atheroscler.Thromb.*, 16, 862-869.

Ohga, E., Nagase, T., Tomita, T., Teramoto, S., Matsuse, T., Katayama, H. et al. (1999). Increased levels of circulating ICAM-1, VCAM-1, and L-selectin in obstructive sleep apnea syndrome. *J.Appl.Physiol*, 87, 10-14.

Ohga, E., Tomita, T., Wada, H., Yamamoto, H., Nagase, T., & Ouchi, Y. (2003). Effects of obstructive sleep apnea on circulating ICAM-1, IL-8, and MCP-1. *J.Appl.Physiol*, 94, 179-184.

Oldenburg, O., Lamp, B., Faber, L., Teschler, H., Horstkotte, D., & Topfer, V. (2007). Sleep-disordered breathing in patients with symptomatic heart failure: a contemporary study of prevalence in and characteristics of 700 patients. *Eur.J.Heart Fail.*, 9, 251-257.

Othman, M., Gordon, S. P., & Iscoe, S. (2010). Repeated inspiratory occlusions in anesthetized rats acutely increase blood coagulability as assessed by thromboelastography. *Respir.Physiol, Neurobiol.*, 171, 61-66.

Ozturk, L., Unal, M., Tamer, L., & Celikoglu, F. (2003). The association of the severity of obstructive sleep apnea with plasma leptin levels. *Arch.Otolaryngol.Head Neck Surg.*, 129, 538-540.

Park, A. M., Nagase, H., Kumar, S. V., & Suzuki, Y. J. (2007). Effects of intermittent hypoxia on the heart. *Antioxid.Redox.Signal.*, 9, 723-729.

Patel, S. R., Malhotra, A., White, D. P., Gottlieb, D. J., & Hu, F. B. (2006). Association between reduced sleep and weight gain in women. *Am.J.Epidemiol.*, 164, 947-954.

Patel, S. R., Palmer, L. J., Larkin, E. K., Jenny, N. S., White, D. P., & Redline, S. (2004). Relationship between obstructive sleep apnea and diurnal leptin rhythms. *Sleep*, 27, 235-239.

Patel, S. R., Zhu, X., Storfer-Isser, A., Mehra, R., Jenny, N. S., Tracy, R. et al. (2009). Sleep duration and biomarkers of inflammation. *Sleep*, 32, 200-204.

Patt, B. T., Jarjoura, D., Haddad, D. N., Sen, C. K., Roy, S., Flavahan, N. A. et al. (2010). Endothelial dysfunction in the microcirculation of patients with obstructive sleep apnea. *Am.J.Respir.Crit. Care. Med.*, 182, 1540-1545.

Peled, N., Kassirer, M., Kramer, M. R., Rogowski, O., Shlomi, D., Fox, B. et al. (2008). Increased erythrocyte adhesiveness and aggregation in obstructive sleep apnea syndrome. *Thromb.Res.*, 121, 631-636.

Phillips, B. G., Kato, M., Narkiewicz, K., Choe, I., & Somers, V. K. (2000). Increases in leptin levels, sympathetic drive, and weight gain in obstructive sleep apnea. *Am.J.Physiol. Heart. Circ.Physiol., 279*, H234-H237.

Phillips, B. G., Narkiewicz, K., Pesek, C. A., Haynes, W. G., Dyken, M. E., & Somers, V. K. (1999). Effects of obstructive sleep apnea on endothelin-1 and blood pressure. *J.Hypertens., 17*, 61-66.

Phipps, P. R., Starritt, E., Caterson, I., & Grunstein, R. R. (2002). Association of serum leptin with hypoventilation in human obesity. *Thorax, 57*, 75-76.

Pichel, F., Zamarron, C., Magan, F., del, C. F., Alvarez-Sala, R., & Suarez, J. R. (2004). Health-related quality of life in patients with obstructive sleep apnea: effects of long-term positive airway pressure treatment. *Respir.Med., 98*, 968-976.

Piemonti, L., Calori, G., Mercalli, A., Lattuada, G., Monti, P., Garancini, M. P. et al. (2003). Fasting plasma leptin, tumor necrosis factor-alpha receptor 2, and monocyte chemoattracting protein 1 concentration in a population of glucose-tolerant and glucose-intolerant women: impact on cardiovascular mortality. *Diabetes Care, 26*, 2883-2889.

Pohl, U. & Busse, R. (1989). Differential vascular sensitivity to luminally and adventitially applied endothelin-1. *J.Cardiovasc.Pharmacol., 13 Suppl 5*, S188-S190.

Polotsky, V. Y., Li, J., Punjabi, N. M., Rubin, A. E., Smith, P. L., Schwartz, A. R. et al. (2003). Intermittent hypoxia increases insulin resistance in genetically obese mice. *J.Physiol, 552*, 253-264.

Prabhakar, N. R., Fields, R. D., Baker, T., & Fletcher, E. C. (2001). Intermittent hypoxia: cell to system. *Am.J.Physiol. Lung. Cell. Mol.Physiol., 281*, L524-L528.

Prentice, A. M. (2006). The emerging epidemic of obesity in developing countries. *Int.J.Epidemiol., 35*, 93-99.

Proulx, K., Richard, D., & Walker, C. D. (2002). Leptin regulates appetite-related neuropeptides in the hypothalamus of developing rats without affecting food intake. *Endocrinology, 143*, 4683-4692.

Punjabi, N. M. & Beamer, B. A. (2007). C-reactive protein is associated with sleep disordered breathing independent of adiposity. *Sleep, 30*, 29-34.

Querido, J. S., Sheel, A. W., Cheema, R., Van, E. S., Mulgrew, A. T., & Ayas, N. T. (2011). Effects of 10 days of modest intermittent hypoxia on circulating measures of inflammation in healthy humans. *Sleep Breath.* Jul 9. [Epub ahead of print]

Quercioli, A., Mach, F., & Montecucco, F. (2010). Inflammation accelerates atherosclerotic processes in obstructive sleep apnea syndrome (OSAS). *Sleep Breath., 14*, 261-269.

Rahangdale, S., Yeh S.Y., Novack, V., Stevenson, K., Barnard M,R., Furman M,I., et al. (2011). The influence of intermittent hypoxemia on platelet activation in obese patients with obstructive sleep apnea. J Clin Sleep Med., 15;7,172-8

Reaven, G. M. (2005). Insulin resistance, the insulin resistance syndrome, and cardiovascular disease. *Panminerva Med., 47*, 201-210.

Reinhart, W. H., Oswald, J., Walter, R., & Kuhn, M. (2002). Blood viscosity and platelet function in patients with obstructive sleep apnea syndrome treated with nasal continuous positive airway pressure. *Clin.Hemorheol.Microcirc., 27*, 201-207.

Remmers, J. E., deGroot, W. J., Sauerland, E. K., & Anch, A. M. (1978). Pathogenesis of upper airway occlusion during sleep. *J.Appl.Physiol, 44*, 931-938.

Resnick, H. E., Jones, K., Ruotolo, G., Jain, A. K., Henderson, J., Lu, W. et al. (2003). Insulin resistance, the metabolic syndrome, and risk of incident cardiovascular disease in nondiabetic american indians: the Strong Heart Study. *Diabetes Care, 26,* 861-867.

Resta, O., Bonfitto, P., Sabato, R., De, P. G., & Barbaro, M. P. (2004). Prevalence of obstructive sleep apnoea in a sample of obese women: effect of menopause. *Diabetes Nutr.Metab., 17,* 296-303.

Ronti, T., Lupattelli, G., & Mannarino, E. (2006). The endocrine function of adipose tissue: an update. *Clin.Endocrinol.(Oxf), 64,* 355-365.

Ross, R. (1999). Atherosclerosis--an inflammatory disease. *N.Engl.J.Med., 340,* 115-126.

Rossi, G. P. & Pitter, G. (2006). Genetic variation in the endothelin system: do polymorphisms affect the therapeutic strategies? *Ann.N.Y.Acad.Sci., 1069,* 34-50.

Ryan, S., Taylor, C. T., & McNicholas, W. T. (2005). Selective activation of inflammatory pathways by intermittent hypoxia in obstructive sleep apnea syndrome. *Circulation, 112,* 2660-2667.

Saarelainen, S. & Hasan, J. (2000). Circulating endothelin-1 and obstructive sleep apnoea. *Eur.Respir.J., 16,* 794-795.

Sanner, B. M., Kollhosser, P., Buechner, N., Zidek, W., & Tepel, M. (2004). Influence of treatment on leptin levels in patients with obstructive sleep apnoea. *Eur.Respir.J., 23,* 601-604.

Schulz, R., Mahmoudi, S., Hattar, K., Sibelius, U., Olschewski, H., Mayer, K. et al. (2000). Enhanced release of superoxide from polymorphonuclear neutrophils in obstructive sleep apnea. Impact of continuous positive airway pressure therapy. *Am.J.Respir.Crit. Care. Med., 162,* 566-570.

Schwartz, A. R., Patil, S. P., Laffan, A. M., Polotsky, V., Schneider, H., & Smith, P. L. (2008). Obesity and obstructive sleep apnea: pathogenic mechanisms and therapeutic approaches. *Proc.Am.Thorac.Soc., 5,* 185-192.

Shahar, E., Redline, S., Young, T., Boland, L. L., Baldwin, C. M., Nieto, F. J. et al. (2003). Hormone replacement therapy and sleep-disordered breathing. *Am.J.Respir.Crit. Care. Med., 167,* 1186-1192.

Shimizu, K., Chin, K., Nakamura, T., Masuzaki, H., Ogawa, Y., Hosokawa, R. et al. (2002). Plasma leptin levels and cardiac sympathetic function in patients with obstructive sleep apnoea-hypopnoea syndrome. *Thorax, 57,* 429-434.

Shimura, R., Tatsumi, K., Nakamura, A., Kasahara, Y., Tanabe, N., Takiguchi, Y. et al. (2005). Fat accumulation, leptin, and hypercapnia in obstructive sleep apnea-hypopnea syndrome. *Chest, 127,* 543-549.

Shinohara, E., Kihara, S., Yamashita, S., Yamane, M., Nishida, M., Arai, T. et al. (1997). Visceral fat accumulation as an important risk factor for obstructive sleep apnoea syndrome in obese subjects. *J.Intern.Med., 241,* 11-18.

Shitrit, D., Peled, N., Shitrit, A. B., Meidan, S., Bendayan, D., Sahar, G. et al. (2005). An association between oxygen desaturation and D-dimer in patients with obstructive sleep apnea syndrome. *Thromb.Haemost., 94,* 544-547.

Snitker, S., Pratley, R. E., Nicolson, M., Tataranni, P. A., & Ravussin, E. (1997). Relationship between muscle sympathetic nerve activity and plasma leptin concentration. *Obes.Res., 5,* 338-340.

Somers, V. K., Mark, A. L., & Abboud, F. M. (1988). Sympathetic activation by hypoxia and hypercapnia--implications for sleep apnea. *Clin.Exp.Hypertens.A, 10 Suppl 1*, 413-422.

Spruyt, K., Sans, C. O., Serpero, L. D., Kheirandish-Gozal, L., & Gozal, D. (2010). Dietary and physical activity patterns in children with obstructive sleep apnea. *J.Pediatr., 156*, 724-30.

Steiropoulos, P., Kotsianidis, I., Nena, E., Tsara, V., Gounari, E., Hatzizisi, O. et al. (2009). Long-term effect of continuous positive airway pressure therapy on inflammation markers of patients with obstructive sleep apnea syndrome. *Sleep, 32*, 537-543.

Svatikova, A., Wolk, R., Shamsuzzaman, A. S., Kara, T., Olson, E. J., & Somers, V. K. (2003). Serum amyloid a in obstructive sleep apnea. *Circulation, 108*, 1451-1454.

Taheri, S., Austin, D., Lin, L., Nieto, F. J., Young, T., & Mignot, E. (2007). Correlates of serum C-reactive protein (CRP)--no association with sleep duration or sleep disordered breathing. *Sleep, 30*, 991-996.

Tamisier, R., Pepin, J. L., Remy, J., Baguet, J. P., Taylor, J. A., Weiss, J. W. et al. (2011). 14 nights of intermittent hypoxia elevate daytime blood pressure and sympathetic activity in healthy humans. *Eur.Respir.J., 37*, 119-128.

Tasali, E., Chapotot, F., Leproult, R., Whitmore, H., & Ehrmann, D. A. (2011). Treatment of obstructive sleep apnea improves cardiometabolic function in young obese women with polycystic ovary syndrome. *J.Clin.Endocrinol.Metab, 96*, 365-374.

Tassone, F., Lanfranco, F., Gianotti, L., Pivetti, S., Navone, F., Rossetto, R. et al. (2003). Obstructive sleep apnoea syndrome impairs insulin sensitivity independently of anthropometric variables. *Clin.Endocrinol.(Oxf), 59*, 374-379.

Tatsumi, K., Kasahara, Y., Kurosu, K., Tanabe, N., Takiguchi, Y., & Kuriyama, T. (2005). Sleep oxygen desaturation and circulating leptin in obstructive sleep apnea-hypopnea syndrome. *Chest, 127*, 716-721.

Teloken, P. E., Smith, E. B., Lodowsky, C., Freedom, T., & Mulhall, J. P. (2006). Defining association between sleep apnea syndrome and erectile dysfunction. *Urology, 67*, 1033-1037.

Theorell-Haglow, J., Berne, C., Janson, C., & Lindberg, E. (2011). The role of obstructive sleep apnea in metabolic syndrome: a population-based study in women. *Sleep Med., 12*, 329-334.

Teramoto, S., Kume, H., Yamamoto, H., Ishii, T., Miyashita, A., Matsuse, T. et al. (2003). Effects of oxygen administration on the circulating vascular endothelial growth factor (VEGF) levels in patients with obstructive sleep apnea syndrome. *Intern.Med., 42*, 681-685.

Teran-Santos, J., Jimenez-Gomez, A., & Cordero-Guevara, J. (1999). The association between sleep apnea and the risk of traffic accidents. Cooperative Group Burgos-Santander. *N.Engl.J.Med., 340*, 847-851.

Tkacova, R., Dorkova, Z., Molcanyiova, A., Radikova, Z., Klimes, I., & Tkac, I. (2008). Cardiovascular risk and insulin resistance in patients with obstructive sleep apnea. *Med.Sci.Monit., 14*, CR438-CR444.

Tokuda, F., Sando, Y., Matsui, H., Koike, H., & Yokoyama, T. (2008). Serum levels of adipocytokines, adiponectin and leptin, in patients with obstructive sleep apnea syndrome. *Intern.Med., 47*, 1843-1849.

Trzepizur, W., Gagnadoux, F., Abraham, P., Rousseau, P., Meslier, N., Saumet, J. L. et al. (2009). Microvascular endothelial function in obstructive sleep apnea: Impact of continuous positive airway pressure and mandibular advancement. *Sleep Med.*, *10*, 746-752.

Tsaoussoglou, M., Bixler, E. O., Calhoun, S., Chrousos, G. P., Sauder, K., & Vgontzas, A. N. (2010). Sleep-disordered breathing in obese children is associated with prevalent excessive daytime sleepiness, inflammation, and metabolic abnormalities. *J.Clin.Endocrinol.Metab*, *95*, 143-150.

Ulukavak, C. T., Kokturk, O., Bukan, N., & Bilgihan, A. (2005). Leptin and ghrelin levels in patients with obstructive sleep apnea syndrome. *Respiration*, *72*, 395-401.

Varol, E., Ozturk, O., Yucel, H., Gonca, T., Has, M., Dogan, A. et al. (2011). The effects of continuous positive airway pressure therapy on mean platelet volume in patients with obstructive sleep apnea. *Platelets. 22, 552-6*

Vatansever, E., Surmen-Gur, E., Ursavas, A., & Karadag, M. (2010). Obstructive sleep apnea causes oxidative damage to plasma lipids and proteins and decreases adiponectin levels. *Sleep Breath. 15, 275-82*

von, K. R. & Dimsdale, J. E. (2003). Hemostatic alterations in patients with obstructive sleep apnea and the implications for cardiovascular disease. *Chest, 124*, 1956-1967.

von, K. R., Loredo, J. S., Ancoli-Israel, S., & Dimsdale, J. E. (2006). Association between sleep apnea severity and blood coagulability: Treatment effects of nasal continuous positive airway pressure. *Sleep Breath., 10*, 139-146.

von, K. R., Loredo, J. S., Ancoli-Israel, S., Mills, P. J., Natarajan, L., & Dimsdale, J. E. (2007). Association between polysomnographic measures of disrupted sleep and prothrombotic factors. *Chest, 131*, 733-739.

von, K. R., Loredo, J. S., Powell, F. L., Adler, K. A., & Dimsdale, J. E. (2005). Short-term isocapnic hypoxia and coagulation activation in patients with sleep apnea. *Clin.Hemorheol.Microcirc., 33*, 369-377.

Wesstrom, J., Ulfberg, J., & Nilsson, S. (2005). Sleep apnea and hormone replacement therapy: a pilot study and a literature review. *Acta Obstet.Gynecol.Scand., 84*, 54-57.

Wilcox, I., McNamara, S. G., Collins, F. L., Grunstein, R. R., & Sullivan, C. E. (1998). "Syndrome Z": the interaction of sleep apnoea, vascular risk factors and heart disease. *Thorax, 53 Suppl 3*, S25-S28.

Wysocka, E., Cofta, S., Cymerys, M., Gozdzik, J., Torlinski, L., & Batura-Gabryel, H. (2008). The impact of the sleep apnea syndrome on oxidant-antioxidant balance in the blood of overweight and obese patients. *J.Physiol Pharmacol., 59 Suppl 6*, 761-769.

Wysocka, E., Cofta, S., Dziegielewska, S., Gozdzik, J., Torlinski, L., & Batura-Gabryel, H. (2009). Adipocytokines in sleep apnea syndrome. *Eur.J.Med.Res., 14 Suppl 4*, 255-258.

Yamamoto, Y., Fujiuchi, S., Hiramatsu, M., Nishigaki, Y., Takeda, A., Fujita, Y. et al. (2008). Resistin is closely related to systemic inflammation in obstructive sleep apnea. *Respiration, 76*, 377-385.

Yokoe, T., Minoguchi, K., Matsuo, H., Oda, N., Minoguchi, H., Yoshino, G. et al. (2003). Elevated levels of C-reactive protein and interleukin-6 in patients with obstructive sleep apnea syndrome are decreased by nasal continuous positive airway pressure. *Circulation, 107*, 1129-1134.

Young, T., Palta, M., Dempsey, J., Skatrud, J., Weber, S., & Badr, S. (1993). The occurrence of sleep-disordered breathing among middle-aged adults. *N.Engl.J.Med.*, *328*, 1230-1235.

Yu, H. J., Lin, B. R., Lee, H. S., Shun, C. T., Yang, C. C., Lai, T. Y. et al. (2005). Sympathetic vesicovascular reflex induced by acute urinary retention evokes proinflammatory and proapoptotic injury in rat liver. *Am.J.Physiol Renal Physiol*, *288*, F1005-F1014.

Zamarron, C., Garcia, P., V, & Riveiro, A. (2008a). Obstructive sleep apnea syndrome is a systemic disease. Current evidence. *Eur.J.Intern.Med.*, *19*, 390-398.

Zamarron, C., Ricoy, J., Riveiro, A., & Gude, F. (2008b). Plasminogen activator inhibitor-1 in obstructive sleep apnea patients with and without hypertension. *Lung*, *186*, 151-156.

Zamarron-Sanz, C., Ricoy-Galbaldon, J., Gude-Sampedro, F., & Riveiro-Riveiro, A. (2006). Plasma levels of vascular endothelial markers in obstructive sleep apnea. *Arch.Med.Res.*, *37*, 552-555.

Zhang, X. L., Yin, K. S., Wang, H., & Su, S. (2006). Serum adiponectin levels in adult male patients with obstructive sleep apnea hypopnea syndrome. *Respiration*, *73*, 73-77.

Zouaoui, B. K., Guillaume, M., Henuzet, C., Delree, P., Cauchie, P., Remacle, C. et al. (2006). Fibrinolysis and cardiovascular risk factors: association with fibrinogen, lipids, and monocyte count. *Eur.J.Intern.Med.*, *17*, 102-108.

# 9

# Mediterranean Diet and Cardiovascular Risk

Javier Delgado-Lista, Ana I. Perez-Caballero, Pablo Perez-Martinez,
Antonio Garcia-Rios, Jose Lopez-Miranda and Francisco Perez-Jimenez
*Unidad de Lipidos y Arteriosclerosis, IMIBIC/Hospital Universitario Reina Sofia,
Universidad de Cordoba, Ciber Fisiopatología Obesidad y Nutrición (CIBEROBN),
Instituto de Salud Carlos III,
Spain*

## 1. Introduction

The Mediterranean diet is becoming a generalized recommended eating pattern worldwide, especially after epidemiological studies showing that adherence to this model is associated with a lower total mortality and cardiovascular diseases. Some of the conditions in which this dietary model has proven to be linked with a lower incidence are coronary events, stroke, hypertension, unfavorable blood glucose control, age cognitive decline or certain types of cancer (D. Giugliano & Esposito, 2008; Kontou et al., 2011; Lopez-Miranda et al., 2010; Solfrizzi et al., 2011; Tangney et al., 2011; Willett, 2006). Although the underlying mechanisms by which this type of diet may exert its beneficial functions are far from being totally understood, current knowledge states that these are beyond the classical cardiovascular risk factors like lipids or the control or blood pressure, and involve, among others, inflammation, oxidative stress, coagulation and endothelial function.

One of the aspects to be taken into account when considering the effects of Mediterranean Diet is the heterogeneity of this concept, comprising different dietary patterns, slightly differing between the different countries in which this diet was originally consumed, because of local foodstuff preferences. The Mediterranean Diet includes a high consumption of food from plant origin (fruits, vegetables, nuts and grains), using olive oil (preferably extra virgin) as the main source of fat, used both as a cooking vehicle as for seasoning, although some other sources of monounsaturated fatty acids as the main dietary fat have been recently proposed. Mediterranean Diet preferred sources of protein are fish and poultry, while red meats are rarely consumed. Additionally, the use of sweets, pastry and dairy products are also of exceptional use. The use of milk and milk derived products, like yoghourt or cheese is moderated in most of the Mediterranean models, although with some country variations, with higher consumers, like the Greek dietary pattern. Finally, in some of the Mediterranean countries (like Spain, France and Italy) there is a common moderate consumption of red wine. These characteristics are summarized in figure 1.

The current interest in this type of food comes from the conjunction of a increasingly scientific evidence of the advantages of its consumption in different health aspects and its high palatability, which validates it for long use purposes, contrarily to other healthy alternatives with low palatability, which are difficult to maintain on a long outlook basis(Panunzio et al., 2011). Supporting the cited scientific evidences on cardiovascular risk, and validated by well designed works(Fuentes et al., 2001; Jansen et al., 2000; Kris-Etherton et al., 1993; Mata et al., 1992), the FDA authorized a health claim on olive oil on coronary heart disease (CFSAN/Office of Nutritional Products, 2004).

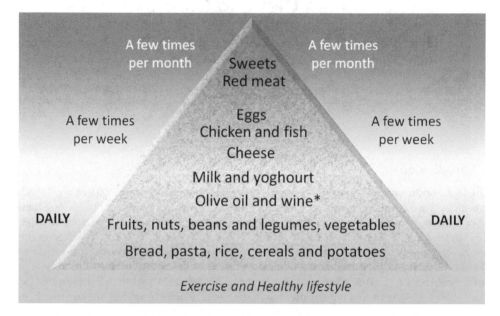

Fig. 1. Schematic representation of a Mediterranean diet pyramid. * Wine is only recommended in those adults that already consume it, or are willing to do it, and always with moderation (lower than 200 cc/day). In no case wine consumption must be started only to comply with the Mediterranean diet.

As stated above, there is a plenty of conditions and physiological features where Mediterranean Diet has shown to be beneficial, from digestive tract motility to neurologic cognitive wellness in the aged persons, or the apparition of some types of cancer (D. Giugliano & Esposito, 2008; Kontou et al., 2011; Lopez-Miranda et al., 2010; Solfrizzi et al., 2011; Tangney et al., 2011; Willett, 2006). However, we will only revise in the present document some of the evidences relating Mediterranean Diet and cardiovascular risk.

Assessing the modification of the cardiovascular risk by diet is a difficult task, specially having into account that cardiovascular risk assessment tools are not strictly uniform. Moreover, some of the increasingly accepted newer cardiovascular risk factors, like inflammation, thrombogenic state, postprandial lipemia, oxidative stress or endothelial function are not still included in the classical risk assessment tools. Finally, assessing the impact of the diet in different geographic locations has the risk of underestimate other diet related circumstances, like the fact of eating at home, eating out, the relative well-being or stress associated meal-time, or other interactions between eating and other behavior factors (like, for example meal-associated smoke consumption). In a recent article, it has been stated that the effects of Mediterranean Diet on total mortality increases when combined with other healthy lifestyle factors, like , nonsmoking, normal weight [BMI (in kg/m(2)): 18.5 to <25], and regular physical activity (van den Brandt, 2011). On the other hand, we cannot forget the interaction between the diet and the genetics of the population investigated, the so called nutrigenetics. The consumption of a nutrient may be more or less healthy in a given population depending on that population genetics(Allayee et al., 2009; Lairon et al., 2009; Lovegrove & Gitau, 2008; Ordovas, 2006; Perez-Martinez et al., 2010a; Perez-Martinez et al., 2011b).

The purpose of this review is to present some evidence of studies which have already demonstrated the benefitial effects of the Mediterranean Diet in the different cardiovascular risk factors, and discuss the underlying mechanisms by which it exerts its effects. We will also review the different studies that link the consumption of this dietary model with a lower prevalence of cardiovascular disease.

## 2. Mediterranean Diet and lipids

The concentration of total cholesterol in plasma, as well as that of its fractions (HDL, LDL) is clearly related to cardiovascular risk, and hence they are included in the most used cardiovascular risk assessment tools, the Frammingham cardiovascular risk tables (N.C.E.P., 2001) and the European SCORE risk tool (HeartScore, 2003). While total cholesterol and LDL cholesterol are directly correlated to the risk, this relationship is reverse with HDL cholesterol. Triglycerides, which were not classically considered when assessing cardiovascular risk, have been recently identified as clear modifiers of cardiovascular risk, even independently of cholesterol, and an enlarged postprandial lipemia (which mainly involves triglyceride and triglyceride rich lipoproteins metabolism) has been identified as one of the major cardiovascular risk factors (Bayturan et al., 2010; Kolovou et al., 2011; Langsted et al., 2011; Lopez-Miranda et al., 2006; Patel et al., 2004; Sarwar et al., 2007; van Wijk et al., 2009; Varbo et al., 2011).

When considering the effects of the different types of diet on plasma lipids, studies have mainly centered on the effects of the fatty components of the diet studied in the lipid profile. For the studies dealing with Mediterranean Diet, this fact has driven to the study of the effects on lipids of olive oil as a food and of monounsaturated fatty acids as dietary fatty acids. With that scope it has been proved that lipid profile becomes healthier when Mediterranean diets rich in monounsaturated fats replace diets rich in saturated fatty acids rich diets, reducing LDL cholesterol, and the ratio total cholesterol/HDL.

The above effects were evaluated and corroborated by the FDA, when it approved the health claim on olive oil in 2004, authorizing the inclusion of the following sentence in the labeling of the olive oil bottles: *Limited and not conclusive scientific evidence suggests that eating about two tablespoons (23 grams) of olive oil daily may reduce the risk of coronary heart disease due to the monounsaturated fat in olive oil. To achieve this possible benefit, olive oil is to replace a similar amount of saturated fat and not increase the total number of calories you eat in a day* (CFSAN/Office of Nutritional Products, 2004).

Furthermore and complementing the favorable effects of olive oil, there has been extensively proven the beneficial effects of vegetables, fruits and pulse when replacing foods rich in saturated fatty acids, like butter, pork or red meat, reducing total cholesterol, triglycerides and LDL cholesterol (Bach-Faig et al., 2006; Lapointe et al., 2005; Mordente et al., 2011;

Pitsavos et al., 2005; Tripoli et al., 2005; Visioli & Galli, 1998; Yubero-Serrano et al., 2011). In addition, LDL resistance to oxidation is augmented when Mediterranean Diet rich in Olive Oil replaces diets rich in saturated fats. It is known that oxidation of LDL cholesterol is a key factor in the development of the atherosclerosis, promoting the formation of foam cells in the sub-endothelial space of the vascular wall. The underlying cause of this latter effect seems to be a combination of the monounsaturated fatty acids from olive oil, the antioxidant power of the minor compounds present in virgin olive oil, like phenols, and the elevated antioxidant capacity of the fruits and vegetables. Furthermore, a recent report from the European Food Safety Authority (EFSA) supports the effects of virgin olive oil phenols on LDL oxidation(EFSA, 2011). Lycopene, a carotenoid abundant in the tomato also deserves a mention, by its biochemical functions including acting as antioxidant scavenger, hypolipaemic agent, or inhibitor of pro-inflammatory and pro-thrombotic factors(Mordente et al., 2011). Additionally, resveratrol, a natural antioxidant present in red wine seems to play a role in this antioxidant effect on LDL cholesterol(Mukamal & Rimm, 2008).

## 3. Mediterranean Diet and blood pressure

The influence of diet on blood pressure is well established. Diets rich in vegetables, like Mediterranean diet, reduce systolic and diastolic blood pressure (Alonso et al., 2006; Gillingham et al., 2011; Masala et al., 2008). These effects have been directly assessed in Mediterranean diet, and again they seem to be due to a combination of the favorable effects of olive oil, vegetables and fish (Alonso et al., 2004; Bondia-Pons et al., 2007; Din et al., 2004; Esposito et al., 2004; Fito et al., 2005; Gillingham et al., 2011; Masala et al., 2008; Perona et al., 2004). In fact, and supporting that the effect of olive oil is independent of the population studied or the dietary pattern, a north-european cohort who consumed olive oil as a part of their habitual diet reduced their blood pressure when switching their main fat source to olive oil(Bondia-Pons et al., 2007). A recent review summarized all the current information on the effects of monounsaturated fatty acids in blood pressure. In overall of the 16 studies analyzed, the authors reported that strong support can be obtained from clinical trials of the blood pressure lowering effects of MUFA rich diets in both normotensive and hypertensive individuals (Gillingham et al., 2011).

Not only the nutrient intake, but also the fiber content influences blood pressure. When adjusted by other possible confounders, the relative high percentage of the Mediterranean Diet is linked to a lower blood pressure (Alonso et al., 2006; Estruch et al., 2009). When studying the micronutrients responsible of these effects, the monounsaturated fats, the phenols from olive oil and vegetables and the n-3 fatty acids from fish seem to be implicated, as well as the relative low sodium levels achieved by vegetables compared to meat and the alcohol present in red wine, among others (Fito et al., 2005; Geleijnse et al., 2002; Masala et al., 2008; B. M. Rasmussen et al., 2006; Shah et al., 2007).

## 4. Mediterranean Diet and smoking effects on cardiovascular disease

Although the smoking habit is detrimental for the health in any dietary habit, the influence of the diet in the deleterious effects of smoking on health has not been widely studied. Epidemiological studies indicate that a high adherence to the Mediterranean Diet model is associated with a reduction of the risk conferred by the smoking habit (Haveman-Nies et al.,

2002; Mitrou et al., 2007). A recent work reviewed this topic in deep (Vardavas et al., 2011), and concludes, that, existing scientific literature indicates that the dietary intake of Mediterranean diet, can act as a positive effect modifier on the impact of smoking on cardiovascular health. When looking for underlying mechanisms, authors postulate two main hypothetical *vias*. Mediterranean Diet is rich in antioxidants. How we explained above, LDL resistance to oxidation in augmented when the person consumes Mediterranean Diet, and, thus, this person could be partially protected to the tobacco-induced LDL-oxidation. On the other hand, the increase of the HDL/total cholesterol provoked by the Mediterranean Diet could partially blunt the development of atherosclerosis caused by the smoking habit (Mitrou et al., 2007).

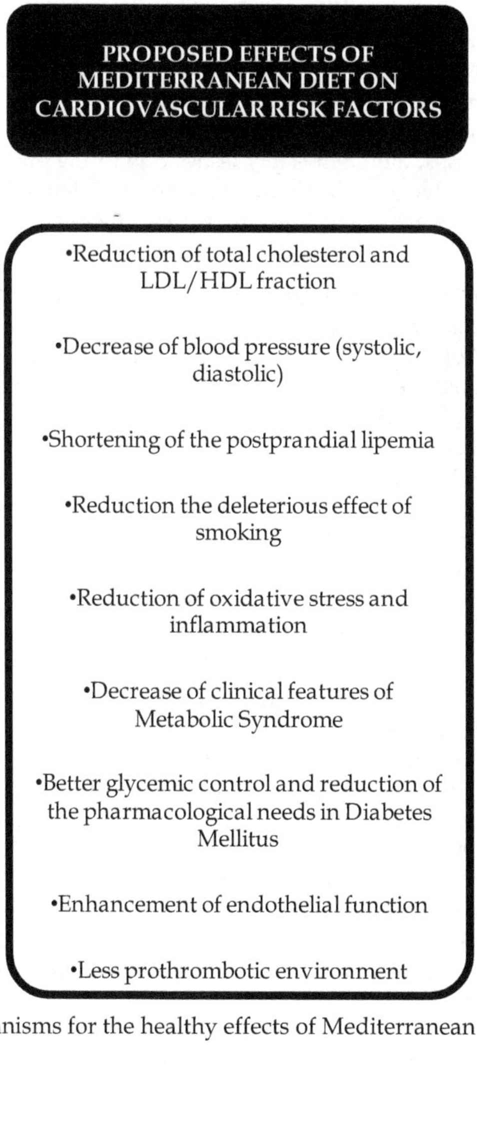

**PROPOSED EFFECTS OF MEDITERRANEAN DIET ON CARDIOVASCULAR RISK FACTORS**

- Reduction of total cholesterol and LDL/HDL fraction

- Decrease of blood pressure (systolic, diastolic)

- Shortening of the postprandial lipemia

- Reduction the deleterious effect of smoking

- Reduction of oxidative stress and inflammation

- Decrease of clinical features of Metabolic Syndrome

- Better glycemic control and reduction of the pharmacological needs in Diabetes Mellitus

- Enhancement of endothelial function

- Less prothrombotic environment

Fig. 2. Proposed mechanisms for the healthy effects of Mediterranean diet on Cardiovascular Disease.

## 5. Mediterranean Diet and hemostasis

Haemostatic system includes platelets and coagulation factors. It is devoted to maintain the optimal blood flow integrity, and to repair the vessels injuries. However, it has been firmly established that an unbalance of this system is a key factor in the development of atherosclerosis(Borissoff et al., 2011). The development of the plaque and its eventual rupture are favored by an increase in plasma of certain coagulation factors and platelet mediators. Diet can modulate the haemostatic equilibrium. Diets rich in fish, (especially blue fish) has an antiaggregant effect, mainly due to its content of n-3 fatty acids, which interferes with platelets metabolism(Renaud & Lanzmann-Petithory, 2002; Seo et al., 2005). Furthermore, the direct effect of n-3 fatty acids reducing cardiovascular events and cardiovascular mortality has been proved both in epidemiological studies and clinical trials, although some recent studies failed to find such advantages(Filion et al., 2010; Harris et al., 2008; Lavie et al., 2009; Mente et al., 2009; Riediger et al., 2009). Currently, the AHA recommends two servings of blue fish a week for general population (to maintain a mean of 500 mg/d), and 1 g/d of marine omega-3 (EPA and DHA) in patients with coronary disease to lower cardiovascular risk, although safety issues due to the presence of harmful metals like mercury in large fish, like tuna or shark currently advices to take this recommendation with caution in pregnant women and little child (Kris-Etherton et al., 2002; Lichtenstein et al., 2006).

The same antiaggregant effect has been also find associated to the intake of olive oil, especially extra virgin olive oil, which has been justified by the presence of oleic acid and the minor components of virgin olive oil, like phenols. The underlying mechanisms for theses effects include tromboxane reduction, decrease of ADP reactivity and ATP release from platelets, decrease of platelet-activating factor (Antonopoulou et al., 2006; Karantonis et al., 2002; Karantonis et al., 2006; Perez-Jimenez et al., 2006; Singh et al., 2008; Sirtori et al., 1986; Smith et al., 2003). Effects of wine, a common element in certain countries consuming Mediterranean Diet have been also examined in some studies, but results are inconclusive. While its moderate consumption decreases some procoagulant species, like fibrinogen, and increase the natural anticoagulant TPA, also increases some proinflammatory markers (ICAM-1, E-Selectin, interleukin-6), and even may lead to an increase in total platelet aggregation (Mezzano & Leighton, 2003; Tozzi Ciancarelli et al., 2011). Hereby, more studies are needed to unveil its overall influence on haemostasis.

The effects of olive oil in haemostasis go beyond platelets, and influences directly the plasma concentration of several procoagulant substances, like FVII (Delgado-Lista et al., 2008; Junker et al., 2001a; Junker et al., 2001b; Mezzano & Leighton, 2003; Mezzano et al., 2003; Smith et al., 2003; Temme et al., 1999; Turpeinen & Mutanen, 1999; Williams, 2001), tissue factor (Bravo-Herrera et al., 2004), fibrinogen (Mezzano & Leighton, 2003), PAI-1 factor (Avellone et al., 1998; Perez-Jimenez, 2005; Perez-Jimenez et al., 1999; Perez-Jimenez et al., 2002) or von Willebrand Factor (Perez-Jimenez et al., 1999; O. Rasmussen et al., 1994), reducing the thrombogenic state when compared to diets rich in saturated fatty acids. Interestingly, these features have been found both in the fasting state and in the postprandial state, and have been also found, although to a lesser extent, associated to the consumption of nuts, other well represented food of Mediterranean diet(Delgado-Lista et al., 2008). These and other evidences of the beneficial influence of components of the Mediterranean diet have been published elsewhere(Delgado-Lista et al., 2011a; Delgado-

Lista et al., 2007; Lopez-Miranda et al., 2007; Mezzano et al., 2003; Mordente et al., 2011). In summary, there are clear evidences on the healthy effects of components of the Mediterranean Diet in reducing the procoagulant and proagreggant species that promote atherosclerosis and eventual coronary events. These foods include extra virgin olive oil, vegetables, nuts and blue fish, and are supported by organizations like the FDA and the AHA(CFSAN/Office of Nutritional Products, 2004; Kris-Etherton et al., 2002).

## 6. Mediterranean Diet and endothelial function

In the new concepts of atherogenesis, the endothelial cells play a pivotal role in controlling the first steps and the final events of atherothombosis. The proper function of the vascular endothelium is essential to maintain a correct vasodilatation, but also to correctly regulate the metabolism of many other players involved in the atherogenesis, like the inflammatory cells, or the platelets. Meals rich in olive oil have a favorable effect on the postprandial vasomotor function of the endothelium, enhancing the vasodilator capacity during this phase, compared to meals rich in saturated fats, but also affect favorably other circulating markers of endothelial function. These effects are carried out, at least partly, by the minor compounds of virgin olive oil (Fuentes et al., 2008; Fuentes et al., 2001; Perez-Jimenez et al., 1999; Perez-Martinez et al., 2010c; Rallidis et al., 2009; Ruano et al., 2005), and may be also mediated by a lesser activation of leukocytes, a lower inflammation, and a higher bioavailability of nitric oxide (Carluccio et al., 2007; Covas, 2007; Davis et al., 2007; Fuentes et al., 2008; Leighton & Urquiaga, 2007; Perez-Jimenez et al., 1999; Perez-Jimenez et al., 2007; Perez-Martinez et al., 2010b; Perona et al., 2006; Schini-Kerth et al., 2010; Serra-Majem et al., 2006; Visioli et al., 2005). Apart from olive oil, other important players in the effects of Mediterranean diet on endothelial function are nuts, fish and vegetables, all contributing to the wellbeing of this organ by promoting a lower proinflammatory, prooxidant environment(Estruch, 2010; Harris et al., 2003; Mena et al., 2009; Nadtochiy & Redman, 2011; Papoutsi et al., 2008). Furthermore, it has been recently shown that people following Mediterranean Diet improve the regenerative capacity of the endothelium(Marin et al., 2011) and that elderly persons may partially blunt the oxidative processes associated to aging by adhering to Mediterranean diet, especially when combined with a rich antioxidant environment(Gutierrez-Mariscal et al., 2011).

## 7. Mediterranean Diet, obesity, metabolic syndrome and type 2 diabetes mellitus

The burden of a epidemic of obesity in modern countries has arisen the importance in public health strategies to search for dietary models reducing the incidence of obesity, and the related metabolic syndrome and type 2 diabetes mellitus, these two latter conditions characterized by a high cardiovascular risk.

Mediterranean Diet is an effective model to replace saturated fat rich diets, when looking for a healthy model to recommend to these persons. In fact, adherence to Mediterranean diet is inversely associated with the clustering of diabetes mellitus, obesity, hypertension and hypercholesterolemia (Sanchez-Tainta et al., 2008). Obesity rates are inversely associated with adherence to the Mediterranean diet on several observational cohorts (Beunza et al., 2010; Bullo et al., 2011; Mendez et al., 2006; Romaguera et al., 2009; Romaguera et al., 2010;

Schroder et al., 2004; Trichopoulou et al., 2005), which has been explained by the higher satiating effect of olive oil rich meals(Schwartz et al., 2008). A recent meta-analysis including 16 randomized clinical trials found Mediterranean Diet as a useful tool to reduce obesity, especially when accompanied by other healthy habits(Esposito et al., 2011). In a similar way, an inverse correlation between the prevalence of Metabolic Syndrome and the adherence to Mediterranean Diet has been extensively reported(Panagiotakos et al., 2004; Tortosa et al., 2007), and some interventional studies have replicated these findings, showing that persons who are submitted to a Mediterranean type diet have a lower probability to show Metabolic Syndrome, even on *ad libitum* dietary regimen (Esposito et al., 2004; Salas-Salvado et al., 2008). These findings are related to the beneficial effects  shown by diets rich in fruits, vegetables, grains, fish and low-fat dairy products, with the additional value of olive oil, which prevents the redistribution of body fat from peripheral to visceral adipose tissue, and partially enhances the postprandial lipid disturbances found in the metabolic syndrome patients(Esmaillzadeh et al., 2007; Jimenez-Gomez et al., 2010; Lutsey et al., 2008; Paniagua et al., 2007b; Pereira et al., 2005). A recent statement from the European Atherosclerosis Society recently recommended the Mediterranean Diet as the tool to combat the Metabolic Syndrome(Stock, 2011) by its capacity to reduce all clinical criteria of the disease, based on a recent meta-analysis that reported that adherence to Mediterranean Diet is related to a decrease in waist circumference by 42 cm, increase in HDL cholesterol by 0.03 mmol/l, decrease of triglycerides by 0.07mmol/l, decrease in blood pressure (2.35/1.58 mm Hg), and decrease in blood glucose by 3.89 mg/dL(Kastorini et al., 2011)

With respect to type 2 diabetes, which is a frequent outcome in patients with sustained Metabolic Syndrome, it is reasonable to infer that Mediterranean Diet might prevent the development of diabetes or might improve the impaired metabolic status of the diabetic persons(D. Giugliano & Esposito, 2008; Perez-Martinez et al., 2011a). In fact, large prospective studies have shown that adherence to Mediterranean Diet is inversely correlated with the risk of presenting type 2 diabetes mellitus (Martinez-Gonzalez et al., 2008; Mozaffarian et al., 2007), which has been eventually corroborated (de Koning et al., 2011; Delgado-Lista et al., 2011b; F. Giugliano et al., 2010). Some authors have published, indeed, that changing from a saturated fat rich diet to a Mediterranean Diet results in a decrease of glycated hemoglobin of around 0.3-2.0%, which is close to the efficacy of some antidiabetic drugs, and allow to reduce pharmacological needs of these patients, which has also been reproduced when comparing Mediterranean Diet with a low fat diet (Elhayany et al., 2010; Itsiopoulos et al., 2010; Reisin, 2010). A recent randomized clinical trial showed that the risk of incident diabetes is reduced by more than 50% when Mediterranean Diet (either with or without supplements of nuts) is compared with the low-fat group (p<0.05)(Salas-Salvado et al., 2011a). Some of the underlying mechanisms by which Mediterranean Diet improves the diabetes control are improving insulin sensitivity and blood lipids(Riccardi et al., 2004), improving postprandial lipemia(Lopez et al., 2008), improving glucose homeostasis  (Paniagua et al., 2007a) or improve the beta-cell insulin secretion (Rojo-Martinez et al., 2006). Furthermore, and linking Mediterranean Diet, type 2 diabetes and cardiovascular risk, it has been recently published that Mediterranean Diet is associated with a better prognosis in total and cardiovascular mortality in type 2 diabetics(Hodge et al., 2010) All the relationships between the Mediterranean Diet, obesity and diabetes have been recently published (Perez-Martinez et al., 2011a; Salas-Salvado et al., 2011b).

## 8. Mediterranean Diet and epidemiological evidences on reduced cardiovascular risk

The adherence to the Mediterranean Diet has been linked to a lower mortality by any cause and by cardiovascular disease in several observational studies, some of them including more than 350000 participants, like the NIH-AARP Diet and Health Study, where a high adherence to this dietary pattern resulted in an hazard ratio of 0.79 for all cause mortality, and of 0.83 for cardiovascular causes, which has been eventually corroborated (Mitrou et al., 2007; Serra-Majem et al., 2006). These data were included in an eventual meta-analysis (including more than 1.5 million persons), where it was stated that a rise of 2 points in a 9 points-scale of adherence to Mediterranean Diet was associated with a reduction of all cause mortality and cardiovascular mortality of about 10% (Sofi et al., 2008), which was eventually replicated in other meta-analysis(Sofi et al., 2010). In another meta-analysis, it has been state that a reduction of 5% of saturated by polyunsaturated fats result in a decrease of coronary risk (hazard ratio 0.87), while if this substitution was done by carbohydrates, there was no effect (Jakobsen et al., 2009). As stated previously, the Mediterranean Diet combines a high consumption of fish and a relative decrease in carbohydrates when compared with the low fat diets, which may combine the favored dietary patterns of the two above meta-analysis. Newer studies corroborate the inverse relationship between adherence to Mediterranean Diet and total mortality and cardiovascular death. High versus low adherence is accompanied was reported to be accompanied by a hazard ratio of 0.79 for total mortality, and 0.66 for cardiovascular death in a set of 40000 persons (Buckland et al., 2011). Furthermore, these effects are also evident in young cohorts. A recent report found a cardiovascular hazard ratio of 0.41 in 13000 young persons (mean age 38) with high versus low adherence to Mediterranean Diet(Martinez-Gonzalez et al., 2011)

Consequences of the non-fatal coronary event may also be limited by the Mediterranean Diet. A recent study has shown that left ventricle systolic dysfunction during hospitalization and the 2-y prognosis after an acute coronary syndrome are associated to the baseline diet. In this study, higher adherence to Mediterranean Diet was associated with less likelihood of developing left ventricle systolic dysfunction at hospitalization, less likelihood of remodeling (ejection fraction <50%) at 3 months of follow-up, and less likelihood of recurrent cardiovascular disease events during the 2 y of follow-up(Chrysohoou et al., 2010)

Other of the underlying mechanisms for the reduced cardiovascular incidence observed in persons eating Mediterranean Diet is by promoting an adequate cardiac rhythm. Although preliminary, there are data supporting that adherence to the Mediterranean Diet is linked to a lower probability of developing atrial fibrillation, and to promote its spontaneous conversion (Mattioli, 2011; Mattioli et al., 2011), and that it improves cardiac autonomic function, as assessed by an increased heart rate variability(Dai et al., 2010)

Cerebrovascular disease is a very common form of presentation of cardiovascular disease, which has not been so studied as coronary heart disease, in relationship with its interaction with diet. A recent study analyzed the impact of Mediterranean Diet on magnetic resonance imaging-assessed cerebrovascular disease. In a random sample of 700 elderly subjects, medium and high adherence to Mediterranean Diet elicited a 22 and 36% lower odds ratio for presenting evidence of infarcts on magnetic resonance imaging with respect to poor adherers (Scarmeas et al., 2011). In fact, adhering to nutritional features of Mediterranean Diet is more effective to act as secondary prevention for stroke than any single medication(Spence, 2010), even provoking the reversion of carotid atherosclerosis(Shai et al., 2010)

## 9. Causal links between Mediterranean Diet and cardiovascular events: The need for randomized clinical trials

With respect to clinical trials, two large dietary intervention trials with diet which used some features of the Mediterranean Diet were performed in Italy and France in the last years of the last century. The DART study evaluated the impact of three different dietary models (rich in fiber, low fat and rich in fish) in clinical outcomes of coronary patients. The use of two servings a week of fish was followed by a reduction of total mortality and cardiovascular death of about 30%, but the effects of other components of the Mediterranean Diet were not assessed (Burr et al., 1989).

The Lyon study evaluated the effect of one so-called Mediterranean Diet on the clinical outcomes of coronary patients. After 4 years of follow up, those who used the Mediterranean Diet lowered the recurrence of cardiovascular events by 50-70% (de Lorgeril et al., 1999). However, it must be said that the investigators used margarine rich in canola oil as their main fat source instead of olive oil, when this is not an usual component of the Mediterranean Diet. The reason for using such product was to provide high amounts of linolenic acid, a n-3 fatty acid of plant origin. Although the rest of the components of the diet that the author used matched the Mediterranean Diet characteristics, the use of the canola oil makes difficult to extrapolate the results to the traditional Mediterranean Diet.

The relative lack of clinical trials exploring cardiovascular outcome, using a complete Mediterranean Diet rich in Olive Oil, has opened the door for new initiatives. The PREDIMED study, close to conclude its follow up aims to compare the effects of a low fat diet with two Mediterranean Diet type diets (one of them enriched in nuts), on clinical cardiovascular endpoints of persons at risk of cardiovascular disease but without clinical disease (primary prevention). Until the final results are released, there have been published preliminary reports. The lower intake of olive oil was correlated with a thicker intima media thickness, a measure of the atherosclerosis in the carotid vessel, and a cardiovascular risk factor (Buil-Cosiales et al., 2008). Other risk factors previously suggested were also confirmed. Mediterranean Diet was followed by a decrease in glucose plasma levels, blood pressure and rises the proportion HDL/total cholesterol (Estruch et al., 2006).

The CordioPrev study aims to explore the effects of a low fat and a Mediterranean Diet in the recurrence of cardiovascular events and cardiovascular mortality in patients with coronary heart disease, exploring also multiple other endpoints, like incidence of cancer, lipids, glucose metabolism or age associated cognitive decline, after 5 years of follow up. This study is still in recruitment stage, and it may unravel the existence of causality in the relationship between Mediterranean Diet and lower recurrence of cardiovascular disease(CordioPrev, 2010).

These and other ongoing studies will help to ascertain if there is causality under the well stablished clinical associations between Mediterranean Diet and cardiovascular disease clinical endpoints.

## 10. Conclusions

Mediterranean Diet has shown beneficial effects in multiple cardiovascular risk factors and underlying mechanisms of atherosclerosis, including a favorable lipid profile, a decrease of blood pressure, a shortening of the postprandial lipemia, a partial reduction in the harmful effects of smoking, a reduction of oxidative stress and inflammation, a reduction in the incidence and control of the clinical features of the Metabolic Syndrome, a better glycemic control, an enhancement of endothelial function, or the creation of a less prothrombotic environment (Figure 2). The results from observational and cohort studies link the high adherence to Mediterranean Diet with a lower total mortality and a decrease in cardiovascular events and cardiovascular mortality. Although it is not the scope of the present chapter, it has also been linked to several other healthy benefits, like a decrease in the incidence of certain types of tumors or a better cognitive function in aged persons.

The underlying mechanisms by which the Mediterranean Diet exerts its pleiotropic effects are difficult to discover, especially having into account that it is a flexible dietary pattern, with local differences depending on the geographical area in which it is studied. However, a combination of the healthy effects of its main components, like the use of Virgin Olive Oil and the high proportion of fruits and vegetables, grains and fish may be in the origin.

Meanwhile the large clinical trials designed to proof causality between Mediterranean Diet and cardiovascular disease publish their results, the effects of this dietary model on the cardiovascular risk factors and on the mechanisms of atherosclerosis, as well as the results from epidemiological studies allow us to infer that Mediterranean Diet may be an optimal dietary model to face the development of cardiovascular diseases.

## 11. Acknowledgments

Supported in part by research grants from the Spanish Ministry of Science and Innovation (AGL 2004-07907, AGL2006-01979, and AGL2009-12270 to J L-M, SAF07-62005 to F P-J and FIS PI10/01041 to P P-M, PI10/02412 to F P-J); Consejería de Economía, Innovación y Ciencia, Proyectos de Investigación de Excelencia, Junta de Andalucía (P06-CTS-01425 to J L-M, CTS5015 and AGR922 to F P-J); Consejería de Salud, Junta de Andalucía (06/128, 07/43, and PI0193/09 to J L-M, 06/129 to F P-J, 06/127 to C M-H, 0118/08 to F F-J, PI-0252/09 to J D-L, and PI-0058/10 to P P-M); Fondo Europeo de Desarrollo Regional (FEDER). The CIBEROBN is an initiative of the Instituto de Salud Carlos III, Madrid, Spain.

## 12. References

Alonso, A., J. J. Beunza, M. Bes-Rastrollo, R. M. Pajares & M. A. Martinez-Gonzalez (2006). "Vegetable protein and fiber from cereal are inversely associated with the risk of hypertension in a Spanish cohort." *Arch Med Res* 37 (6): 778-786.

Alonso, A., C. de la Fuente, A. M. Martin-Arnau, J. de Irala, J. A. Martinez & M. A. Martinez-Gonzalez (2004). "Fruit and vegetable consumption is inversely associated with blood pressure in a Mediterranean population with a high vegetable-fat intake: the Seguimiento Universidad de Navarra (SUN) Study." *Br J Nutr* 92 (2): 311-319.

Allayee, H., N. Roth & H. N. Hodis (2009). "Polyunsaturated fatty acids and cardiovascular disease: implications for nutrigenetics." *J Nutrigenet Nutrigenomics* 2 (3): 140-148.

Antonopoulou, S., E. Fragopoulou, H. C. Karantonis, E. Mitsou, M. Sitara, J. Rementzis, A. Mourelatos, A. Ginis & C. Phenekos (2006). "Effect of traditional Greek Mediterranean meals on platelet aggregation in normal subjects and in patients with type 2 diabetes mellitus." *J Med Food* 9 (3): 356-362.

Avellone, G., R. Cordova, L. Scalffidi & G. Bompiani (1998). "Effects of Mediterranean diet on lipid, coagulative and fibrinolytic parameters in two randomly selected population samples in Western Sicily." *Nutr Metab Cardiovasc Dis* 8: 287-296.

Bach-Faig, A., D. Geleva, J. L. Carrasco, L. Ribas-Barba & L. Serra-Majem (2006). "Evaluating associations between Mediterranean diet adherence indexes and biomarkers of diet and disease." *Public Health Nutr* 9 (8A): 1110-1117.

Bayturan, O., E. M. Tuzcu, A. Lavoie, T. Hu, K. Wolski, P. Schoenhagen, S. Kapadia, S. E. Nissen & S. J. Nicholls (2010). "The metabolic syndrome, its component risk factors, and progression of coronary atherosclerosis." *Arch Intern Med* 170 (5): 478-484.

Beunza, J. J., E. Toledo, F. B. Hu, M. Bes-Rastrollo, M. Serrano-Martinez, A. Sanchez-Villegas, J. A. Martinez & M. A. Martinez-Gonzalez (2010). "Adherence to the Mediterranean diet, long-term weight change, and incident overweight or obesity: the Seguimiento Universidad de Navarra (SUN) cohort." *Am J Clin Nutr* 92 (6): 1484-1493.

Bondia-Pons, I., H. Schroder, M. I. Covas, A. I. Castellote, J. Kaikkonen, H. E. Poulsen, A. V. Gaddi, A. Machowetz, H. Kiesewetter & M. C. Lopez-Sabater (2007). "Moderate consumption of olive oil by healthy European men reduces systolic blood pressure in non-Mediterranean participants." *J Nutr* 137 (1): 84-87.

Borissoff, J. I., H. M. Spronk & H. ten Cate (2011). "The hemostatic system as a modulator of atherosclerosis." *N Engl J Med* 364 (18): 1746-1760.

Bravo-Herrera, M. D., J. Lopez-Miranda, C. Marin, P. Gomez, M. J. Gomez, J. A. Moreno, P. Perez-Martinez, A. Blanco, Y. Jimenez-Gomez & F. Perez-Jimenez (2004). "Tissue factor expression is decreased in monocytes obtained from blood during Mediterranean or high carbohydrate diets." *Nutr Metab Cardiovasc Dis* 14 (3): 128-132.

Buckland, G., A. Agudo, N. Travier, J. Maria Huerta, L. Cirera, M. J. Tormo, C. Navarro, M. Dolores Chirlaque, C. Moreno-Iribas, E. Ardanaz, A. Barricarte, J. Etxeberria, P. Marin, J. Ramon Quiros, M. L. Redondo, N. Larranaga, P. Amiano, M. Dorronsoro, L. Arriola, M. Basterretxea, M. J. Sanchez, E. Molina & C. A. Gonzalez (2011). "Adherence to the Mediterranean diet reduces mortality in the Spanish cohort of the European Prospective Investigation into Cancer and Nutrition (EPIC-Spain)." *Br J Nutr*: 1-11.

Buil-Cosiales, P., P. Irimia, N. Berrade, A. Garcia-Arellano, M. Riverol, M. Murie-Fernandez, E. Martinez-Vila, M. A. Martinez-Gonzalez & M. Serrano-Martinez (2008). "Carotid intima-media thickness is inversely associated with olive oil consumption." *Atherosclerosis* 196 (2): 742-748.

Bullo, M., M. Garcia-Aloy, M. A. Martinez-Gonzalez, D. Corella, J. D. Fernandez-Ballart, M. Fiol, E. Gomez-Gracia, R. Estruch, M. Ortega-Calvo, S. Francisco, G. Flores-Mateo, L. Serra-Majem, X. Pinto, M. I. Covas, E. Ros, R. Lamuela-Raventos & J. Salas-Salvado (2011). "Association between a healthy lifestyle and general obesity and abdominal obesity in an elderly population at high cardiovascular risk." *Prev Med*.

Burr, M. L., A. M. Fehily, J. F. Gilbert, S. Rogers, R. M. Holliday, P. M. Sweetnam, P. C. Elwood & N. M. Deadman (1989). "Effects of changes in fat, fish, and fibre intakes on death and myocardial reinfarction: diet and reinfarction trial (DART)." *Lancet* 2 (8666): 757-761.

Carluccio, M. A., M. Massaro, E. Scoditti & R. De Caterina (2007). "Vasculoprotective potential of olive oil components." *Mol Nutr Food Res* 51 (10): 1225-1234.

CFSAN/Office of Nutritional Products, L. a. D. S. (2004) "Letter Responding to Health Claim Petition dated August 28, 2003: Monounsaturated Fatty Acids from Olive Oil and Coronary Heart Disease (Docket No 2003Q-0559)." http://www.cfsan.fda.gov/~dms/qhcolive.html#ref.

CordioPrev (2010). "(www.cordioprev.org/en)."

Covas, M. I. (2007). "Olive oil and the cardiovascular system." *Pharmacol Res* 55 (3): 175-186.

Chrysohoou, C., D. B. Panagiotakos, P. Aggelopoulos, C. M. Kastorini, I. Kehagia, C. Pitsavos & C. Stefanadis (2010). "The Mediterranean diet contributes to the preservation of left ventricular systolic function and to the long-term favorable prognosis of patients who have had an acute coronary event." *Am J Clin Nutr* 92 (1): 47-54.

Dai, J., R. Lampert, P. W. Wilson, J. Goldberg, T. R. Ziegler & V. Vaccarino (2010). "Mediterranean dietary pattern is associated with improved cardiac autonomic function among middle-aged men: a twin study." *Circ Cardiovasc Qual Outcomes* 3 (4): 366-373.

Davis, N., S. Katz & J. Wylie-Rosett (2007). "The effect of diet on endothelial function." *Cardiol Rev* 15 (2): 62-66.

de Koning, L., S. E. Chiuve, T. T. Fung, W. C. Willett, E. B. Rimm & F. B. Hu (2011). "Diet-quality scores and the risk of type 2 diabetes in men." *Diabetes Care* 34 (5): 1150-1156.

de Lorgeril, M., P. Salen, J. L. Martin, I. Monjaud, J. Delaye & N. Mamelle (1999). "Mediterranean diet, traditional risk factors, and the rate of cardiovascular complications after myocardial infarction: final report of the Lyon Diet Heart Study." *Circulation* 99 (6): 779-785.

Delgado-Lista, J., A. Garcia-Rios, P. Perez-Martinez, J. Lopez-Miranda & F. Perez-Jimenez (2011a). "Olive oil and haemostasis: platelet function, thrombogenesis and fibrinolysis." *Curr Pharm Des* 17 (8): 778-785.

Delgado-Lista, J., A. Garcia-Rios, P. Perez-Martinez, J. Solivera, E. M. Yubero-Serrano, F. Fuentes, L. D. Parnell, J. Shen, P. Gomez, Y. Jimenez-Gomez, M. J. Gomez-Luna, C. Marin, S. E. Belisle, F. Rodriguez-Cantalejo, S. N. Meydani, J. M. Ordovas, F. Perez-Jimenez & J. Lopez-Miranda (2011b). "Interleukin 1B variant -1473G/C (rs1143623) influences triglyceride and interleukin 6 metabolism." *J Clin Endocrinol Metab* 96 (5): E816-820.

Delgado-Lista, J., J. Lopez-Miranda, B. Cortes, P. Perez-Martinez, A. Lozano, R. Gomez-Luna, P. Gomez, M. J. Gomez, J. Criado, F. Fuentes & F. Perez-Jimenez (2008). "Chronic dietary fat intake modifies the postprandial response of hemostatic markers to a single fatty test meal." *Am J Clin Nutr* 87 (2): 317-322.

Delgado-Lista, J., J. Lopez-Miranda, P. Perez-Martinez, J. Ruano, F. Fuentes & F. Perez-Jimenez (2007). "Olive Oil and Hemostasis." *Current Nutrition & Food Science* 3 (1): 175-182.

Din, J. N., D. E. Newby & A. D. Flapan (2004). "Omega 3 fatty acids and cardiovascular disease--fishing for a natural treatment." *Bmj* 328 (7430): 30-35.

EFSA (2011). "Scientific Opinion on the substantiation of health claims related to polyphenols in olive and protection of LDL particles from oxidative damage (ID 1333, 1638, 1639, 1696, 2865), maintenance of normal blood HDL cholesterol concentrations (ID 1639), maintenance of normal blood pressure (ID 3781), "anti-inflammatory properties" (ID 1882), "contributes to the upper respiratory tract health" (ID 3468), "can help to maintain a normal function of gastrointestinal tract" (3779), and "contributes to body defences against external agents" (ID 3467) pursuant to Article 13(1) of Regulation (EC) No 1924/2006." *EFSA journal* 9 (4): 2033-2058.

Elhayany, A., A. Lustman, R. Abel, J. Attal-Singer & S. Vinker (2010). "A low carbohydrate Mediterranean diet improves cardiovascular risk factors and diabetes control among overweight patients with type 2 diabetes mellitus: a 1-year prospective randomized intervention study." *Diabetes Obes Metab* 12 (3): 204-209.

Esmaillzadeh, A., M. Kimiagar, Y. Mehrabi, L. Azadbakht, F. B. Hu & W. C. Willett (2007). "Dietary patterns, insulin resistance, and prevalence of the metabolic syndrome in women." *Am J Clin Nutr* 85 (3): 910-918.

Esposito, K., C. M. Kastorini, D. B. Panagiotakos & D. Giugliano (2011). "Mediterranean diet and weight loss: meta-analysis of randomized controlled trials." *Metab Syndr Relat Disord* 9 (1): 1-12.

Esposito, K., R. Marfella, M. Ciotola, C. Di Palo, F. Giugliano, G. Giugliano, M. D'Armiento, F. D'Andrea & D. Giugliano (2004). "Effect of a mediterranean-style diet on endothelial dysfunction and markers of vascular inflammation in the metabolic syndrome: a randomized trial." *JAMA* 292 (12): 1440-1446.

Estruch, R. (2010). "Anti-inflammatory effects of the Mediterranean diet: the experience of the PREDIMED study." *Proc Nutr Soc* 69 (3): 333-340.

Estruch, R., M. A. Martinez-Gonzalez, D. Corella, J. Basora-Gallisa, V. Ruiz-Gutierrez, M. I. Covas, M. Fiol, E. Gomez-Gracia, M. C. Lopez-Sabater, R. Escoda, M. A. Pena, J. Diez-Espino, C. Lahoz, J. Lapetra, G. Saez & E. Ros (2009). "Effects of dietary fiber intake on risk factors for cardiovascular disease in subjects at high risk." *J Epidemiol Community Health*.

Estruch, R., M. A. Martinez-Gonzalez, D. Corella, J. Salas-Salvado, V. Ruiz-Gutierrez, M. I. Covas, M. Fiol, E. Gomez-Gracia, M. C. Lopez-Sabater, E. Vinyoles, F. Aros, M. Conde, C. Lahoz, J. Lapetra, G. Saez & E. Ros (2006). "Effects of a Mediterranean-style diet on cardiovascular risk factors: a randomized trial." *Ann Intern Med* 145 (1): 1-11.

Filion, K. B., F. El Khoury, M. Bielinski, I. Schiller, N. Dendukuri & J. M. Brophy (2010). "Omega-3 fatty acids in high-risk cardiovascular patients: a meta-analysis of randomized controlled trials." *BMC Cardiovasc Disord* 10: 24.

Fito, M., M. Cladellas, R. de la Torre, J. Marti, M. Alcantara, M. Pujadas-Bastardes, J. Marrugat, J. Bruguera, M. C. Lopez-Sabater, J. Vila & M. I. Covas (2005). "Antioxidant effect of virgin olive oil in patients with stable coronary heart disease: a randomized, crossover, controlled, clinical trial." *Atherosclerosis* 181 (1): 149-158.

Fuentes, F., J. Lopez-Miranda, P. Perez-Martinez, Y. Jimenez, C. Marin, P. Gomez, J. M. Fernandez, J. Caballero, J. Delgado-Lista & F. Perez-Jimenez (2008). "Chronic effects of a high-fat diet enriched with virgin olive oil and a low-fat diet enriched with alpha-linolenic acid on postprandial endothelial function in healthy men." *Br J Nutr* 100 (1): 159-165.

Fuentes, F., J. Lopez-Miranda, E. Sanchez, F. Sanchez, J. Paez, E. Paz-Rojas, C. Marin, P. Gomez, J. Jimenez-Pereperez, J. M. Ordovas & F. Perez-Jimenez (2001). "Mediterranean and low-fat diets improve endothelial function in hypercholesterolemic men." *Ann Intern Med* 134 (12): 1115-1119.

Gasparyan, A. Y., L. Ayvazyan, D. P. Mikhailidis & G. D. Kitas (2011). "Mean platelet volume: a link between thrombosis and inflammation?" *Curr Pharm Des* 17 (1): 47-58.

Geleijnse, J. M., E. J. Giltay, D. E. Grobbee, A. R. Donders & F. J. Kok (2002). "Blood pressure response to fish oil supplementation: metaregression analysis of randomized trials." *J Hypertens* 20 (8): 1493-1499.

Gillingham, L. G., S. Harris-Janz & P. J. Jones (2011). "Dietary monounsaturated fatty acids are protective against metabolic syndrome and cardiovascular disease risk factors." *Lipids* 46 (3): 209-228.

Giugliano, D. & K. Esposito (2008). "Mediterranean diet and metabolic diseases." *Curr Opin Lipidol* 19 (1): 63-68.

Giugliano, F., M. I. Maiorino, G. Bellastella, R. Autorino, M. De Sio, D. Giugliano & K. Esposito (2010). "Adherence to Mediterranean diet and erectile dysfunction in men with type 2 diabetes." *J Sex Med* 7 (5): 1911-1917.

Gutierrez-Mariscal, F. M., P. Perez-Martinez, J. Delgado-Lista, E. M. Yubero-Serrano, A. Camargo, N. Delgado-Casado, C. Cruz-Teno, M. Santos-Gonzalez, F. Rodriguez-Cantalejo, J. P. Castano, J. M. Villalba-Montoro, F. Fuentes, F. Perez-Jimenez & J. Lopez-Miranda (2011). "Mediterranean diet supplemented with coenzyme Q10 induces postprandial changes in p53 in response to oxidative DNA damage in elderly subjects." *Age (Dordr)*.

Harris, W. S., P. M. Kris-Etherton & K. A. Harris (2008). "Intakes of long-chain omega-3 fatty acid associated with reduced risk for death from coronary heart disease in healthy adults." *Curr Atheroscler Rep* 10 (6): 503-509.

Harris, W. S., Y. Park & W. L. Isley (2003). "Cardiovascular disease and long-chain omega-3 fatty acids." *Curr Opin Lipidol* 14 (1): 9-14.

Haveman-Nies, A., L. P. de Groot, J. Burema, J. A. Cruz, M. Osler & W. A. van Staveren (2002). "Dietary quality and lifestyle factors in relation to 10-year mortality in older Europeans: the SENECA study." *Am J Epidemiol* 156 (10): 962-968.

HeartScore (2003). "http://www.heartscore.org."

Hodge, A. M., D. R. English, C. Itsiopoulos, K. O'Dea & G. G. Giles (2010). "Does a Mediterranean diet reduce the mortality risk associated with diabetes: Evidence from the Melbourne Collaborative Cohort Study." *Nutr Metab Cardiovasc Dis*.

Itsiopoulos, C., L. Brazionis, M. Kaimakamis, M. Cameron, J. D. Best, K. O'Dea & K. Rowley (2010). "Can the Mediterranean diet lower HbA1c in type 2 diabetes? Results from a randomized cross-over study." *Nutr Metab Cardiovasc Dis*.

Jakobsen, M. U., E. J. O'Reilly, B. L. Heitmann, M. A. Pereira, K. Balter, G. E. Fraser, U. Goldbourt, G. Hallmans, P. Knekt, S. Liu, P. Pietinen, D. Spiegelman, J. Stevens, J. Virtamo, W. C. Willett & A. Ascherio (2009). "Major types of dietary fat and risk of coronary heart disease: a pooled analysis of 11 cohort studies." *Am J Clin Nutr* 89 (5): 1425-1432.

Jansen, S., J. Lopez-Miranda, P. Castro, F. Lopez-Segura, C. Marin, J. M. Ordovas, E. Paz, J. Jimenez-Pereperez, F. Fuentes & F. Perez-Jimenez (2000). "Low-fat and high-monounsaturated fatty acid diets decrease plasma cholesterol ester transfer protein concentrations in young, healthy, normolipemic men." *Am J Clin Nutr* 72 (1): 36-41.

Jimenez-Gomez, Y., C. Marin, P. Peerez-Martinez, J. Hartwich, M. Malczewska-Malec, I. Golabek, B. Kiec-Wilk, C. Cruz-Teno, F. Rodriguez, P. Gomez, M. J. Gomez-Luna, C. Defoort, M. J. Gibney, F. Perez-Jimenez, H. M. Roche & J. Lopez-Miranda (2010). "A low-fat, high-complex carbohydrate diet supplemented with long-chain (n-3) fatty acids alters the postprandial lipoprotein profile in patients with metabolic syndrome." *J Nutr* 140 (9): 1595-1601.

Junker, R., M. Kratz, M. Neufeld, M. Erren, J. R. Nofer, H. Schulte, U. Nowak-Gottl, G. Assmann & U. Wahrburg (2001a). "Effects of diets containing olive oil, sunflower oil, or rapeseed oil on the hemostatic system." *Thromb Haemost* 85 (2): 280-286.

Junker, R., B. Pieke, H. Schulte, R. Nofer, M. Neufeld, G. Assmann & U. Wahrburg (2001b). "Changes in hemostasis during treatment of hypertriglyceridemia with a diet rich in monounsaturated and n-3 polyunsaturated fatty acids in comparison with a low-fat diet." *Thromb Res* 101 (5): 355-366.

Karantonis, H. C., S. Antonopoulou & C. A. Demopoulos (2002). "Antithrombotic lipid minor constituents from vegetable oils. Comparison between olive oils and others." *J Agric Food Chem* 50 (5): 1150-1160.

Karantonis, H. C., S. Antonopoulou, D. N. Perrea, D. P. Sokolis, S. E. Theocharis, N. Kavantzas, D. G. Iliopoulos & C. A. Demopoulos (2006). "In vivo antiatherogenic properties of olive oil and its constituent lipid classes in hyperlipidemic rabbits." *Nutr Metab Cardiovasc Dis* 16 (3): 174-185.

Kastorini, C. M., H. J. Milionis, K. Esposito, D. Giugliano, J. A. Goudevenos & D. B. Panagiotakos (2011). "The effect of Mediterranean diet on metabolic syndrome and its components: a meta-analysis of 50 studies and 534,906 individuals." *J Am Coll Cardiol* 57 (11): 1299-1313.

Kolovou, G. D., D. P. Mikhailidis, J. Kovar, D. Lairon, B. G. Nordestgaard, T. C. Ooi, P. Perez-Martinez, H. Bilianou, K. Anagnostopoulou & G. Panotopoulos (2011). "Assessment and clinical relevance of non-fasting and postprandial triglycerides: an expert panel statement." *Curr Vasc Pharmacol* 9 (3): 258-270.

Kontou, N., T. Psaltopoulou, D. Panagiotakos, M. A. Dimopoulos & A. Linos (2011). "The Mediterranean Diet in Cancer Prevention: A Review." *J Med Food*.

Kris-Etherton, P. M., J. Derr, D. C. Mitchell, V. A. Mustad, M. E. Russell, E. T. McDonnell, D. Salabsky & T. A. Pearson (1993). "The role of fatty acid saturation on plasma lipids, lipoproteins, and apolipoproteins: I. Effects of whole food diets high in cocoa butter, olive oil, soybean oil, dairy butter, and milk chocolate on the plasma lipids of young men." *Metabolism* 42 (1): 121-129.

Kris-Etherton, P. M., W. S. Harris & L. J. Appel (2002). "Fish consumption, fish oil, omega-3 fatty acids, and cardiovascular disease." *Circulation* 106 (21): 2747-2757.

Lairon, D., C. Defoort, J. C. Martin, M. J. Amiot-Carlin, M. Gastaldi & R. Planells (2009). "Nutrigenetics: links between genetic background and response to Mediterranean-type diets." *Public health nutrition* 12 (9A): 1601-1606.

Langsted, A., J. J. Freiberg, A. Tybjaerg-Hansen, P. Schnohr, G. B. Jensen & B. G. Nordestgaard (2011). "Nonfasting cholesterol and triglycerides and association with risk of myocardial infarction and total mortality: the Copenhagen City Heart Study with 31 years of follow-up." *J Intern Med* 270 (1): 65-75.

Lapointe, A., J. Goulet, C. Couillard, B. Lamarche & S. Lemieux (2005). "A nutritional intervention promoting the Mediterranean food pattern is associated with a decrease in circulating oxidized LDL particles in healthy women from the Quebec City metropolitan area." *J Nutr* 135 (3): 410-415.

Lavie, C. J., R. V. Milani, M. R. Mehra & H. O. Ventura (2009). "Omega-3 polyunsaturated fatty acids and cardiovascular diseases." *J Am Coll Cardiol* 54 (7): 585-594.

Leighton, F. & I. Urquiaga (2007). "Endothelial nitric oxide synthase as a mediator of the positive health effects of Mediterranean diets and wine against metabolic syndrome." *World Rev Nutr Diet* 97: 33-51.

Lichtenstein, A. H., L. J. Appel, M. Brands, M. Carnethon, S. Daniels, H. A. Franch, B. Franklin, P. Kris-Etherton, W. S. Harris, B. Howard, N. Karanja, M. Lefevre, L. Rudel, F. Sacks, L. Van Horn, M. Winston & J. Wylie-Rosett (2006). "Diet and lifestyle recommendations revision 2006: a scientific statement from the American Heart Association Nutrition Committee." *Circulation* 114 (1): 82-96.

Lopez-Miranda, J., J. Delgado-Lista, P. Perez-Martinez, Y. Jimenez-Gomez, F. Fuentes, J. Ruano & C. Marin (2007). "Olive oil and the haemostatic system." *Mol Nutr Food Res* 51 (10): 1249-1259.

Lopez-Miranda, J., F. Perez-Jimenez, E. Ros, R. De Caterina, L. Badimon, M. I. Covas, E. Escrich, J. M. Ordovas, F. Soriguer, R. Abia, C. A. de la Lastra, M. Battino, D. Corella, J. Chamorro-Quiros, J. Delgado-Lista, D. Giugliano, K. Esposito, R. Estruch, J. M. Fernandez-Real, J. J. Gaforio, C. La Vecchia, D. Lairon, F. Lopez-Segura, P. Mata, J. A. Menendez, F. J. Muriana, J. Osada, D. B. Panagiotakos, J. A. Paniagua, P. Perez-Martinez, J. Perona, M. A. Peinado, M. Pineda-Priego, H. E. Poulsen, J. L. Quiles, M. C. Ramirez-Tortosa, J. Ruano, L. Serra-Majem, R. Sola, M. Solanas, V. Solfrizzi, R. de la Torre-Fornell, A. Trichopoulou, M. Uceda, J. M. Villalba-Montoro, J. R. Villar-Ortiz, F. Visioli & N. Yiannakouris (2010). "Olive oil and health: summary of the II international conference on olive oil and health consensus report, Jaen and Cordoba (Spain) 2008." *Nutr Metab Cardiovasc Dis* 20 (4): 284-294.

Lopez-Miranda, J., P. Perez-Martinez, C. Marin, J. A. Moreno, P. Gomez & F. Perez-Jimenez (2006). "Postprandial lipoprotein metabolism, genes and risk of cardiovascular disease." *Curr Opin Lipidol* 17 (2): 132-138.

Lopez, S., B. Bermudez, Y. M. Pacheco, J. Villar, R. Abia & F. J. Muriana (2008). "Distinctive postprandial modulation of beta cell function and insulin sensitivity by dietary fats: monounsaturated compared with saturated fatty acids." *Am J Clin Nutr* 88 (3): 638-644.

Lovegrove, J. A. & R. Gitau (2008). "Nutrigenetics and CVD: what does the future hold?" *The Proceedings of the Nutrition Society* 67 (2): 206-213.

Lutsey, P. L., L. M. Steffen & J. Stevens (2008). "Dietary intake and the development of the metabolic syndrome: the Atherosclerosis Risk in Communities study." *Circulation* 117 (6): 754-761.

Marin, C., R. Ramirez, J. Delgado-Lista, E. M. Yubero-Serrano, P. Perez-Martinez, J. Carracedo, A. Garcia-Rios, F. Rodriguez, F. M. Gutierrez-Mariscal, P. Gomez, F. Perez-Jimenez & J. Lopez-Miranda (2011). "Mediterranean diet reduces endothelial damage and improves the regenerative capacity of endothelium." *Am J Clin Nutr* 93 (2): 267-274.

Martinez-Gonzalez, M. A., C. de la Fuente-Arrillaga, J. M. Nunez-Cordoba, F. J. Basterra-Gortari, J. J. Beunza, Z. Vazquez, S. Benito, A. Tortosa & M. Bes-Rastrollo (2008). "Adherence to Mediterranean diet and risk of developing diabetes: prospective cohort study." *Bmj* 336 (7657): 1348-1351.

Martinez-Gonzalez, M. A., M. Garcia-Lopez, M. Bes-Rastrollo, E. Toledo, E. H. Martinez-Lapiscina, M. Delgado-Rodriguez, Z. Vazquez, S. Benito & J. J. Beunza (2011). "Mediterranean diet and the incidence of cardiovascular disease: a Spanish cohort." *Nutr Metab Cardiovasc Dis* 21 (4): 237-244.

Masala, G., B. Bendinelli, D. Versari, C. Saieva, M. Ceroti, F. Santagiuliana, S. Caini, S. Salvini, F. Sera, S. Taddei, L. Ghiadoni & D. Palli (2008). "Anthropometric and dietary determinants of blood pressure in over 7000 Mediterranean women: the European Prospective Investigation into Cancer and Nutrition-Florence cohort." *J Hypertens* 26 (11): 2112-2120.

Mata, P., J. A. Garrido, J. M. Ordovas, E. Blazquez, L. A. Alvarez-Sala, M. J. Rubio, R. Alonso & M. de Oya (1992). "Effect of dietary monounsaturated fatty acids on plasma lipoproteins and apolipoproteins in women." *Am J Clin Nutr* 56 (1): 77-83.

Mattioli, A. V. (2011). "Lifestyle and atrial fibrillation." *Expert Rev Cardiovasc Ther* 9 (7): 895-902.

Mattioli, A. V., C. Miloro, S. Pennella, P. Pedrazzi & A. Farinetti (2011). "Adherence to Mediterranean diet and intake of antioxidants influence spontaneous conversion of atrial fibrillation." *Nutr Metab Cardiovasc Dis.*

Mena, M. P., E. Sacanella, M. Vazquez-Agell, M. Morales, M. Fito, R. Escoda, M. Serrano-Martinez, J. Salas-Salvado, N. Benages, R. Casas, R. M. Lamuela-Raventos, F. Masanes, E. Ros & R. Estruch (2009). "Inhibition of circulating immune cell activation: a molecular antiinflammatory effect of the Mediterranean diet." *Am J Clin Nutr* 89 (1): 248-256.

Mendez, M. A., B. M. Popkin, P. Jakszyn, A. Berenguer, M. J. Tormo, M. J. Sanchez, J. R. Quiros, G. Pera, C. Navarro, C. Martinez, N. Larranaga, M. Dorronsoro, M. D. Chirlaque, A. Barricarte, E. Ardanaz, P. Amiano, A. Agudo & C. A. Gonzalez (2006). "Adherence to a Mediterranean diet is associated with reduced 3-year incidence of obesity." *J Nutr* 136 (11): 2934-2938.

Mente, A., L. de Koning, H. S. Shannon & S. S. Anand (2009). "A systematic review of the evidence supporting a causal link between dietary factors and coronary heart disease." *Arch Intern Med* 169 (7): 659-669.

Mezzano, D. & F. Leighton (2003). "Haemostatic cardiovascular risk factors: differential effects of red wine and diet on healthy young." *Pathophysiol Haemost Thromb* 33 (5-6): 472-478.

Mezzano, D., F. Leighton, P. Strobel, C. Martinez, G. Marshall, A. Cuevas, O. Castillo, O. Panes, B. Munoz, J. Rozowski & J. Pereira (2003). "Mediterranean diet, but not red wine, is associated with beneficial changes in primary haemostasis." *Eur J Clin Nutr* 57 (3): 439-446.

Mitrou, P. N., V. Kipnis, A. C. Thiebaut, J. Reedy, A. F. Subar, E. Wirfalt, A. Flood, T. Mouw, A. R. Hollenbeck, M. F. Leitzmann & A. Schatzkin (2007). "Mediterranean dietary pattern and prediction of all-cause mortality in a US population: results from the NIH-AARP Diet and Health Study." *Arch Intern Med* 167 (22): 2461-2468.

Mordente, A., B. Guantario, E. Meucci, A. Silvestrini, E. Lombardi, G. E. Martorana, B. Giardina & V. Bohm (2011). "Lycopene and cardiovascular diseases: an update." *Curr Med Chem* 18 (8): 1146-1163.

Mozaffarian, D., R. Marfisi, G. Levantesi, M. G. Silletta, L. Tavazzi, G. Tognoni, F. Valagussa & R. Marchioli (2007). "Incidence of new-onset diabetes and impaired fasting glucose in patients with recent myocardial infarction and the effect of clinical and lifestyle risk factors." *Lancet* 370 (9588): 667-675.

Mukamal, K. J. & E. B. Rimm (2008). "Alcohol consumption: risks and benefits." *Curr Atheroscler Rep* 10 (6): 536-543.

N.C.E.P. (2001). "http://www.nhlbi.nih.gov/guidelines/cholesterol/atglance.pdf."

Nadtochiy, S. M. & E. K. Redman (2011). "Mediterranean diet and cardioprotection: the role of nitrite, polyunsaturated fatty acids, and polyphenols." *Nutrition* 27 (7-8): 733-744.

Ordovas, J. M. (2006). "Nutrigenetics, plasma lipids, and cardiovascular risk." *Journal of the American Dietetic Association* 106 (7): 1074-1081; quiz 1083.

Panagiotakos, D. B., C. Pitsavos, C. Chrysohoou, J. Skoumas, D. Tousoulis, M. Toutouza, P. Toutouzas & C. Stefanadis (2004). "Impact of lifestyle habits on the prevalence of the metabolic syndrome among Greek adults from the ATTICA study." *Am Heart J* 147 (1): 106-112.

Paniagua, J. A., A. G. de la Sacristana, E. Sanchez, I. Romero, A. Vidal-Puig, F. J. Berral, A. Escribano, M. J. Moyano, P. Perez-Martinez, J. Lopez-Miranda & F. Perez-Jimenez (2007a). "A MUFA-rich diet improves posprandial glucose, lipid and GLP-1 responses in insulin-resistant subjects." *J Am Coll Nutr* 26 (5): 434-444.

Paniagua, J. A., A. Gallego de la Sacristana, I. Romero, A. Vidal-Puig, J. M. Latre, E. Sanchez, P. Perez-Martinez, J. Lopez-Miranda & F. Perez-Jimenez (2007b). "Monounsaturated fat-rich diet prevents central body fat distribution and decreases postprandial adiponectin expression induced by a carbohydrate-rich diet in insulin-resistant subjects." *Diabetes Care* 30 (7): 1717-1723.

Panunzio, M. F., R. Caporizzi, A. Antoniciello, E. P. Cela, L. R. Ferguson & P. D'Ambrosio (2011). "Randomized, controlled nutrition education trial promotes a Mediterranean diet and improves anthropometric, dietary, and metabolic parameters in adults." *Ann Ig* 23 (1): 13-25.

Papoutsi, Z., E. Kassi, I. Chinou, M. Halabalaki, L. A. Skaltsounis & P. Moutsatsou (2008). "Walnut extract (Juglans regia L.) and its component ellagic acid exhibit anti-inflammatory activity in human aorta endothelial cells and osteoblastic activity in the cell line KS483." *Br J Nutr* 99 (4): 715-722.

Patel, A., F. Barzi, K. Jamrozik, T. H. Lam, H. Ueshima, G. Whitlock & M. Woodward (2004). "Serum triglycerides as a risk factor for cardiovascular diseases in the Asia-Pacific region." *Circulation* 110 (17): 2678-2686.

Pereira, M. A., A. I. Kartashov, C. B. Ebbeling, L. Van Horn, M. L. Slattery, D. R. Jacobs, Jr. & D. S. Ludwig (2005). "Fast-food habits, weight gain, and insulin resistance (the CARDIA study): 15-year prospective analysis." *Lancet* 365 (9453): 36-42.

Perez-Jimenez, F. (2005). "International conference on the healthy effect of virgin olive oil." *Eur J Clin Invest* 35 (7): 421-424.

Perez-Jimenez, F., P. Castro, J. Lopez-Miranda, E. Paz-Rojas, A. Blanco, F. Lopez-Segura, F. Velasco, C. Marin, F. Fuentes & J. M. Ordovas (1999). "Circulating levels of endothelial function are modulated by dietary monounsaturated fat." *Atherosclerosis* 145 (2): 351-358.

Perez-Jimenez, F., J. D. Lista, P. Perez-Martinez, F. Lopez-Segura, F. Fuentes, B. Cortes, A. Lozano & J. Lopez-Miranda (2006). "Olive oil and haemostasis: a review on its healthy effects." *Public Health Nutr* 9 (8A): 1083-1088.

Perez-Jimenez, F., J. Lopez-Miranda & P. Mata (2002). "Protective effect of dietary monounsaturated fat on arteriosclerosis: beyond cholesterol." *Atherosclerosis* 163 (2): 385-398.

Perez-Jimenez, F., J. Ruano, P. Perez-Martinez, F. Lopez-Segura & J. Lopez-Miranda (2007). "The influence of olive oil on human health: not a question of fat alone." *Mol Nutr Food Res* 51 (10): 1199-1208.

Perez-Martinez, P., J. Delgado-Lista, F. Perez-Jimenez & J. Lopez-Miranda (2010a). "Update on genetics of postprandial lipemia." *Atheroscler Suppl* 11 (1): 39-43.

Perez-Martinez, P., J. M. Garcia-Quintana, E. M. Yubero-Serrano, I. Tasset-Cuevas, I. Tunez, A. Garcia-Rios, J. Delgado-Lista, C. Marin, F. Perez-Jimenez, H. M. Roche & J. Lopez-Miranda (2010b). "Postprandial oxidative stress is modified by dietary fat: evidence from a human intervention study." *Clin Sci (Lond)* 119 (6): 251-261.

Perez-Martinez, P., A. Garcia-Rios, J. Delgado-Lista, F. Perez-Jimenez & J. Lopez-Miranda (2011a). "Mediterranean diet rich in olive oil and obesity, metabolic syndrome and diabetes mellitus." *Curr Pharm Des* 17 (8): 769-777.

Perez-Martinez, P., A. Garcia-Rios, J. Delgado-Lista, F. Perez-Jimenez & J. Lopez-Miranda (2011b). "Nutrigenetics of the postprandial lipoprotein metabolism: evidences from human intervention studies." *Curr Vasc Pharmacol* 9 (3): 287-291.

Perez-Martinez, P., M. Moreno-Conde, C. Cruz-Teno, J. Ruano, F. Fuentes, J. Delgado-Lista, A. Garcia-Rios, C. Marin, M. J. Gomez-Luna, F. Perez-Jimenez, H. M. Roche & J. Lopez-Miranda (2010c). "Dietary fat differentially influences regulatory endothelial function during the postprandial state in patients with metabolic syndrome: from the LIPGENE study." *Atherosclerosis* 209 (2): 533-538.

Perona, J. S., R. Cabello-Moruno & V. Ruiz-Gutierrez (2006). "The role of virgin olive oil components in the modulation of endothelial function." *J Nutr Biochem* 17 (7): 429-445.

Perona, J. S., J. Canizares, E. Montero, J. M. Sanchez-Dominguez, A. Catala & V. Ruiz-Gutierrez (2004). "Virgin olive oil reduces blood pressure in hypertensive elderly subjects." *Clin Nutr* 23 (5): 1113-1121.

Pitsavos, C., D. B. Panagiotakos, N. Tzima, C. Chrysohoou, M. Economou, A. Zampelas & C. Stefanadis (2005). "Adherence to the Mediterranean diet is associated with total antioxidant capacity in healthy adults: the ATTICA study." *Am J Clin Nutr* 82 (3): 694-699.

Purnak, T., C. Efe, O. Yuksel, Y. Beyazit, E. Ozaslan & E. Altiparmak (2011). "Mean platelet volume could be a promising biomarker to monitor dietary compliance in celiac disease." *Ups J Med Sci* 116 (3): 208-211.

Rallidis, L. S., J. Lekakis, A. Kolomvotsou, A. Zampelas, G. Vamvakou, S. Efstathiou, G. Dimitriadis, S. A. Raptis & D. T. Kremastinos (2009). "Close adherence to a Mediterranean diet improves endothelial function in subjects with abdominal obesity." *Am J Clin Nutr* 90 (2): 263-268.

Rasmussen, B. M., B. Vessby, M. Uusitupa, L. Berglund, E. Pedersen, G. Riccardi, A. A. Rivellese, L. Tapsell & K. Hermansen (2006). "Effects of dietary saturated, monounsaturated, and n-3 fatty acids on blood pressure in healthy subjects." *Am J Clin Nutr* 83 (2): 221-226.

Rasmussen, O., C. Thomsen, J. Ingerslev & K. Hermansen (1994). "Decrease in von Willebrand factor levels after a high-monounsaturated-fat diet in non-insulin-dependent diabetic subjects." *Metabolism* 43 (11): 1406-1409.

Reisin, E. (2010). "The benefit of the Mediterranean-style diet in patients with newly diagnosed diabetes." *Curr Hypertens Rep* 12 (2): 56-58.

Renaud, S. & D. Lanzmann-Petithory (2002). "Dietary fats and coronary heart disease pathogenesis." *Curr Atheroscler Rep* 4 (6): 419-424.

Riccardi, G., R. Giacco & A. A. Rivellese (2004). "Dietary fat, insulin sensitivity and the metabolic syndrome." *Clin Nutr* 23 (4): 447-456.

Riediger, N. D., R. A. Othman, M. Suh & M. H. Moghadasian (2009). "A systemic review of the roles of n-3 fatty acids in health and disease." *J Am Diet Assoc* 109 (4): 668-679.

Rojo-Martinez, G., I. Esteva, M. S. Ruiz de Adana, J. M. Garcia-Almeida, F. Tinahones, F. Cardona, S. Morcillo, E. Garcia-Escobar, E. Garcia-Fuentes & F. Soriguer (2006). "Dietary fatty acids and insulin secretion: a population-based study." *Eur J Clin Nutr* 60 (10): 1195-1200.

Romaguera, D., T. Norat, T. Mouw, A. M. May, C. Bamia, N. Slimani, N. Travier, H. Besson, J. Luan, N. Wareham, S. Rinaldi, E. Couto, F. Clavel-Chapelon, M. C. Boutron-Ruault, V. Cottet, D. Palli, C. Agnoli, S. Panico, R. Tumino, P. Vineis, A. Agudo, L. Rodriguez, M. J. Sanchez, P. Amiano, A. Barricarte, J. M. Huerta, T. J. Key, E. A. Spencer, H. B. Bueno-de-Mesquita, F. L. Buchner, P. Orfanos, A. Naska, A. Trichopoulou, S. Rohrmann, R. Kaaks, M. Bergmann, H. Boeing, I. Johansson, V. Hellstrom, J. Manjer, E. Wirfalt, M. Uhre Jacobsen, K. Overvad, A. Tjonneland, J. Halkjaer, E. Lund, T. Braaten, D. Engeset, A. Odysseos, E. Riboli & P. H. Peeters (2009). "Adherence to the Mediterranean diet is associated with lower abdominal adiposity in European men and women." *J Nutr* 139 (9): 1728-1737.

Romaguera, D., T. Norat, A. C. Vergnaud, T. Mouw, A. M. May, A. Agudo, G. Buckland, N. Slimani, S. Rinaldi, E. Couto, F. Clavel-Chapelon, M. C. Boutron-Ruault, V. Cottet, S. Rohrmann, B. Teucher, M. Bergmann, H. Boeing, A. Tjonneland, J. Halkjaer, M. U. Jakobsen, C. C. Dahm, N. Travier, L. Rodriguez, M. J. Sanchez, P. Amiano, A. Barricarte, J. M. Huerta, J. Luan, N. Wareham, T. J. Key, E. A. Spencer, P. Orfanos, A. Naska, A. Trichopoulou, D. Palli, C. Agnoli, A. Mattiello, R. Tumino, P. Vineis, H. B. Bueno-de-Mesquita, F. L. Buchner, J. Manjer, E. Wirfalt, I. Johansson, V. Hellstrom, E. Lund, T. Braaten, D. Engeset, A. Odysseos, E. Riboli & P. H. Peeters (2010). "Mediterranean dietary patterns and prospective weight change in participants of the EPIC-PANACEA project." *Am J Clin Nutr* 92 (4): 912-921.

Ruano, J., J. Lopez-Miranda, F. Fuentes, J. A. Moreno, C. Bellido, P. Perez-Martinez, A. Lozano, P. Gomez, Y. Jimenez & F. Perez Jimenez (2005). "Phenolic content of virgin olive oil improves ischemic reactive hyperemia in hypercholesterolemic patients." *J Am Coll Cardiol* 46 (10): 1864-1868.

Salas-Salvado, J., M. Bullo, N. Babio, M. A. Martinez-Gonzalez, N. Ibarrola-Jurado, J. Basora, R. Estruch, M. I. Covas, D. Corella, F. Aros, V. Ruiz-Gutierrez & E. Ros (2011a). "Reduction in the incidence of type 2 diabetes with the Mediterranean diet: results of the PREDIMED-Reus nutrition intervention randomized trial." *Diabetes Care* 34 (1): 14-19.

Salas-Salvado, J., J. Fernandez-Ballart, E. Ros, M. A. Martinez-Gonzalez, M. Fito, R. Estruch, D. Corella, M. Fiol, E. Gomez-Gracia, F. Aros, G. Flores, J. Lapetra, R. Lamuela-Raventos, V. Ruiz-Gutierrez, M. Bullo, J. Basora & M. I. Covas (2008). "Effect of a Mediterranean diet supplemented with nuts on metabolic syndrome status: one-year results of the PREDIMED randomized trial." *Arch Intern Med* 168 (22): 2449-2458.

Salas-Salvado, J., M. A. Martinez-Gonzalez, M. Bullo & E. Ros (2011b). "The role of diet in the prevention of type 2 diabetes." *Nutr Metab Cardiovasc Dis*.

Sanchez-Tainta, A., R. Estruch, M. Bullo, D. Corella, E. Gomez-Gracia, M. Fiol, J. Algorta, M. I. Covas, J. Lapetra, I. Zazpe, V. Ruiz-Gutierrez, E. Ros & M. A. Martinez-Gonzalez (2008). "Adherence to a Mediterranean-type diet and reduced prevalence of clustered cardiovascular risk factors in a cohort of 3,204 high-risk patients." *Eur J Cardiovasc Prev Rehabil* 15 (5): 589-593.

Sarwar, N., J. Danesh, G. Eiriksdottir, G. Sigurdsson, N. Wareham, S. Bingham, S. M. Boekholdt, K. T. Khaw & V. Gudnason (2007). "Triglycerides and the risk of coronary heart disease: 10,158 incident cases among 262,525 participants in 29 Western prospective studies." *Circulation* 115 (4): 450-458.

Scarmeas, N., J. A. Luchsinger, Y. Stern, Y. Gu, J. He, C. DeCarli, T. Brown & A. M. Brickman (2011). "Mediterranean diet and magnetic resonance imaging-assessed cerebrovascular disease." *Ann Neurol* 69 (2): 257-268.

Schini-Kerth, V. B., C. Auger, N. Etienne-Selloum & T. Chataigneau (2010). "Polyphenol-induced endothelium-dependent relaxations role of NO and EDHF." *Adv Pharmacol* 60: 133-175.

Schroder, H., J. Marrugat, J. Vila, M. I. Covas & R. Elosua (2004). "Adherence to the traditional mediterranean diet is inversely associated with body mass index and obesity in a spanish population." *J Nutr* 134 (12): 3355-3361.

Schwartz, G. J., J. Fu, G. Astarita, X. Li, S. Gaetani, P. Campolongo, V. Cuomo & D. Piomelli (2008). "The lipid messenger OEA links dietary fat intake to satiety." *Cell Metab* 8 (4): 281-288.

Seo, T., W. S. Blaner & R. J. Deckelbaum (2005). "Omega-3 fatty acids: molecular approaches to optimal biological outcomes." *Curr Opin Lipidol* 16 (1): 11-18.

Serra-Majem, L., B. Roman & R. Estruch (2006). "Scientific evidence of interventions using the Mediterranean diet: a systematic review." *Nutr Rev* 64 (2 Pt 2): S27-47.

Shah, M., B. Adams-Huet & A. Garg (2007). "Effect of high-carbohydrate or high-cis-monounsaturated fat diets on blood pressure: a meta-analysis of intervention trials." *Am J Clin Nutr* 85 (5): 1251-1256.

Shai, I., J. D. Spence, D. Schwarzfuchs, Y. Henkin, G. Parraga, A. Rudich, A. Fenster, C. Mallett, N. Liel-Cohen, A. Tirosh, A. Bolotin, J. Thiery, G. M. Fiedler, M. Bluher, M.

Stumvoll & M. J. Stampfer (2010). "Dietary intervention to reverse carotid atherosclerosis." *Circulation* 121 (10): 1200-1208.

Singh, I., M. Mok, A. M. Christensen, A. H. Turner & J. A. Hawley (2008). "The effects of polyphenols in olive leaves on platelet function." *Nutr Metab Cardiovasc Dis* 18 (2): 127-132.

Sirtori, C. R., E. Tremoli, E. Gatti, G. Montanari, M. Sirtori, S. Colli, G. Gianfranceschi, P. Maderna, C. Z. Dentone, G. Testolin & et al. (1986). "Controlled evaluation of fat intake in the Mediterranean diet: comparative activities of olive oil and corn oil on plasma lipids and platelets in high-risk patients." *Am J Clin Nutr* 44 (5): 635-642.

Slavka, G., T. Perkmann, H. Haslacher, S. Greisenegger, C. Marsik, O. F. Wagner & G. Endler (2011). "Mean platelet volume may represent a predictive parameter for overall vascular mortality and ischemic heart disease." *Arterioscler Thromb Vasc Biol* 31 (5): 1215-1218.

Smith, R. D., C. N. Kelly, B. A. Fielding, D. Hauton, K. D. Silva, M. C. Nydahl, G. J. Miller & C. M. Williams (2003). "Long-term monounsaturated fatty acid diets reduce platelet aggregation in healthy young subjects." *Br J Nutr* 90 (3): 597-606.

Sofi, F., R. Abbate, G. F. Gensini & A. Casini (2010). "Accruing evidence about benefits of adherence to the Mediterranean diet on health: an updated systematic review and meta-analysis." *Am J Clin Nutr*.

Sofi, F., F. Cesari, R. Abbate, G. F. Gensini & A. Casini (2008). "Adherence to Mediterranean diet and health status: meta-analysis." *Bmj* 337: a1344.

Solfrizzi, V., F. Panza, V. Frisardi, D. Seripa, G. Logroscino, B. P. Imbimbo & A. Pilotto (2011). "Diet and Alzheimer's disease risk factors or prevention: the current evidence." *Expert Rev Neurother* 11 (5): 677-708.

Spence, J. D. (2010). "Secondary stroke prevention." *Nat Rev Neurol* 6 (9): 477-486.

Stock, J. (2011). "Mediterranean diet for combating the metabolic syndrome." *Atherosclerosis*.

Tangney, C. C., M. J. Kwasny, H. Li, R. S. Wilson, D. A. Evans & M. C. Morris (2011). "Adherence to a Mediterranean-type dietary pattern and cognitive decline in a community population." *Am J Clin Nutr* 93 (3): 601-607.

Tekbas, E., A. F. Kara, Z. Ariturk, H. Cil, Y. Islamoglu, M. A. Elbey, S. Soydinc & M. S. Ulgen (2011). "Mean platelet volume in predicting short- and long-term morbidity and mortality in patients with or without ST-segment elevation myocardial infarction." *Scand J Clin Lab Invest*.

Temme, E. H., R. P. Mensink & G. Hornstra (1999). "Effects of diets enriched in lauric, palmitic or oleic acids on blood coagulation and fibrinolysis." *Thromb Haemost* 81 (2): 259-263.

Tortosa, A., M. Bes-Rastrollo, A. Sanchez-Villegas, F. J. Basterra-Gortari, J. M. Nunez-Cordoba & M. A. Martinez-Gonzalez (2007). "Mediterranean diet inversely associated with the incidence of metabolic syndrome: the SUN prospective cohort." *Diabetes Care* 30 (11): 2957-2959.

Tozzi Ciancarelli, M. G., C. Di Massimo, D. De Amicis, I. Ciancarelli & A. Carolei (2011). "Moderate consumption of red wine and human platelet responsiveness." *Thromb Res* 128 (2): 124-129.

Trichopoulou, A., A. Naska, P. Orfanos & D. Trichopoulos (2005). "Mediterranean diet in relation to body mass index and waist-to-hip ratio: the Greek European Prospective Investigation into Cancer and Nutrition Study." *Am J Clin Nutr* 82 (5): 935-940.

Tripoli, E., M. Giammanco, G. Tabacchi, D. Di Majo, S. Giammanco & M. La Guardia (2005). "The phenolic compounds of olive oil: structure, biological activity and beneficial effects on human health." *Nutr Res Rev* 18: 98-112.

Turpeinen, A. M. & M. Mutanen (1999). "Similar effects of diets high in oleic or linoleic acids on coagulation and fibrinolytic factors in healthy humans." *Nutr Metab Cardiovasc Dis* 9 (2): 65-72.

van den Brandt, P. A. (2011). "The impact of a Mediterranean diet and healthy lifestyle on premature mortality in men and women." *Am J Clin Nutr.*

van Wijk, D. F., E. S. Stroes & J. J. Kastelein (2009). "Lipid measures and cardiovascular disease prediction." *Dis Markers* 26 (5-6): 209-216.

Varbo, A., B. G. Nordestgaard, A. Tybjaerg-Hansen, P. Schnohr, G. B. Jensen & M. Benn (2011). "Nonfasting triglycerides, cholesterol, and ischemic stroke in the general population." *Ann Neurol* 69 (4): 628-634.

Vardavas, C. I., A. D. Flouris, A. Tsatsakis, A. G. Kafatos & W. H. Saris (2011). "Does adherence to the Mediterranean diet have a protective effect against active and passive smoking?" *Public Health* 125 (3): 121-128.

Visioli, F., D. Caruso, S. Grande, R. Bosisio, M. Villa, G. Galli, C. Sirtori & C. Galli (2005). "Virgin Olive Oil Study (VOLOS): vasoprotective potential of extra virgin olive oil in mildly dyslipidemic patients." *Eur J Nutr* 44 (2): 121-127.

Visioli, F. & C. Galli (1998). "The effect of minor constituents of olive oil on cardiovascular disease: new findings." *Nutr Rev* 56 (5 Pt 1): 142-147.

Wang, R. T., Y. Li, X. Y. Zhu & Y. N. Zhang (2011). "Increased mean platelet volume is associated with arterial stiffness." *Platelets* 22 (6): 447-451.

Willett, W. C. (2006). "The Mediterranean diet: science and practice." *Public Health Nutr* 9 (1A): 105-110.

Williams, C. M. (2001). "Beneficial nutritional properties of olive oil: implications for postprandial lipoproteins and factor VII." *Nutr Metab Cardiovasc Dis* 11 (4 Suppl): 51-56.

Yubero-Serrano, E. M., A. Garcia-Rios, J. Delgado-Lista, N. Delgado-Casado, P. Perez-Martinez, F. Rodriguez-Cantalejo, F. Fuentes, C. Cruz-Teno, I. Tunez, I. Tasset-Cuevas, F. J. Tinahones, F. Perez-Jimenez & J. Lopez-Miranda (2011). "Postprandial effects of the Mediterranean diet on oxidant and antioxidant status in elderly men and women." *J Am Geriatr Soc* 59 (5): 938-940.

# 10

# Dietary Supplements and Cardiovascular Disease: What is the Evidence and What Should We Recommend?

Satoshi Kashiwagi and Paul L. Huang

*Cardiovascular Research Center and Cardiology Division, Massachusetts General Hospital and Harvard Medical School, Charlestown, MA, USA*

## 1. Introduction

### 1.1 Importance of cardiovascular disease and scope of this chapter

Cardiovascular disease, diabetes, and obesity are important causes of morbidity and mortality. Cardiovascular disease affects 80 million Americans and is the leading cause of death (Lloyd-Jones et al., 2009). Diabetes and obesity are also increasing at alarming rates, and together, the three conditions have a significant impact on public health (Ogden et al., 2006). Cardiovascular disease, diabetes and obesity can be influenced by lifestyle changes, including diet and physical activity (McCullough et al., 2000). The American Heart Association recommends a diet rich in vegetables and fruits, whole grains, high-fiber foods, with lean meats and poultry, moderate consumption of fish, an emphasis on fat-free or low fat dairy products, and limiting the amount of saturated fat, trans fat and cholesterol (Lichtenstein et al., 2006).

Among natural products found in food, fish oils, vitamin E, and soy isoflavones have been studied for their effects on cardiovascular disease. Many of these compounds are available as food supplements. There is a great interest among the public and in the lay press about the use of these compounds to treat or prevent disease. The scope of this chapter is to review the evidence for the effects of these compounds on cardiovascular disease, so that physicians and patients may better understand their health effects, in an effort to reduce the risk for cardiovascular disease, diabetes and obesity.

### 1.2 Types of evidence: Epidemiologic, mechanistic, and randomized clinical trials

It is important to realize the different kinds of evidence in support of health benefits of natural products. One type of evidence is *epidemiologic evidence*. Epidemiologic information may offer the first suggestion that certain natural products in the diet may influence the risk and course of chronic diseases like cardiovascular disease, diabetes, and cancer. Cross-cultural studies might indicate that populations that have high or low intake of certain compounds have different incidence of cardiovascular disease. This does not prove that supplementation with these compounds would necessarily change the course of cardiovascular disease. Genetic and environmental factors may all contribute to the effects observed in the epidemiologic studies. Cohort studies, which follow groups of people and their intake of certain compounds, also provide suggestive evidence for their effects.

A second type of evidence comes from *mechanistic studies* in the laboratory or in animal models. Here, the natural products or compounds in question are added to cells or enzyme reactions, to see what their effects are. Studies may be done in animal models of human disease, for example apoE knockout mice that develop diet-induced atherosclerosis. They may be carried out on blood vessels from animals to see whether the compounds affect vascular function. Mechanistic studies help determine the possible molecular and cellular mechanisms and pathways involved in biological function. However, just because a compound has an effect in these experiments or animals models does not mean that taking them will necessarily reduce disease in people. Many of these experiments are done *in vitro*, not *in vivo*.

A third type of evidence comes from *randomized controlled clinical trials*. In these trials, compounds are administered to a large population, which is then followed for clearly defined disease events. Randomized clinical trials offer the strongest scientific evidence for or against health benefits. These studies often use pure compounds or standardized preparations. Often, compounds for which epidemiologic studies suggest benefit, and mechanistic studies show effects, fail to do so in large randomized clinical trials. There have also been surprising results of increased disease risk from certain natural products, suggesting the need for caution and for ongoing studies to obtain evidence of the best possible quality. It is important to approach results of studies with a critical eye, and to always consider the quality of the information and how strongly it supports an effect.

In this article, three specific classes of compounds—omega-3 fatty acids, vitamin E, and soy isoflavones—are reviewed. Evidence for their biological effects are presented, categorized separately according to type of evidence: epidemiological studies, mechanistic studies, and where available, randomized controlled trials. It is hoped that this review will provide the basis for evidence-based recommendations to patients regarding these compounds and food supplements.

## 2. Fish oils: Omega-3 fatty acids

### 2.1 Structure and food sources

While many fatty acids serve as energy stores that are broken down by the body to generate energy, *omega-3* and *omega-6* fatty acids are two types of polyunsaturated fatty acids that serve as precursors to biologically active molecules, including prostaglandins, leukotrienes, and thromboxanes. This role gives them particular importance in the diet.

Polyunsaturated fatty acids are a family of long-chain (typically 18-24 carbon atoms) fatty acids containing two or more double bonds. Omega-3 and omega-6 refer to the position of the last double bond. The convention in chemical nomenclature is to label the COOH carbon as the first carbon, and the one furthest from this as the last, or *omega*, carbon. Thus, omega-3 fatty acids contain a double bond three carbons from the end of the molecule furthest from the COOH group. Given that the length of the hydrocarbon chain is variable, the length is sometimes referred to as "n," so omega-3 fatty acids are also known as n-3 fatty acids, and omega-6 fatty acids as n-6 fatty acids.

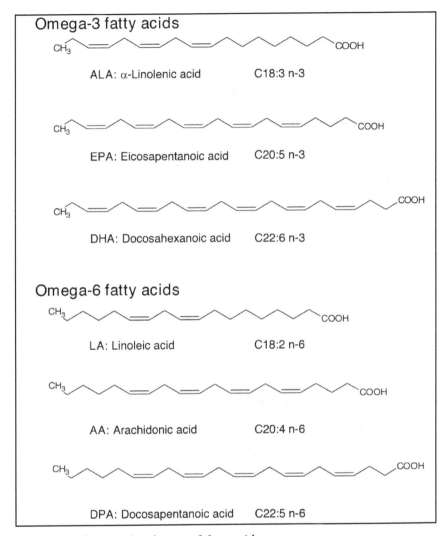

Fig. 1. Structures of omega-6 and omega-3 fatty acids
Omega-3 fatty acids differ from omega-6 fatty acids by the location of their first double bond from the methyl ($CH_3$) end of the fatty acid. Omega-3 fatty acids include α-linolenic acid (ALA), eicosapentanoic acid (EPA), and docosahexanoic acid (DHA). Omega-6 fatty acids include linoleic acid (LA), arachidonic acid (AA), and docosapentanoic acid (DPA). In the chemical names, the number of carbon atoms is given first, separated by a colon from the number of double bonds, followed by the position of the first double bond.

The structures of omega-3 and omega-6 fatty acids are shown in Figure 1. Representative omega-3 fatty acids are α-linolenic acid (ALA), eicosapentanoic acid (EPA), and docosahexanoic acid (DHA). Of these, the parent omega-3 fatty acid is ALA, an 18 carbon fatty acid with three double bonds, the last of which is located between carbons 15 and 16 (the n-3 position). Therefore, in shorthand, ALA is C18:3 n-3. ALA serves as the precursor to the omega-3 fatty acids EPA (C20:5 n-3) and DHA (C22:6 n-3) by the addition of carbons to the chain (elongation) and by the replacement of single bonds by double bonds (desaturation). Likewise, representative omega-6 fatty acids are linoleic acid (LA), arachidonic acid (AA), and docosapentanoic acid. LA is an 18 carbon fatty acid with two double bonds, with the last one located at the n-6 position (C18:2 n-6). LA serves as a precursor to AA (C20:4 n-6) and docosapentanoic acid (C22:5 n-6), which are formed by elongation and desaturation.

The parent fatty acids of the omega-3 family (ALA) and omega-6 family (LA) cannot be made by the human body, so they are *essential* fatty acids. They must be supplied in the diet. LA is found in vegetable oils like soybean and canola, and also in nuts, seeds, vegetables, legumes, grains, and fruit. ALA is found in vegetable sources like flaxseed, but only 5% of ALA is converted to DHA and EPA. The richest sources of DHA and EPA are fish and fish oils.

## 2.2 Biological roles of omega-3 and omega-6 fatty acids

Omega-3 and -6 fatty acids are important biologically because they influence production of prostaglandins, leukotrienes, and thromboxanes. These mediators affect many diverse processes, and are involved in inflammation, pain, and thrombosis (Calder, 2006). Moreover, omega-3 and omega-6 fatty acids are separate families that cannot be interconverted by the human body. Because they compete for the same enzymes, the ratio of omega-3 to omega-6 fatty acids in the diet influences the relative amounts of prostaglandins and leukotrienes that are synthesized from arachidonic acid.

## 2.3 Epidemiologic data on fish oils and cardiovascular disease

Epidemiologic data from fish-eating populations like the Greenland Inuits established a link between fish oil consumption and lower incidence of cardiovascular disease (Dyerberg et al., 1975). Fish oil consumption was also linked with low levels of triglycerides, plasma cholesterol and very low-density lipoproteins (VLDL) and high levels of high-density lipoproteins (HDL), all of which would protect against cardiovascular disease.

## 2.4 Mechanistic studies

Omega-3 fatty acids may influence cardiovascular disease through effects on lipid profiles, eicosanoid pathways, and susceptibility to arrythmias.

### 2.4.1 Lipid profiles

Omega-3 fatty acids decrease plasma cholesterol concentrations in animal models (Fernandez & West, 2005). They increase hepatic LDL receptor number and LDL turnover *in vivo* (Fernandez & McNamar, 1989, Fernandez et al., 1992), and bind to peroxisome proliferator activated receptors (PPARs), liver X receptors (LXRs), hepatic nuclear factor-4 (HNF-4), and sterol regulatory element binding proteins (SREBPs) (Jump, 2002). Omega-3 fatty acids suppress SREBP-1 expression, leading to decreased lipogenesis and VLDL secretion (Field et al., 2003), increased LPL activity (Illingworth & Schmidt, 1993), and decreased apoC3 levels (Shachter, 2001). They also decrease lipogenesis and VLDL secretion while increasing reverse cholesterol transport (Vasandani et al., 2002).

### 2.4.2 Eicosanoid metabolism

Omega-3 and omega-6 fatty acids are precursors to a broad array of structurally diverse and potent bioactive lipids, including eicosanoids, prostaglandins, and thromboxanes. Eicosanoids are produced from arachidonic acid, EPA, and dihomolinolenic acid when these fatty acids are released from membranes by phospholipase $A_2$ (Zhou & Nilsson, 2001). The availability of these eicosanoid precursors depends on dietary levels of these molecules, as well as the parent fatty acids of each family: ALA for omega-3 fatty acids, and LA for omega-6 fatty acids. Because omega-6 and omega-3 fatty acids cannot be interconverted, their relative ratios are important.

Arachidonic acid, an omega-6 fatty acid, is a precursor of prostaglandins, leukotrienes and related compounds that mediate inflammation. Because omega-3 fatty acids compete with omega-6 fatty acid metabolism, increased consumption of omega-3 fatty acids (particularly DHA and EPA) results in the partial replacement of arachidonic acid in cell membranes by EPA and DHA, and a decrease in the production of biological mediators derived from AA. Intake of 6 g DHA/d decreased production of prostaglandin $E_2$ by 60% and leukotriene $B_4$ by 75% in endotoxin-stimulated mononuclear cells (Kelley et al., 1999). Other studies have shown a shift in the relative amounts of prostaglandin $I_2$ and thromboxane $A_2$, resulting in vasodilation and reduced thrombosis (von Schacky et al., 1985, Goodnight et al., 1989). Omega-3 fatty acids, particularly DHA and EPA in fish oil, may themselves reduce expression of ICAM-1 on the surface of stimulated blood monocytes (Hughes et al., 1996), and decrease hydrogen peroxide production (Fisher et al., 1990).

### 2.4.3 Antiarrhythmic effects

DHA and EPA may be preferentially incorporated into membrane phospholipids, accounting for an antiarrhythmic effect after dietary intake (Nair et al., 1999). These fatty acids directly influence conduction of several membrane ion channels (Leaf et al., 2003), inhibit voltage-gated sodium currents and L-type calcium currents (Kang et al., 1995), and shift the steady-state inactivation potential to more negative values in cardiomyocytes. These results provide an electrophysiological basis for antiarrhythmic effects.

### 2.5 Clinical studies

Dietary intake of omega-3 fatty acids, particularly DHA and EPA found in fatty fish or fish-oil supplements, reduces risk of CVD (Kris-Etherton et al., 2002, Wang et al., 2006). The strongest evidence comes from the Italian GISSI trial (1999), a secondary prevention study in over 11,000 patients with recent myocardial infarction. Supplementation with 0.85 g EPA and DHA per day reduced all-cause mortality by 21%, cardiac death by 35%, and sudden death by 45%. No effect was found on stroke. In contrast, a Norwegian study of 300 patients following MI, randomized to a higher intake of omega-3 fatty acids (3.4 g EPA and DPA per day), failed to show a difference in CVD events, but there was a high background of fish oil intake in both groups. Several other small studies suggested beneficial trends in CVD and PVD, but these were not statistically significant (Sacks et al., 1995, Nilsen et al., 2001).

In these studies, patients with implantable cardiac defibrillators (ICD) were excluded. Several randomized controlled trials, ranging in size from 200 to over 500 patients, studied fish oil consumption in patients with ICDs (Raitt et al., 2005,Brouwer et al., 2006). These studies showed no change in mortality from fish oil consumption. It is possible that the beneficial effects of fish oils may not be observed in the ICD population, because these patients all have defibrillators and therefore cardiac arrhythmic sudden death would be removed from both groups.

Primary prevention trials, which study patients in the general population who do not have known heart disease, have not shown as strong an effect as the GISSI trial. Most primary prevention data on fish oils comes from large cohort studies from China, Japan, and the United States (Dolecek, 1992, Nagata et al., 2002) and others. In aggregate, these studies included over 343,000 subjects, and showed reductions in all-cause mortality, cardiac mortality, and sudden death. Interestingly, in one of these studies (Mozaffarian et al., 2003), the protection was found with tuna and other nonfried fish, while consumption of fried fish or fried fish sandwiches was associated with increased cardiovascular events.

## 3. Vitamin E

### 3.1 Structure and food sources

Vitamin E is a fat-soluble vitamin that exists in at least eight naturally occurring forms, as shown in Figure 2. Tocotrienols differ from tocopherols by the presence of three double bonds in their isoprenoid side chains. The $\alpha$-, $\beta$-, $\gamma$-, and $\delta$- forms are defined by the identity of the R groups on the chromanol rings. Vitamin E found naturally in food is primarily $\gamma$-tocopherol, but $\alpha$-tocopherol is the predominant form found in supplements, and is also the most biologically active form.

Vitamin E is an essential vitamin because it cannot be synthesized by the body. Sources of vitamin E include nuts and seeds, such as almonds, peanuts, sunflower seeds, and filberts.

Tocopherols are similar in structure to tocotrienols, except that tocotrienols have three double bonds in the phytyl side chains. There are three positions on the chromanol ring, denoted $R_1$, $R_2$, and $R_3$. The particular identity of the tocopherol or tocotrienol is determined by the identities of these side chains. Vitamin E found naturally in food is primarily $\gamma$-tocopherol. $\alpha$-tocopherol, which is the most biologically active, is the predominant form found in supplements.

Vitamin E is also found in vegetable oils (soy, corn or sunflower), and their derivatives (margarine), cereals and grains. Vitamin E is found in potato chips and tomato products because of the vegetable oils that they contain.

### 3.2 Biological roles of vitamin E

Vitamin E is an antioxidant, because it breaks chain reactions that are propagated by free radicals. Vitamin E is present in biological membranes, and serves as an important lipid soluble antioxidant. It reacts with oxidant molecules and protects cell membranes from lipid peroxidation by trapping peroxyl radicals. One molecule of $\alpha$-tocopherol per 1,000 phospholipids can protect cellular membranes. $\alpha$-tocopherol can also be regenerated from its tocopheroxyl radical by an electron donor like vitamin C.

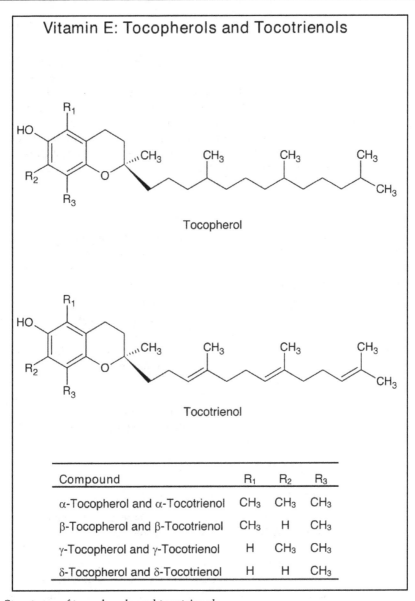

Fig. 2. Structures of tocopherols and tocotrienols

## 3.3 Epidemiologic data on vitamin E and cardiovascular disease

High intake of vitamin E is epidemiologically associated with lower cardiovascular disease risk. The World Health Organization/Monica project performed cross-cultural analysis on vitamin intake in populations with different incidence of coronary heart disease mortality. Differences in cardiovascular mortality were primarily attributable to plasma levels of vitamin E in middle-aged men representing 16 European study populations (Gey et al., 1991).

Several cohort studies showed similar results. The US Nurse's Health Study followed a cohort of 87,245 female nurses between the ages of 34 and 59 years, over an eight year period. Supplementation with α-tocopherol for at least two years was associated with reduced risk of cardiovascular disease (Stampfer et al., 1993). Incidence of heart disease was 30-40% lower in those with the highest intakes of vitamin E. Another cohort study followed 39,910 male health professionals between the ages of 40 and 75. Consumption of more than 60 IU/d of vitamin E was associated with a 40% relative risk reduction of cardiovascular disease (Rimm et al., 1993). Vitamin E intake from food was inversely associated with CVD risk in 34,486 postmenopausal women (Kushi et al., 1996).

### 3.4 Mechanistic studies

In *ex vivo* human studies, monocytes isolated from healthy human subjects supplemented with α-tocopherol showed decreased LDL oxidation (Devaraj et al., 1996). In other studies, vitamin E supplementation failed to affect lipid oxidation, including isoprostanes and 4-hydroxynonenal (breakdown products of fatty acid autooxidation) (Meagher et al., 2001).

One animal study showed that vitamin E intake inversely correlates with atherosclerotic lesions and liver peroxidation in apoE knockout mice (Ferre et al., 2001). In another study, vitamin E and coenzyme Q (CoQ) supplementation significantly reduced tissue lipid hydroperoxide formation and limited the development of atherosclerosis in apoE knockout mice (Thomas et al., 2001). However, still other studies found that vitamin E did not reduce atherosclerosis in apoE knockout mice (Paul et al., 2001), or fatty streak formation in C57/Bl6 mice (Munday et al., 1998). The degree of lipid oxidation in vascular tissue also failed to correlate with the extent of the lesions in apoE knockout mice (Wu et al., 2006). Thus, animal studies do not show uniform benefit of vitamin E supplementation in preventing LDL oxidation or reducing atherosclerosis.

### 3.5 Clinical trials on vitamin E

### 3.5.1 Vitamin E and cardiovascular disease

Some clinical trials suggest a benefit of vitamin E in reducing cardiovascular disease. The Cambridge Heart Antioxidant Study (CHAOS) randomized 2,002 patients with coronary disease to α-tocopherol (400 to 800 IU) or placebo. The vitamin E treated groups showed 1.9 fold reductions in cardiovascular death and nonfatal myocardial infarction (Stephens et al., 1996). The Secondary Prevention with Antioxidants of Cardiovascular Disease in End-stage Renal Disease (SPACE) trial randomized 192 renal failure patients undergoing hemodialysis to 800 IU vitamin E or placebo. The vitamin E treated group showed a significant decrease in both fatal and nonfatal cardiovascular endpoints (Boaz et al., 2000).

Other clinical trials failed to show benefit. In the GISSI study, 11,324 patients were given omega-3 fatty acids, vitamin E at 300 mg per day, both, or neither, and followed over a 3½ year period. Two-way analysis did not show any reduction in fatal or nonfatal cardiovascular events from vitamin E supplementation (Marchioli et al., 2002), (1999). The Heart Outcomes Prevention Evaluation (HOPE) trial was a multinational study of over 9,500 patients with known cardiovascular disease, randomized to the angiotensin converting enzyme inhibitor ramipril, natural source vitamin E at 400 IU per day, both, or neither. Over a 4½ year follow-up, there was no reduction in fatal or nonfatal cardiovascular events in the vitamin E treated groups (Yusuf et al., 2000). In an extension study (HOPE –TOO), almost 4000 subjects continued to take vitamin E or placebo for an additional 2½ years (Lonn et al., 2005). Despite this 7 year total follow-up period, there was no significant protection against cardiovascular disease, stroke, or death.

Of concern, the HOPE-TOO study showed a higher incidence of heart failure in the treated group. In the Women's Angiographic Vitamin and Estrogen Study, 423 post-menopausal women with coronary disease took supplements with 400 IU vitamin E or placebo (Waters et al., 2002). Not only did women taking vitamin E not show cardiovascular benefit, but there was an increase in all-cause mortality. In the Physicians Health Study II, 15,000 health physicians age 50 or over were randomized to α-tocopherol (400 IU), 500 mg vitamin C, both, or placebo (Sesso et al., 2008). Over a follow-up period of 8 years, neither vitamin E nor vitamin C resulted in a decrease in cardiovascular events, stroke, or cardiovascular mortality. In contrast, α-tocopherol was associated with an increase in hemorrhagic stroke. Taking the results of all of these results together, including a meta-analysis (Miller et al., 2005), vitamin E is not recommended for the purpose of reducing cardiovascular risk.

### 3.5.2 Vitamin E and diabetes

Oxidative stress and inflammation have been implicated in the pathogenesis of diabetes(Ho & Bray, 1999). Vitamin E treatment (600 mg per day) improved insulin-mediated glucose disposal in 36 healthy, nondiabetic volunteers (Facchini et al., 2000). A prospective cohort study showed that plasma concentration of α-tocopherol was inversely related to fasting plasma glucose concentration and oxidative stress markers in 101 women at high risk of type 2 diabetes in Finland (Ylonen et al., 2003). In secondary prevention trials, 600 mg/day of vitamin E supplementation significantly decreased markers of oxidative stress and improved brachial artery reactivity in 40 patients with diabetes (Paolisso et al., 2000). However, the Insulin Resistance and Atherosclerosis Study (IRAS) cohort study showed no protective effect for either reported intake of vitamin E or plasma concentration of α-tocopherol in 895 nondiabetic adults (Mayer-Davis et al., 2002). In another study, high levels of α-tocopherol and β-carotene were associated with decreased risk of non-insulin dependent diabetes mellitus, but the association disappeared after adjustment for cardiovascular risk factors (Reunanen et al., 1998). Whether vitamin E influences the development of diabetes is not clear and warrants further investigation.

## 4. Phytoestrogens

### 4.1 Structure and food sources of phytoestrogens

Phytoestrogens are flavonoids that have similar chemical structure to estrogen. They include isoflavones, coumestans, and lignans (Kurzer & Xu, 1997). Figure 3 shows a comparison of the chemical structures of estradiol (a naturally occurring human estrogen), genistein (an isoflavone), and coumestrol (a coumestan). A number of these compounds have been identified in fruits, vegetables, and whole grains commonly consumed as food. Soybeans, clover and alfalfa sprouts, and oilseeds (such as flaxseed) are the most significant dietary sources.

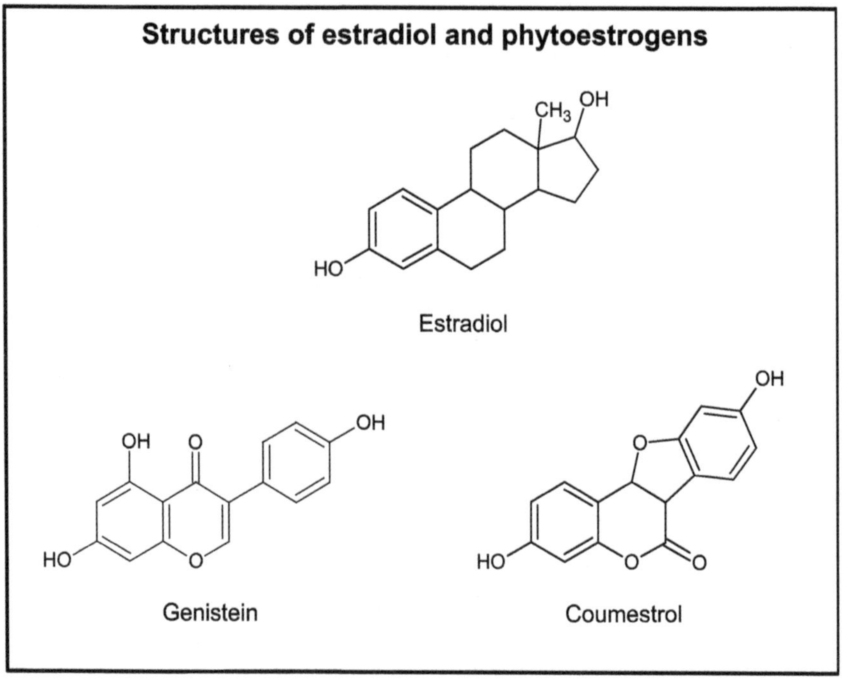

Fig. 3. Structures of isoflavones and coumestans compared with estrogen
The structure of estradiol, a natural estrogen, is shown along with the structures of genistein, a prototypic isoflavone found in soy, and coumestrol, a prototypic coumestan.

## 4.2 Epidemiology data on phytoestrogens and cardiovascular disease

While typical isoflavone intake is less than 1 mg per day in Western countries, intakes of 20-50 mg per day are common in Asian countries such as China and Japan, where soy is a traditional staple food (Adlercreutz & Mazur, 1997). These countries also have shown reduced incidence of cardiovascular disease compared with Western countries, an effect that is diminishing as Western eating habits and diets are adopted.

## 4.3 Biological activities of phytoestrogens

Dietary phytoestrogens may play an important role in prevention of menopausal symptoms, osteoporosis, cancer, and cardiovascular disease. The major mechanisms of biological action for the phytoestrogens are those mediated by estrogen receptors (estrogenic and antiestrogenic effects), effects on tyrosine kinase and DNA topoisomerase activities, suppression of angiogenesis, and antioxidant effects.

Although not as active as 17β-estradiol, phytoestrogens compete with estradiol for binding to estrogen receptors (ER), particularly ERβ (Kuiper et al., 1998). ERβ, present in high concentrations in ovary and testis, binds phytoestrogens with higher affinity, and may mediate some of their biological effects (Kuiper et al., 1998). Alternatively, soy isoflavones may be natural selective estrogen receptor modulators (SERMs) with both agonist and antagonist activities (Setchell, 2001).

Soy isoflavones decrease total cholesterol, LDL, and triglycerides, and increase HDL levels (Clarkson et al., 2001). They also lower blood pressure and improve endothelial reactivity (Teede et al., 2001, Steinberg et al., 2003). Supplementation of isoflavones derived from red clover containing genistein, daidzein, biochanin, and formononetin significantly improved arterial compliance in elderly men and women (Nestel et al., 1999).

Several studies reveal the potential of phytoestrogens to induce hormone-dependent cancers (e.g. breast and endometrium) (McMichael-Phillips et al., 1998), leading to safety concerns. Because of this, a maximum daily intake level for phytoestrogens has been suggested in several countries (Sirtori et al., 2005).

---

**Summary of key points**

**Omega-3 fatty acids**

- Important omega-3 fatty acids include EPA and DHA
- Mechanisms for omega-3 fatty acids include
  -reduced inflammation due to decreased prostaglandin and leukotriene synthesis
  -reduced thrombosis and platelet aggregation
  -direct antiarrythmic effects in cell membranes
- Large studies confirm that omega-3 fatty acid intake reduces cardiovascular disease and sudden death
- The American Heart Association recommends eating fish twice a week, and daily intake of 1 g EPA and DHA to reduce cardiovascular disease

**Vitamin E**

- Vitamin E is an essential fat soluble vitamin that is an antioxidant
- Animal studies do not uniformly show beneficial effects
- Vitamin E reduced cardiovascular risk in two studies (CHAOS and SPACE), but not in others (GISSI, HOPE-TOO)
- Vitamin E supplementation has been associated with higher incidence of heart failure, so routine supplementation with vitamin E is *not* recommended

**Phytoestrogens**

- Phytoestrogens, including soy isoflavones, are plant compounds with chemical structures that resemble estrogens
- Mechanisms include improved lipid profiles and improved endothelial reactivity
- Phytoestrogens may induce hormone dependent cancers (breast and endometrial), leading to recommendations on maximum daily intake

## 5. Conclusions and evidence-based recommendations

Omega-3 fatty acids have been clearly shown in epidemiological studies and clinical trials to reduce the incidence of cardiovascular disease. Thus, the American Heart Association recommends eating fish (particularly fatty fish) at least twice a week. They also recommend foods rich in ALA (flaxseed, canola, and soybean oils; flaxseed and walnuts). For patients with documented coronary heart disease, the recommended level of consumption is 1 g of EPA+DHA per day, either from fish (preferably), or supplementation. For subjects with elevated triglyceride levels, 2-4 grams of EPA+DHA is recommended as supplementation (Kris-Etherton et al., 2002).

At this time, the evidence does not justify the use of vitamin E supplements for CVD risk reduction, both because of lack of evidence for benefit and possible adverse effect reflected in the increases in all-cause mortality and hemorrhagic stroke. However, a balanced diet with emphasis on antioxidant-rich fruits, vegetables, and whole grains is recommended (Kris-Etherton et al., 2004). Whether antioxidant vitamin supplements including vitamin E influence the development of diabetes, in which oxidative stress plays an important role, is not clear and warrants further investigation.

Supplementing the diet with soy protein has failed to confirm phytoestrogens as the responsible agent for beneficial cardiovascular effects. Furthermore, soy phytoestrogens may increase carcinogenesis. Thus, isoflavone supplements are not currently recommended (Sacks et al., 2006). Soy foods may still be beneficial to cardiovascular and overall health because of their high content of polyunsaturated fats, fiber, vitamins, and minerals and low content of saturated fat (Krauss et al., 2000).

Epidemiologic evidence has suggested an array of potentially beneficial compounds in foods. While there have been many mechanistic studies in the laboratory or in animal models, large scale randomized controlled clinical trials are necessary to prove or disprove their effects on health and safety, particularly in light of possible toxicities. Until the results of such studies are available, a diet consistent with American Heart Association recommendations (Kris-Etherton et al., 2004), with emphasis on antioxidant-rich fruits, vegetables, and whole grains, appears to be the most sensible approach.

## 6. Acknowledgements

PLH acknowledges grant support from Public Health Service grant R01-NS33335 from the National Institute of Neurologic Diseases and Stroke, and grant R01-HL048426 from the National Heart Lung and Blood Institute.

## 7. References

Adlercreutz, H. and W. Mazur. (1997). Phyto-oestrogens and Western diseases. *Ann Med,* Vol. 29, pp. 95-120.

Boaz, M., S. Smetana, et al. (2000). Secondary prevention with antioxidants of cardiovascular disease in endstage renal disease (SPACE): randomised placebo-controlled trial. *Lancet,* Vol. 356, pp. 1213-8.

Brouwer, I. A., P. L. Zock, et al. (2006). Effect of fish oil on ventricular tachyarrhythmia and death in patients with implantable cardioverter defibrillators: the Study on Omega-

3 Fatty Acids and Ventricular Arrhythmia (SOFA) randomized trial. *Jama*, Vol. 295, pp. 2613-9.

Calder, P. C. (2006). n-3 polyunsaturated fatty acids, inflammation, and inflammatory diseases. *Am J Clin Nutr*, Vol. 83, pp. 1505S-1519S.

Clarkson, T. B., M. S. Anthony, et al. (2001). Inhibition of postmenopausal atherosclerosis progression: a comparison of the effects of conjugated equine estrogens and soy phytoestrogens. *J Clin Endocrinol Metab*, Vol. 86, pp. 41-7.

Devaraj, S., D. Li, et al. (1996). The effects of alpha tocopherol supplementation on monocyte function. Decreased lipid oxidation, interleukin 1 beta secretion, and monocyte adhesion to endothelium. *J Clin Invest*, Vol. 98, pp. 756-63.

Dolecek, T. A. (1992). Epidemiological evidence of relationships between dietary polyunsaturated fatty acids and mortality in the multiple risk factor intervention trial. *Proc Soc Exp Biol Med*, Vol. 200, pp. 177-82.

Dyerberg, J., H. O. Bang, et al. (1975). Fatty acid composition of the plasma lipids in Greenland Eskimos. *Am J Clin Nutr*, Vol. 28, pp. 958-66.

Facchini, F. S., M. H. Humphreys, et al. (2000). Relation between insulin resistance and plasma concentrations of lipid hydroperoxides, carotenoids, and tocopherols. *Am J Clin Nutr*, Vol. 72, pp. 776-9.

Fernandez, M. L., E. C. Lin, et al. (1992). Differential effects of saturated fatty acids on low density lipoprotein metabolism in the guinea pig. *J Lipid Res*, Vol. 33, pp. 1833-42.

Fernandez, M. L. and D. J. McNamar. (1989). Dietary fat-mediated changes in hepatic apoprotein B/E receptor in the guinea pig: effect of polyunsaturated, monounsaturated, and saturated fat. *Metabolism*, Vol. 38, pp. 1094-102.

Fernandez, M. L. and K. L. West. (2005). Mechanisms by which dietary fatty acids modulate plasma lipids. *J Nutr*, Vol. 135, pp. 2075-8.

Ferre, N., J. Camps, et al. (2001). Effects of high-fat, low-cholesterol diets on hepatic lipid peroxidation and antioxidants in apolipoprotein E-deficient mice. *Mol Cell Biochem*, Vol. 218, pp. 165-9.

Field, F. J., E. Born, et al. (2003). Fatty acid flux suppresses fatty acid synthesis in hamster intestine independently of SREBP-1 expression. *J Lipid Res*, Vol. 44, pp. 1199-208.

Fisher, M., P. H. Levine, et al. (1990). Dietary n-3 fatty acid supplementation reduces superoxide production and chemiluminescence in a monocyte-enriched preparation of leukocytes. *Am J Clin Nutr*, Vol. 51, pp. 804-8.

Gey, K. F., P. Puska, et al. (1991). Inverse correlation between plasma vitamin E and mortality from ischemic heart disease in cross-cultural epidemiology. *Am J Clin Nutr*, Vol. 53, pp. 326S-334S.

GISSI. (1999). Dietary supplementation with n-3 polyunsaturated fatty acids and vitamin E after myocardial infarction: results of the GISSI-Prevenzione trial. Gruppo Italiano per lo Studio della Sopravvivenza nell'Infarto miocardico. *Lancet*, Vol. 354, pp. 447-55.

Goodnight, S. H., M. Fisher, et al. (1989). Assessment of the therapeutic use of dietary fish oil in atherosclerotic vascular disease and thrombosis. *Chest*, Vol. 95, pp. 19S-25S.

Ho, E. and T. M. Bray. (1999). Antioxidants, NFkappaB activation, and diabetogenesis. *Proc Soc Exp Biol Med*, Vol. 222, pp. 205-13.

Hughes, D. A., A. C. Pinder, et al. (1996). Fish oil supplementation inhibits the expression of major histocompatibility complex class II molecules and adhesion molecules on human monocytes. *Am J Clin Nutr*, Vol. 63, pp. 267-72.

Illingworth, D. R. and E. B. Schmidt. (1993). The influence of dietary n-3 fatty acids on plasma lipids and lipoproteins. *Ann N Y Acad Sci*, Vol. 676, pp. 60-9.

Jump, D. B. (2002). Dietary polyunsaturated fatty acids and regulation of gene transcription. *Curr Opin Lipidol*, Vol. 13, pp. 155-64.

Kang, J. X., Y. F. Xiao, et al. (1995). Free, long-chain, polyunsaturated fatty acids reduce membrane electrical excitability in neonatal rat cardiac myocytes. *Proc Natl Acad Sci U S A*, Vol. 92, pp. 3997-4001.

Kelley, D. S., P. C. Taylor, et al. (1999). Docosahexaenoic acid ingestion inhibits natural killer cell activity and production of inflammatory mediators in young healthy men. *Lipids*, Vol. 34, pp. 317-24.

Krauss, R. M., R. H. Eckel, et al. (2000). AHA Dietary Guidelines: revision 2000: A statement for healthcare professionals from the Nutrition Committee of the American Heart Association. *Circulation*, Vol. 102, pp. 2284-99.

Kris-Etherton, P. M., W. S. Harris, et al. (2002). Fish consumption, fish oil, omega-3 fatty acids, and cardiovascular disease. *Circulation*, Vol. 106, pp. 2747-57.

Kris-Etherton, P. M., A. H. Lichtenstein, et al. (2004). Antioxidant vitamin supplements and cardiovascular disease. *Circulation*, Vol. 110, pp. 637-41.

Kuiper, G. G., J. G. Lemmen, et al. (1998). Interaction of estrogenic chemicals and phytoestrogens with estrogen receptor beta. *Endocrinology*, Vol. 139, pp. 4252-63.

Kurzer, M. S. and X. Xu. (1997). Dietary phytoestrogens. *Annu Rev Nutr*, Vol. 17, pp. 353-81.

Kushi, L. H., A. R. Folsom, et al. (1996). Dietary antioxidant vitamins and death from coronary heart disease in postmenopausal women. *N Engl J Med*, Vol. 334, pp. 1156-62.

Leaf, A., J. X. Kang, et al. (2003). Clinical prevention of sudden cardiac death by n-3 polyunsaturated fatty acids and mechanism of prevention of arrhythmias by n-3 fish oils. *Circulation*, Vol. 107, pp. 2646-52.

Lichtenstein, A. H., L. J. Appel, et al. (2006). Diet and lifestyle recommendations revision 2006: a scientific statement from the American Heart Association Nutrition Committee. *Circulation*, Vol. 114, pp. 82-96.

Lloyd-Jones, D., R. Adams, et al. (2009). Heart disease and stroke statistics--2009 update: a report from the American Heart Association Statistics Committee and Stroke Statistics Subcommittee. *Circulation*, Vol. 119, pp. 480-6.

Lonn, E., J. Bosch, et al. (2005). Effects of long-term vitamin E supplementation on cardiovascular events and cancer: a randomized controlled trial. *Jama*, Vol. 293, pp. 1338-47.

Marchioli, R., F. Barzi, et al. (2002). Early protection against sudden death by n-3 polyunsaturated fatty acids after myocardial infarction: time-course analysis of the results of the Gruppo Italiano per lo Studio della Sopravvivenza nell'Infarto Miocardico (GISSI)-Prevenzione. *Circulation*, Vol. 105, pp. 1897-903.

Mayer-Davis, E. J., T. Costacou, et al. (2002). Plasma and dietary vitamin E in relation to incidence of type 2 diabetes: The Insulin Resistance and Atherosclerosis Study (IRAS). *Diabetes Care*, Vol. 25, pp. 2172-7.

McCullough, M. L., D. Feskanich, et al. (2000). Adherence to the Dietary Guidelines for Americans and risk of major chronic disease in men. *Am J Clin Nutr,* Vol. 72, pp. 1223-31.

McMichael-Phillips, D. F., C. Harding, et al. (1998). Effects of soy-protein supplementation on epithelial proliferation in the histologically normal human breast. *Am J Clin Nutr,* Vol. 68, pp. 1431S-1435S.

Meagher, E. A., O. P. Barry, et al. (2001). Effects of vitamin E on lipid peroxidation in healthy persons. *Jama,* Vol. 285, pp. 1178-82.

Miller, E. R., 3rd, R. Pastor-Barriuso, et al. (2005). Meta-analysis: high-dosage vitamin E supplementation may increase all-cause mortality. *Ann Intern Med,* Vol. 142, pp. 37-46.

Mozaffarian, D., R. N. Lemaitre, et al. (2003). Cardiac benefits of fish consumption may depend on the type of fish meal consumed: the Cardiovascular Health Study. *Circulation,* Vol. 107, pp. 1372-7.

Munday, J. S., K. G. Thompson, et al. (1998). Dietary antioxidants do not reduce fatty streak formation in the C57BL/6 mouse atherosclerosis model. *Arterioscler Thromb Vasc Biol,* Vol. 18, pp. 114-9.

Nagata, C., N. Takatsuka, et al. (2002). Soy and fish oil intake and mortality in a Japanese community. *Am J Epidemiol,* Vol. 156, pp. 824-31.

Nair, S. S., J. Leitch, et al. (1999). Cardiac (n-3) non-esterified fatty acids are selectively increased in fish oil-fed pigs following myocardial ischemia. *J Nutr,* Vol. 129, pp. 1518-23.

Nestel, P. J., S. Pomeroy, et al. (1999). Isoflavones from red clover improve systemic arterial compliance but not plasma lipids in menopausal women. *J Clin Endocrinol Metab,* Vol. 84, pp. 895-8.

Nilsen, D. W., G. Albrektsen, et al. (2001). Effects of a high-dose concentrate of n-3 fatty acids or corn oil introduced early after an acute myocardial infarction on serum triacylglycerol and HDL cholesterol. *Am J Clin Nutr,* Vol. 74, pp. 50-6.

Ogden, C. L., M. D. Carroll, et al. (2006). Prevalence of overweight and obesity in the United States, 1999-2004. *Jama,* Vol. 295, pp. 1549-55.

Paolisso, G., M. R. Tagliamonte, et al. (2000). Chronic vitamin E administration improves brachial reactivity and increases intracellular magnesium concentration in type II diabetic patients. *J Clin Endocrinol Metab,* Vol. 85, pp. 109-15.

Paul, A., L. Calleja, et al. (2001). Supplementation with vitamin E and/or zinc does not attenuate atherosclerosis in apolipoprotein E-deficient mice fed a high-fat, high-cholesterol diet. *Int J Vitam Nutr Res,* Vol. 71, pp. 45-52.

Raitt, M. H., W. E. Connor, et al. (2005). Fish oil supplementation and risk of ventricular tachycardia and ventricular fibrillation in patients with implantable defibrillators: a randomized controlled trial. *Jama,* Vol. 293, pp. 2884-91.

Reunanen, A., P. Knekt, et al. (1998). Serum antioxidants and risk of non-insulin dependent diabetes mellitus. *Eur J Clin Nutr,* Vol. 52, pp. 89-93.

Rimm, E. B., M. J. Stampfer, et al. (1993). Vitamin E consumption and the risk of coronary heart disease in men. *N Engl J Med,* Vol. 328, pp. 1450-6.

Sacks, F. M., A. Lichtenstein, et al. (2006). Soy protein, isoflavones, and cardiovascular health: an American Heart Association Science Advisory for professionals from the Nutrition Committee. *Circulation,* Vol. 113, pp. 1034-44.

Sacks, F. M., P. H. Stone, et al. (1995). Controlled trial of fish oil for regression of human coronary atherosclerosis. HARP Research Group. *J Am Coll Cardiol,* Vol. 25, pp. 1492-8.

Sesso, H. D., J. E. Buring, et al. (2008). Vitamins E and C in the prevention of cardiovascular disease in men: the Physicians' Health Study II randomized controlled trial. *Jama*, Vol. 300, pp. 2123-33.

Setchell, K. D. (2001). Soy isoflavones--benefits and risks from nature's selective estrogen receptor modulators (SERMs). *J Am Coll Nutr*, Vol. 20, pp. 354S-362S; discussion 381S-383S.

Shachter, N. S. (2001). Apolipoproteins C-I and C-III as important modulators of lipoprotein metabolism. *Curr Opin Lipidol*, Vol. 12, pp. 297-304.

Sirtori, C. R., A. Arnoldi, et al. (2005). Phytoestrogens: end of a tale? *Ann Med*, Vol. 37, pp. 423-38.

Stampfer, M. J., C. H. Hennekens, et al. (1993). Vitamin E consumption and the risk of coronary disease in women. *N Engl J Med*, Vol. 328, pp. 1444-9.

Steinberg, F. M., N. L. Guthrie, et al. (2003). Soy protein with isoflavones has favorable effects on endothelial function that are independent of lipid and antioxidant effects in healthy postmenopausal women. *Am J Clin Nutr*, Vol. 78, pp. 123-30.

Stephens, N. G., A. Parsons, et al. (1996). Randomised controlled trial of vitamin E in patients with coronary disease: Cambridge Heart Antioxidant Study (CHAOS). *Lancet*, Vol. 347, pp. 781-6.

Teede, H. J., F. S. Dalais, et al. (2001). Dietary soy has both beneficial and potentially adverse cardiovascular effects: a placebo-controlled study in men and postmenopausal women. *J Clin Endocrinol Metab*, Vol. 86, pp. 3053-60.

Thomas, S. R., S. B. Leichtweis, et al. (2001). Dietary cosupplementation with vitamin E and coenzyme Q(10) inhibits atherosclerosis in apolipoprotein E gene knockout mice. *Arterioscler Thromb Vasc Biol*, Vol. 21, pp. 585-93.

Vasandani, C., A. I. Kafrouni, et al. (2002). Upregulation of hepatic LDL transport by n-3 fatty acids in LDL receptor knockout mice. *J Lipid Res*, Vol. 43, pp. 772-84.

von Schacky, C., S. Fischer, et al. (1985). Long-term effects of dietary marine omega-3 fatty acids upon plasma and cellular lipids, platelet function, and eicosanoid formation in humans. *J Clin Invest*, Vol. 76, pp. 1626-31.

Wang, C., W. S. Harris, et al. (2006). n-3 Fatty acids from fish or fish-oil supplements, but not alpha-linolenic acid, benefit cardiovascular disease outcomes in primary- and secondary-prevention studies: a systematic review. *Am J Clin Nutr*, Vol. 84, pp. 5-17.

Waters, D. D., E. L. Alderman, et al. (2002). Effects of hormone replacement therapy and antioxidant vitamin supplements on coronary atherosclerosis in postmenopausal women: a randomized controlled trial. *Jama*, Vol. 288, pp. 2432-40.

Wu, B. J., K. Kathir, et al. (2006). Antioxidants protect from atherosclerosis by a heme oxygenase-1 pathway that is independent of free radical scavenging. *J Exp Med*, Vol. 203, pp. 1117-27.

Ylonen, K., G. Alfthan, et al. (2003). Dietary intakes and plasma concentrations of carotenoids and tocopherols in relation to glucose metabolism in subjects at high risk of type 2 diabetes: the Botnia Dietary Study. *Am J Clin Nutr*, Vol. 77, pp. 1434-41.

Yusuf, S., G. Dagenais, et al. (2000). Vitamin E supplementation and cardiovascular events in high-risk patients. The Heart Outcomes Prevention Evaluation Study Investigators. *N Engl J Med*, Vol. 342, pp. 154-60.

Zhou, L. and A. Nilsson. (2001). Sources of eicosanoid precursor fatty acid pools in tissues. *J Lipid Res*, Vol. 42, pp. 1521-42.

# Permissions

The contributors of this book come from diverse backgrounds, making this book a truly international effort. This book will bring forth new frontiers with its revolutionizing research information and detailed analysis of the nascent developments around the world.

We would like to thank Armen Yuri Gasparyan and George D. Kitas, for lending their expertise to make the book truly unique. They have played a crucial role in the development of this book. Without their invaluable contribution this book wouldn't have been possible. They have made vital efforts to compile up to date information on the varied aspects of this subject to make this book a valuable addition to the collection of many professionals and students.

This book was conceptualized with the vision of imparting up-to-date information and advanced data in this field. To ensure the same, a matchless editorial board was set up. Every individual on the board went through rigorous rounds of assessment to prove their worth. After which they invested a large part of their time researching and compiling the most relevant data for our readers. Conferences and sessions were held from time to time between the editorial board and the contributing authors to present the data in the most comprehensible form. The editorial team has worked tirelessly to provide valuable and valid information to help people across the globe.

Every chapter published in this book has been scrutinized by our experts. Their significance has been extensively debated. The topics covered herein carry significant findings which will fuel the growth of the discipline. They may even be implemented as practical applications or may be referred to as a beginning point for another development. Chapters in this book were first published by InTech; hereby published with permission under the Creative Commons Attribution License or equivalent.

The editorial board has been involved in producing this book since its inception. They have spent rigorous hours researching and exploring the diverse topics which have resulted in the successful publishing of this book. They have passed on their knowledge of decades through this book. To expedite this challenging task, the publisher supported the team at every step. A small team of assistant editors was also appointed to further simplify the editing procedure and attain best results for the readers.

Our editorial team has been hand-picked from every corner of the world. Their multi-ethnicity adds dynamic inputs to the discussions which result in innovative outcomes. These outcomes are then further discussed with the researchers and contributors who give their valuable feedback and opinion regarding the same. The feedback is then collaborated with the researches and they are edited in a comprehensive manner to aid the understanding of the subject.

Apart from the editorial board, the designing team has also invested a significant amount of their time in understanding the subject and creating the most relevant covers. They scrutinized every image to scout for the most suitable representation of the subject and create an appropriate cover for the book.

The publishing team has been involved in this book since its early stages. They were actively engaged in every process, be it collecting the data, connecting with the contributors or procuring relevant information. The team has been an ardent support to the editorial, designing and production team. Their endless efforts to recruit the best for this project, has resulted in the accomplishment of this book. They are a veteran in the field of academics and their pool of knowledge is as vast as their experience in printing. Their expertise and guidance has proved useful at every step. Their uncompromising quality standards have made this book an exceptional effort. Their encouragement from time to time has been an inspiration for everyone.

The publisher and the editorial board hope that this book will prove to be a valuable piece of knowledge for researchers, students, practitioners and scholars across the globe.

# List of Contributors

**Annette Schmidt**
Leibniz-Institute of Arteriosclerosis Research at the University of Muenster, Germany

**Taina Hintsa, Tom Rosenström and Liisa Keltikangas-Järvinen**
IBS, Unit of Personality Work and Health Psychology, University of Helsinki, Finland

**Mirka Hintsanen**
IBS, Unit of Personality Work and Health Psychology, University of Helsinki, Finland
Helsinki Collegium for Advanced Studies, University of Helsinki, Finland

**Adel Berbari and Abdo Jurjus**
American University of Beirut, Lebanon

**Aldo Pende and Andrea Denegri**
Clinic of Internal Medicine, Department of Internal Medicine, University of Genoa School of Medicine, Genoa, Italy

**Chiara Leuzzi, Raffaella Marzullo, Emma Tarabini Castellani and Maria Grazia Modena**
Department of Cardiovascular Disease, Women's Clinic, University of Modena and Reggio Emilia, Italy

**Anna Skoczynska and Marta Skoczynska**
Wroclaw Medical University, Poland

**Nicolás Terrados**
Regional Sports Medicine Unit of the Principality of Asturias, Avilés, Spain
Department of Functional Biology, The University of Oviedo, Asturias, Spain

**Eduardo Iglesias-Gutiérrez**
Department of Functional Biology, The University of Oviedo, Asturias, Spain

**Carlos Zamarrón and Emilio Morete**
Servicio de Neumología, Hospital Clínico Universitario, Santiago, Spain

**Felix del Campo Matias**
Hospital Universitario Rio Hortega, Valladolid, Spain

**Javier Delgado-Lista, Ana I. Perez-Caballero, Pablo Perez-Martinez, Antonio Garcia-Rios, Jose Lopez-Miranda and Francisco Perez-Jimenez**
Unidad de Lipidos y Arteriosclerosis, IMIBIC/Hospital Universitario Reina Sofia, Universidad de Cordoba, Ciber Fisiopatología Obesidad y Nutrición (CIBEROBN), Instituto de Salud Carlos III, Spain

**Satoshi Kashiwagi and Paul L. Huang**
Cardiovascular Research Center and Cardiology Division, Massachusetts General Hospital and Harvard Medical School, Charlestown, MA, USA

Printed in the USA
CPSIA information can be obtained
at www.ICGtesting.com
JSHW011411221024
72173JS00003B/507